LIPPINCO̶T̶T̶
of NURSIN̶G̶ ̶P̶R̶A̶C̶TICE
Series

ALARMING SIGNS & SYMPTOMS

◆

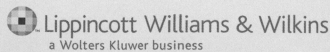 Lippincott Williams & Wilkins
a Wolters Kluwer business

Philadelphia · Baltimore · New York · London
Buenos Aires · Hong Kong · Sydney · Tokyo

STAFF

Executive Publisher
Judith A. Schilling McCann, RN, MSN

Editorial Director
H. Nancy Holmes

Clinical Director
Joan M. Robinson, RN, MSN

Senior Art Director
Arlene Putterman

Editorial Project Manager
William Welsh

Clinical Project Manager
Carol A. Saunderson, RN, BA, BS

Editor
Elizabeth Jacqueline Mills

Clinical Editors
Tamara M. Kear, RN, MSN,CNN;
Carol Knauff, RN, MSN, CCRN

Copy Editors
Kimberly Bilotta (supervisor),
Amy Furman, Dona Perkins,
Carolyn Petersen, Irene Pontarelli,
Pamela Wingrod

Designer
Debra Moloshok (book design
and project manager)

Digital Composition Services
Diane Paluba (manager),
Joyce Rossi Biletz, Donna S. Morris

Manufacturing
Patricia K. Dorshaw (director),
Beth J. Welsh

Editorial Assistants
Megan L. Aldinger, Karen J. Kirk,
Linda K. Ruhf

Indexer
Barbara Hodgson

LMNPSS010206

**Library of Congress
Cataloging-in-Publication Data**

Alarming signs & symptoms.
    p. ; cm. — (Lippincott manual of nursing practice series)
  Includes bibliographical references and index.
  1. Nursing assessment — Handbooks, manuals, etc. 2. Drug interactions — Handbooks, manuals, etc. 3. Bioterrorism — Handbooks, manuals, etc. 4. Symptoms — Handbooks, manuals, etc. I. Lippincott Williams & Wilkins. II. Title: Alarming signs and symptoms. III. Series.
  [DNLM: 1. Nursing Assessment--methods — Handbooks. 2. Bioterrorism--Handbooks. 3. Drug Interactions — Handbooks. 4. Herb-Drug Interactions — Handbooks. 5. Pharmacokinetics — Handbooks. WY 49 A322 2006]
  RT48.A43 2006
  616.07'5 — dc22
  ISBN 1-58255-624-5 (alk. paper)   2005032621

CONTENTS

CONTRIBUTORS
AND CONSULTANTS

◆

Deirdre Herr Byers, RN, BSN, CCRN
Staff Nurse
Southeast Georgia Health System
Brunswick

Colleen Davenport, RN, MSN
Staff Nurse
Wrangell (Alaska) Medical Center

Anna Easter, ACNP, PhD, CNS(M/S)
Nurse Practitioner
Central Arkansas Veteran's Hospital
Little Rock

Julia Anne Isen, FNP-C, BSN, MS
Family Nurse Practitioner
University of California at San Francisco
    Medical Center

Cynthia Julian, RN, BSN
Clinical Coordinator
Ancillary Care Management
Omaha

Carol T. Lemay, RN
Staff Nurse
University of Massachusetts Amherst

Valerie Lyttle, RN, BSN, CEN
Patient Care Manager
Auburn (Wash.) Regional Medical Center

William J. Pawlyshyn, RN, BSN, MS, MN,
    ANP-C
Nurse Practitioner
Cape Cod Ears, Nose & Throat Specialists
Hyannis, Mass.

Catherine Pence, RN, MSN, CCRN
Assistant Professor
Northern Kentucky University
Highland Heights

Marg Poling, RN, BScN, PHCNP, Pall, MN
Palliative Care Nurse Practitioner
Victorian Order of Nurse's Thunder Bay
Ontario

Sherry L. Rogman, RN
Emergency Department Charge Nurse
Bryan/LGH Memorial Hospital
Lincoln, Nebr.

Donna Scemons, RN, MSN, FNP-C, CNS,
    CWOCN
President
Healthcare Systems, Inc.
Castaic, Calif.

Lisa Wolf, RN, BSN
Clinical Educator
Mount Carmel Health
Columbus, Ohio

Dawn M. Zwick, RN, MSN, CRNP
Faculty
Kent (Ohio) State University

Abdominal pain

Abdominal pain usually results from a GI disorder, but can also be caused by drug use, ingestion of toxins, or disorders of the reproductive, genitourinary (GU), musculoskeletal, or vascular systems. At times, such pain signals life-threatening complications.

Abdominal pain arises from the abdominopelvic viscera, the parietal peritoneum, or the capsules of the liver, kidney, or spleen. It may be acute or chronic, diffuse or localized. Visceral pain develops slowly into a deep, dull, aching pain that's poorly localized in the epigastric, periumbilical, or lower midabdominal (hypogastric) region. In contrast, somatic (parietal, peritoneal) pain produces a sharp, more intense, and well-localized discomfort that rapidly follows the insult. Movement or coughing aggravates somatic pain. (See *Abdominal pain: Types and locations,* page 2.)

Pain may also be referred to the abdomen from another site with the same nerve supply. This sharp, well-localized, referred pain is felt in the skin or deeper tissues and may coexist with skin and muscle hypersensitivity to painful stimuli.

Mechanisms that produce abdominal pain include stretching or tension of the gut wall, traction on the peritoneum or mesentery, vigorous intestinal contraction, inflammation, ischemia, and sensory nerve irritation.

Act now *If the patient is experiencing sudden and severe abdominal pain, quickly take his vital signs and palpate pulses below the waist. Stay alert for signs of hypovolemic shock, such as tachycardia and hypotension. Establish I.V. access.*

Emergency surgery may be required if the patient also has mottled skin below the waist and a pulsating epigastric mass or rebound tenderness and rigidity.

ASSESSMENT
History

If the patient's condition permits, obtain his history. Ask whether he has had this type of pain before. Because some patients report abdominal pain as indigestion or gas pain, it's important to ask the patient to describe his pain in detail. For example, is it dull, sharp, stabbing, or burning? Ask him where the pain is located and whether it radiates to other areas. If a language barrier exists between you and the patient, use a pain rating scale with visual cues such as faces.

Ask the patient about factors that relieve the pain or make it worse. For example, do movement, coughing, exertion, vomiting, eating, elimination, or walking relieve the pain or worsen it? Ask him when the pain began and whether it's intermittent or constant. If pain is intermittent, ask about the duration of a typical episode.

Intermittent, cramping abdominal pain suggests obstruction of a hollow organ. Constant, steady abdominal pain suggests organ perforation, ischemia, or inflammation or blood in the peritoneal cavity.

Ask the patient about substance abuse and a history of vascular, GI, GU, or reproductive disorders. Ask the female patient about the date of her last menses, changes in her menstrual pattern, or dyspareunia.

ABDOMINAL PAIN: TYPES AND LOCATIONS

AFFECTED ORGAN	VISCERAL PAIN	PARIETAL PAIN	REFERRED PAIN
Appendix	Periumbilical area	Right lower quadrant	Right lower quadrant
Distal colon	Hypogastrium and left flank for descending colon	Over affected site	Left lower quadrant and back (rare)
Gallbladder	Middle epigastrium	Right upper quadrant	Right subscapular area
Liver	Middle epigastrium	Right upper quadrant	Right shoulder
Ovaries, fallopian tubes, and uterus	Hypogastrium and groin	Over affected site	Inner thighs
Pancreas	Middle epigastrium and left upper quadrant	Middle epigastrium and left upper quadrant	Back and left shoulder
Proximal colon	Periumbilical area and right flank for ascending colon	Over affected site	Right lower quadrant and back (rare)
Small intestine	Periumbilical area	Over affected site	Midback (rare)
Stomach	Middle epigastrium	Middle epigastrium and left upper quadrant	Shoulders
Ureters	Costovertebral angle	Over affected site	Groin; scrotum in men, labia in women (rare)

Ask the patient about appetite changes. Ask about the onset and frequency of nausea or vomiting. Has he experienced increased flatulence, constipation, diarrhea, or changes in stool consistency? When was the patient's last bowel movement? Ask about urinary frequency, urgency, or pain. Is the urine cloudy or pink?

Physical examination

Obtain the patient's vital signs, and assess skin turgor and mucous membranes. Inspect his abdomen for distention or visible peristaltic waves and, if indicated, measure his abdominal girth.

Auscultate for bowel sounds in all four quadrants for at least 10 to 15 seconds and characterize their motility. Listen for systolic bruits in such locations as the abdominal aorta, renal artery, or iliac artery. (See *Auscultating for vascular sounds.*)

Percuss all quadrants, noting the percussion sounds.

 Alert *Abdominal percussion or palpation is contraindicated in patients with suspected*

abdominal aortic aneurysm, those who have received abdominal organ transplants, and children with suspected Wilms' tumor. If performing abdominal percussion or palpation in patients with suspected appendicitis, use extreme caution to avoid precipitating a rupture.

Palpate the entire abdomen for masses, rigidity, and tenderness. Involuntary rigidity is generally asymmetrical, evident on inspiration and expiration, unaffected by relaxation techniques, and painful when the patient sits up using his abdominal muscles alone. Check for costovertebral angle (CVA) tenderness, abdominal tenderness with guarding, and rebound tenderness. Peritonitis and appendicitis can cause rebound tenderness. Because appendicitis may be accompanied by increased abdominal wall resistance and guarding, perform the maneuver for rebound tenderness *only once* — repeating the maneuver can rupture an inflamed appendix. (See *Eliciting rebound tenderness,* page 4.)

Pediatric pointers

Because a child commonly has difficulty describing abdominal pain, you should pay close attention to nonverbal cues, such as wincing, lethargy, or unusual positioning such as a side-lying position with knees flexed to the abdomen. Observing the child while he coughs, walks, or climbs may also offer diagnostic clues. Remember that a parent's description of the child's complaints is a subjective interpretation of what the parent believes is wrong. In a child, abdominal pain can signal a disorder with greater severity or different associated signs than in an adult. Appendicitis, for example, has higher rupture and mortality in children, and vomiting may be the only other sign. Acute pyelonephritis may cause abdominal pain, vomiting, and diarrhea in children without the classic urologic signs found in adults. Peptic ulcer causes nocturnal pain and colic, which, unlike peptic ulcer in adults, may not be relieved by food.

Abdominal pain in children can also result from lactose intolerance, allergic-tension-fatigue syndrome, volvulus, Meckel's diverticulum, intussusception, mesenteric adenitis, diabetes mellitus, juvenile rheumatoid arthritis, and such uncommon disorders as heavy metal poisoning.

Geriatric pointers

Advanced age may decrease the manifestations of acute abdominal disease. Pain may be less severe, fever less pronounced, and signs of peritoneal inflammation diminished or absent. The influence of mental status changes also provide misleading findings.

MEDICAL CAUSES

See *Abdominal pain: Causes and associated findings,* pages 6 to 11.

● *Abdominal aortic aneurysm (dissecting).* Initially, life-threatening abdominal aortic aneurysm may produce dull lower abdominal, lower back, or severe chest pain. Typically, it produces constant upper abdominal pain, which may worsen when the patient lies down and may abate when he leans forward or sits up. Palpation may reveal an epigastric mass that pulsates before rupture but not after it.

Other findings may include mottled skin below the waist, absent femoral and pedal pulses, lower blood pressure in the legs than in the arms, mild to moderate abdominal

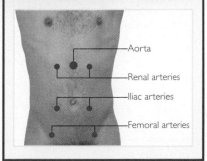

AUSCULTATING FOR VASCULAR SOUNDS

Use the bell of the stethoscope to auscultate for vascular sounds at the sites shown in the illustration.

Aorta
Renal arteries
Iliac arteries
Femoral arteries

tenderness with guarding, and abdominal rigidity. Signs of shock, such as tachycardia and tachypnea, may appear.

● *Abdominal cancer.* Abdominal pain usually occurs late in abdominal cancer. It may be accompanied by anorexia, weight loss, weakness, depression, and an abdominal mass and distention.

● *Adrenal crisis.* Severe abdominal pain appears early, along with nausea, vomiting, dehydration, profound weakness, anorexia, and fever. Later signs are progressive loss of consciousness; hypotension; tachycardia; oliguria; cool, clammy skin; and increased motor activity, which may progress to delirium or seizures.

● *Anthrax, GI.* Anthrax is an acute infectious disease caused by the gram-positive, spore-forming bacterium Bacillus anthracis. Although the disease most commonly occurs in wild and domestic grazing animals, such as cattle, sheep, and goats, the spores can live in the soil for many years. The disease can occur in humans exposed to infected animals, tissue from infected animals, or biological warfare. Most natural cases occur in agricultural regions worldwide. Anthrax may occur in cutaneous, inhaled, or GI forms.

Eating contaminated meat from an infected animal causes GI anthrax. Initial signs and symptoms include loss of appetite, nausea, vomiting, and fever. Late signs and symptoms include abdominal pain, severe bloody diarrhea, and hematemesis.

ELICITING REBOUND TENDERNESS

To elicit rebound tenderness, help the patient into a supine position, and push your fingers deeply and steadily into his abdomen (as shown). Then quickly release the pressure. Pain that results from the rebound of palpated tissue — rebound tenderness — indicates peritoneal inflammation or peritonitis.

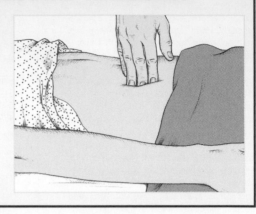

- **Appendicitis.** With appendicitis, a life-threatening disorder, pain initially occurs in the epigastric or umbilical region. Anorexia, nausea, or vomiting may occur after the onset of pain. Pain localizes at McBurney's point in the right lower quadrant and is accompanied by abdominal rigidity, increasing tenderness (especially over McBurney's point), rebound tenderness, and retractive respirations. Later signs and symptoms include malaise, constipation (or diarrhea), low-grade fever, and tachycardia.
- **Cholecystitis.** Severe pain in the right upper quadrant may arise suddenly or increase gradually over several hours, usually after meals. It may radiate to the right shoulder, chest, or back. Accompanying the pain are anorexia, nausea, vomiting, fever, abdominal rigidity, tenderness, pallor, and diaphoresis. Murphy's sign (inspiratory arrest elicited when the examiner palpates the right upper quadrant as the patient takes a deep breath) is common.
- **Cholelithiasis.** Patients may suffer sudden, severe, and paroxysmal pain in the right upper quadrant lasting several minutes to several hours. The pain may radiate to the epigastrium, back, or shoulder blades. The pain is accompanied by anorexia, nausea, vomiting (sometimes bilious), diaphoresis, restlessness, and abdominal tenderness with guarding over the gallbladder or biliary duct. The patient may also experience fatty food intolerance and frequent indigestion.
- **Cirrhosis.** Dull abdominal aching occurs early and is usually accompanied by anorexia, indigestion, nausea, vomiting, constipation, or diarrhea. Subsequent right upper quadrant pain worsens when the patient sits up or leans forward. Associated signs include fever, ascites, leg edema, weight gain, hepatomegaly, jaundice, severe pruritus, bleeding tendencies, palmar erythema, and spider angiomas. Gynecomastia and testicular atrophy may also be present.
- **Crohn's disease.** An acute attack causes severe cramping pain in the lower abdomen, typically preceded by weeks or months of milder cramping pain. Crohn's disease may also cause diarrhea, hyperactive bowel sounds, dehydration, weight loss, fever, abdominal tenderness with guarding, and possibly a palpable mass in the lower quadrant. Abdominal pain is usually relieved by defecation. Milder chronic signs and symptoms include right lower quadrant pain with diarrhea, steatorrhea, and weight loss. Complications include perirectal or vaginal fistulas.
- **Cystitis.** Abdominal pain and tenderness are usually suprapubic. Associated signs and symptoms include malaise, flank pain, low back pain, nausea, vomiting, urinary frequency and urgency, nocturia, dysuria, fever, and chills.
- **Diabetic ketoacidosis.** Rarely, severe, sharp, shooting, and girdling pain may persist for several days. Fruity breath odor, a weak and rapid pulse, Kussmaul's respirations, poor skin turgor, polyuria, polydipsia, nocturia, hypotension, decreased bowel sounds, and confusion also occur.

- *Diverticulitis.* Mild cases usually produce intermittent, diffuse left lower quadrant pain, which is sometimes relieved by defecation or passage of flatus and worsened by eating. Other signs and symptoms include nausea, constipation or diarrhea, low-grade fever and, in many cases, a palpable abdominal mass that's usually tender, firm, and fixed. Rupture causes severe left lower quadrant pain, abdominal rigidity, and possibly signs and symptoms of sepsis and shock (high fever, chills, and hypotension).
- *Duodenal ulcer.* Localized abdominal pain — described as steady, gnawing, burning, aching, or hunger like — may occur high in the midepigastrium, slightly off center, and usually on the right. The pain usually doesn't radiate unless pancreatic penetration occurs. It typically begins 2 to 4 hours after a meal and may cause nocturnal awakening. Ingestion of food or antacids brings relief until the cycle starts again, but it also may produce weight gain. Other symptoms include changes in bowel habits and heartburn or retrosternal burning.
- *Ectopic pregnancy.* Lower abdominal pain may be sharp, dull, or cramping, and constant or intermittent in ectopic pregnancy — a potentially life-threatening disorder. Vaginal bleeding, nausea, and vomiting may occur, along with urinary frequency, a tender adnexal mass, and a 1- to 2-month history of amenorrhea. Rupture of the fallopian tube produces sharp lower abdominal pain, which may radiate to the shoulders and neck and become extreme with cervical or adnexal palpation. Signs of shock (such as pallor, tachycardia, and hypotension) may also appear.
- *Endometriosis.* Constant, severe pain in the lower abdomen usually begins 5 to 7 days before the start of menses and may be aggravated by defecation. Depending on the location of the ectopic tissue, the pain may be accompanied by constipation, abdominal tenderness, dysmenorrhea, dyspareunia, and deep sacral pain.
- **Escherichia coli *O157:H7*.** *E. coli* O157:H7 is an aerobic, gram-negative bacillus that causes food-borne illness. Most strains of *E. coli* are harmless; some are present in the normal intestinal flora of healthy humans and animals. *E. coli* O157:H7, one of hundreds of strains of the bacterium, is capable of producing a powerful toxin and can cause severe illness. Eating undercooked beef or other foods contaminated with the bacteria causes the disease. Signs and symptoms include watery or bloody diarrhea, nausea, vomiting, fever, and abdominal cramps. Elderly people and children younger than age 5 may develop hemolytic uremic syndrome, which may ultimately lead to acute renal failure.
- *Gastric ulcer.* Diffuse, gnawing, burning pain in the left upper quadrant or epigastric area commonly occurs 1 to 2 hours after meals; it may be relieved by ingestion of food or antacids. Vague bloating and nausea after eating are common. Indigestion, weight change, anorexia, and episodes of GI bleeding may also occur.
- *Gastritis.* With acute gastritis, the patient experiences a rapid onset of abdominal pain that can range from mild epigastric discomfort to burning pain in the left upper quadrant. Other typical features include belching, fever, malaise, anorexia, nausea, bloody or coffee-ground vomitus, and melena. However, significant bleeding is unusual unless the patient has hemorrhagic gastritis.
- *Gastroenteritis.* Cramping or colicky abdominal pain, which can be diffuse, originates in the left upper quadrant and radiates or migrates to the other quadrants, usually in a peristaltic manner. It's accompanied by diarrhea, hyperactive bowel sounds, headache, myalgia, nausea, and vomiting.
- *Heart failure.* Right upper quadrant pain commonly accompanies the hallmarks of heart failure: jugular vein distention, dyspnea, tachycardia, and peripheral edema. Other findings include nausea, vomiting, ascites, productive cough, crackles, cool extremities, and cyanotic nail beds. Clinical signs are numerous and vary according to the stage of the disease and amount of cardiovascular impairment.
- *Hepatic abscess.* Steady, severe abdominal pain in the right upper quadrant or midepigastrium typically accompanies hepatic abscess, a rare disorder; however, right upper quadrant tenderness is the most important finding. Other signs and symptoms are anorexia, diarrhea, nausea, fever, diaphoresis, elevated right hemidiaphragm and, in rare cases, vomiting.
- *Hepatic amebiasis.* Hepatic amebiasis, which is rare in the United States, causes relatively severe right upper quadrant pain as well as tenderness over the liver and, possi-

(Text continues on page 10.)

ABDOMINAL PAIN:
CAUSES AND ASSOCIATED FINDINGS

MAJOR ASSOCIATED SIGNS AND SYMPTOMS

COMMON CAUSES	Abdominal distention	Abdominal mass	Abdominal rigidity	Abdominal tenderness	Amenorrhea	Anorexia	Bowel sounds, absent	Bowel sounds, hyperactive	Bowel sounds, hypoactive	Breath odor, fruity	Chest pain	
Abdominal aortic aneurysm (dissecting)		●	●	●							●	
Abdominal cancer	●	●				●						
Abdominal trauma			●	●			●		●			
Adrenal crisis						●						
Anthrax, GI						●						
Appendicitis			●	●		●						
Cholecystitis			●	●		●					●	
Cholelithiasis				●		●						
Cirrhosis	●					●						
Crohn's disease		●		●				●				
Cystitis				●								
Diabetic ketoacidosis										●		
Diverticulitis		●	●									
Duodenal ulcer											●	
Ectopic pregnancy		●			●							
Endometriosis				●								
Escherichia coli O157:H7												
Gastric ulcer						●						
Gastritis						●						
Gastroenteritis								●				
Heart failure	●											
Hepatic abscess				●		●						

Constipation	Costovertebral angle tenderness	Cough	Diarrhea	Dyspnea	Fever	Kussmaul's respirations	Nausea	Oliguria or anuria	Skin lesions	Skin mottling	Tachycardia	Tachypnea	Urinary frequency	Vomiting	Weakness	Weight change
										●	●	●				
															●	●
											●			●		
					●		●	●			●			●	●	
			●		●		●							●		
●			●		●		●				●			●		
					●		●							●		
					●		●							●		
●			●		●		●							●		●
			●		●											●
					●		●						●	●		
											●					
●					●		●									
																●
							●				●		●	●		
●																
			●		●		●							●		
							●									●
					●		●							●		●
				●			●							●		
		●		●			●				●			●		
			●		●		●							●		

(continued)

MAJOR ASSOCIATED SIGNS AND SYMPTOMS

COMMON CAUSES	Abdominal distention	Abdominal mass	Abdominal rigidity	Abdominal tenderness	Amenorrhea	Anorexia	Bowel sounds, absent	Bowel sounds, hyperactive	Bowel sounds, hypoactive	Breath odor, fruity	Chest pain	
Hepatic amebiasis				●								
Hepatitis				●		●						
Herpes zoster				●							●	
Insect toxins			●									
Intestinal obstruction	●			●			●	●	●			
Irritable bowel syndrome	●			●								
Listeriosis												
Mesenteric artery ischemia			●	●		●						
Myocardial infarction											●	
Ovarian cyst	●	●		●	●							
Pancreatitis			●	●					●			
Pelvic inflammatory disease		●		●								
Perforated ulcer			●	●			●					
Peritonitis	●		●	●			●		●			
Pleurisy											●	
Pneumonia			●	●							●	
Pneumothorax											●	
Prostatitis												
Pyelonephritis (acute)				●								
Renal calculi												
Sickle cell crisis											●	
Smallpox (variola major)												

Constipation	Costovertebral angle tenderness	Cough	Diarrhea	Dyspnea	Fever	Kussmaul's respirations	Nausea	Oliguria or anuria	Skin lesions	Skin mottling	Tachycardia	Tachypnea	Urinary frequency	Vomiting	Weakness	Weight change
					•										•	•
							•							•		
					•				•							
					•		•							•		
•							•				•			•		
•			•				•									
			•		•		•							•		
•			•								•	•		•		
				•			•							•	•	
					•		•				•			•		
					•		•				•			•		
					•		•							•		
					•						•					
					•						•	•		•		
								•				•				
		•		•	•											
				•							•	•				
					•								•			
	•				•		•							•	•	•
	•				•		•							•		
				•											•	
					•			•								

(continued)

MAJOR ASSOCIATED SIGNS AND SYMPTOMS

COMMON CAUSES	Abdominal distention	Abdominal mass	Abdominal rigidity	Abdominal tenderness	Amenorrhea	Anorexia	Bowel sounds, absent	Bowel sounds, hyperactive	Bowel sounds, hypoactive	Breath odor, fruity	Chest pain
Splenic infarction											●
Systemic lupus erythematosus	●			●		●					●
Ulcerative colitis				●		●			●		
Uremia				●		●				●	

bly, the right shoulder. Accompanying signs and symptoms include fever, weakness, weight loss, chills, diaphoresis, and jaundiced or brownish skin.

● *Hepatitis.* Liver enlargement from any type of hepatitis causes discomfort or dull pain and tenderness in the right upper quadrant. Associated signs and symptoms may include dark urine, clay-colored stools, nausea, vomiting, anorexia, jaundice, malaise, and pruritus.

● *Herpes zoster.* Herpes zoster of the thoracic, lumbar, or sacral nerves can cause localized abdominal and chest pain in the areas served by these nerves. Pain, tenderness, and fever can precede or accompany erythematous papules that rapidly evolve into grouped vesicles. Although rare, herpes zoster can also affect the viscera of the abdominal cavity, causing adhesions and chronic pain.

● *Insect toxins.* Generalized, cramping abdominal pain usually occurs, along with low-grade fever, nausea, vomiting, abdominal rigidity, tremors, and localized pain and swelling.

● *Intestinal obstruction.* Short episodes of intense, colicky, cramping pain alternate with pain-free intervals in intestinal obstruction, a life-threatening disorder. Accompanying signs and symptoms may include obstipation, pain-induced agitation, visible peristaltic waves, and abdominal distention, tenderness, and guarding. The patient may also exhibit high-pitched, tinkling, or hyperactive sounds proximal to the obstruction; distally, sounds may be hypoactive or absent. In jejunal and duodenal obstruction, nausea and bilious vomiting occur early. In distal small-or large-bowel obstruction, nausea and vomiting are commonly feculent. Bowel sounds are absent in complete obstruction. Late-stage obstruction produces signs of hypovolemic shock, such as hypotension and tachycardia.

● *Irritable bowel syndrome.* Lower abdominal cramping or pain is aggravated by eating coarse or raw foods and may be alleviated by defecation or passage of flatus. Related findings include abdominal tenderness, diurnal diarrhea alternating with constipation or normal bowel function, and small stools with visible mucus. Dyspepsia, nausea, and abdominal distention with a feeling of incomplete evacuation may also occur. Stress, anxiety, and emotional lability may intensify the symptoms.

● *Listeriosis.* Listeriosis is a serious infection caused by eating food contaminated with the bacterium *Listeria monocytogenes.* This illness primarily affects pregnant women, neonates, and those with weakened immune systems. Signs and symptoms include fever, myalgia, abdominal pain, nausea, vomiting, and diar-

Constipation	Costovertebral angle tenderness	Cough	Diarrhea	Dyspnea	Fever	Kussmaul's respirations	Nausea	Oliguria or anuria	Skin lesions	Skin mottling	Tachycardia	Tachypnea	Urinary frequency	Vomiting	Weakness	Weight change
					●									●		
			●		●		●							●		●
			●				●	●						●		

rhea. If the infection spreads to the nervous system, meningitis may develop; signs and symptoms include fever, headache, nuchal rigidity, and a change in the level of consciousness (LOC). Infections during pregnancy may lead to premature delivery, infection of the neonate, or stillbirth.

● *Mesenteric artery ischemia.* Initially, the abdomen is soft and tender, with decreased bowel sounds. Associated findings include vomiting, anorexia, alternating periods of diarrhea and constipation and, in late stages, extreme abdominal tenderness with rigidity, tachycardia, tachypnea, absence of bowel sounds, and cool, clammy skin.

Always suspect mesenteric artery ischemia in patients older than age 50 with chronic heart failure, cardiac arrhythmias, cardiovascular infarct, or hypotension who develop sudden, severe abdominal pain after 2 to 3 days of colicky periumbilical pain and diarrhea.

● *Myocardial infarction (MI).* Substernal chest pain may radiate to the abdomen in an MI, a life-threatening disorder. Associated signs and symptoms include weakness, diaphoresis, nausea, vomiting, anxiety, syncope, jugular vein distention, and dyspnea.

● *Ovarian cyst.* Torsion or hemorrhage causes pain and tenderness in the right or left lower quadrant. Sharp and severe if the patient suddenly stands or stoops, the pain becomes brief and intermittent if the torsion self-corrects or dull and diffuse after several hours if it doesn't. Pain may be accompanied by slight fever, mild nausea and vomiting, abdominal tenderness, a palpable abdominal mass and, possibly, amenorrhea. Abdominal distention may occur if the cyst is large. Peritoneal irritation causes high fever and severe nausea and vomiting; these symptoms also occur with rupture and ensuing peritonitis.

● *Pancreatitis.* Life-threatening acute pancreatitis produces fulminating, continuous upper abdominal pain that may radiate to both flanks and the back. To relieve this pain, the patient may bend forward, draw his knees to his chest, or move about restlessly. Early findings include abdominal tenderness, nausea, vomiting, fever, pallor, tachycardia and, in some patients, abdominal rigidity, rebound tenderness, and hypoactive bowel sounds. Turner's sign (ecchymosis of the abdomen or flank) or Cullen's sign (a bluish tinge around the umbilicus) signals hemorrhagic pancreatitis. Jaundice may occur as inflammation subsides.

Chronic pancreatitis produces severe left upper quadrant or epigastric pain that radiates to the back. Abdominal tenderness, a midepigastric mass, jaundice, fever, and splenomegaly may occur. Steatorrhea, weight loss, poor digestion, and diabetes mellitus are common.

- **Pelvic inflammatory disease.** Pain in the right or left lower quadrant ranges from vague discomfort worsened by movement to deep, severe, and progressive pain. Metrorrhagia occasionally precedes or accompanies the onset of pain. Extreme pain accompanies cervical or adnexal palpation. Associated findings include abdominal tenderness, a palpable abdominal or pelvic mass, fever, occasional chills, nausea, vomiting, urinary discomfort, and abnormal vaginal bleeding or purulent vaginal discharge.
- **Perforated ulcer.** With a perforated ulcer — a life-threatening disorder — sudden, severe, and prostrating epigastric pain may radiate through the abdomen to the back or right shoulder. Other signs and symptoms include boardlike abdominal rigidity, tenderness with guarding, generalized rebound tenderness, absent bowel sounds, grunting and shallow respirations and, in many cases, fever, tachycardia, hypotension, and syncope.
- **Peritonitis.** In peritonitis, a life-threatening disorder, sudden and severe pain can be diffuse or localized in the area of the underlying disorder; movement worsens the pain. The degree of abdominal tenderness usually varies according to the extent of disease. Typical findings include fever, chills, nausea, vomiting, hypoactive or absent bowel sounds, rebound tenderness and guarding, hyperalgesia, tachycardia, hypotension, tachypnea, and abdominal tenderness, distention, and rigidity. Positive psoas and obturator signs also occur.
- **Pleurisy.** Pleurisy may produce upper abdominal or costal margin pain referred from the chest. Characteristic sharp, stabbing chest pain increases with inspiration and movement. Many patients have a pleural friction rub and rapid, shallow breathing; some develop a low-grade fever.
- **Pneumonia.** Lower-lobe pneumonia can cause pleuritic chest pain and referred, severe upper abdominal pain, tenderness, and rigidity that diminish with inspiration. It can also cause fever, shaking chills, achiness, headache, blood-tinged or rusty sputum, dyspnea, and a dry, hacking cough. Accompanying signs include crackles, egophony, decreased breath sounds, and dullness on percussion.
- **Pneumothorax.** Potentially life threatening, pneumothorax can cause pain across the upper abdomen and costal margin; this pain

is referred from the chest. Characteristic chest pain arises suddenly and worsens with deep inspiration or movement. Accompanying signs and symptoms include anxiety, dyspnea, cyanosis, decreased or absent breath sounds over the affected area, tachypnea, and tachycardia. Watch for asymmetrical chest movements on inspiration.
- **Prostatitis.** Vague abdominal pain or discomfort in the lower abdomen, groin, perineum, or rectum may develop. Other findings include dysuria, urinary frequency and urgency, fever, chills, low back pain, myalgia, arthralgia, and nocturia. Scrotal pain, penile pain, and pain on ejaculation may occur in chronic cases.
- **Pyelonephritis (acute).** Progressive lower quadrant pain in one or both sides, flank pain, and costovertebral angle tenderness characterize acute pyelonephritis. Pain may radiate to the lower midabdomen or groin. Additional signs and symptoms include abdominal and back tenderness, high fever, shaking chills, nausea, vomiting, and urinary frequency and urgency.
- **Renal calculi.** Depending on the location of calculi, severe abdominal or back pain may occur. However, the classic symptom is severe, colicky pain that travels from the costovertebral angle to the flank, suprapubic region, and external genitalia. The pain may be excruciating or dull and constant. Pain-induced agitation, nausea, vomiting, abdominal distention, fever, chills, hypertension, and urinary urgency with hematuria and dysuria may occur.
- **Sickle cell crisis.** Sudden, severe abdominal pain may accompany chest, back, hand, or foot pain. Associated signs and symptoms include weakness, aching joints, dyspnea, and scleral jaundice.
- **Smallpox (variola major).** Worldwide eradication of smallpox was achieved in 1977. The United States and Russia have the only documented storage sites for the virus, and the virus is considered a potential agent for biological warfare. Initial signs and symptoms include high fever, malaise, prostration, severe headache, backache, and abdominal pain. A maculopapular rash develops on the mucosa of the mouth, pharynx, face, and forearms and spreads to the trunk and legs. Within 2 days, the rash becomes vesicular and, later, pustular. The lesions, which develop simultaneously rather than gradually increasing in number, occur more frequently

on the face and extremities. The pustules are round, firm, and embedded in the skin. After 8 to 9 days, the pustules form a crust. Later, the scab separates from the skin, leaving a pitted scar. In fatal cases, death results from encephalitis, extensive bleeding, or secondary infection.

• *Splenic infarction.* Fulminating pain in the left upper quadrant occurs with chest pain that may worsen on inspiration. Pain commonly radiates to the left shoulder with splinting of the left diaphragm, abdominal guarding and, occasionally, a splenic friction rub.

• *Systemic lupus erythematosus.* Generalized abdominal pain is unusual but may occur after meals. Butterfly rash, photosensitivity, alopecia, mucous membrane ulcers, and nondeforming arthritis are characteristic. Other common signs and symptoms include anorexia, vomiting, abdominal tenderness with guarding, abdominal distention after meals, fatigue, fever, and weight loss. Precordial chest pain and a pericardial rub may also occur.

• *Ulcerative colitis.* Ulcerative colitis may begin with vague abdominal discomfort that leads to cramping lower abdominal pain. As ulcerative colitis progresses, the pain may become steady and diffuse, increasing with movement and coughing. The most common symptom — recurrent and possibly severe diarrhea with blood, pus, and mucus — may relieve the pain. The abdomen may feel soft, squashy, and extremely tender. High-pitched, infrequent bowel sounds may accompany nausea, vomiting, anorexia, weight loss, and mild, intermittent fever.

• *Uremia.* Characterized by generalized or periumbilical pain that shifts and varies in intensity, uremia causes diverse GI signs and symptoms, including nausea, anorexia, vomiting, and diarrhea. Abdominal tenderness that changes in location and intensity may occur, along with vision disturbances, bleeding, headache, decreased LOC, vertigo, and oliguria or anuria. Chest pain may occur secondary to pericardial effusion. Localized or diffuse pruritus is common.

OTHER CAUSES

• *Abdominal trauma.* Generalized or localized abdominal pain occurs with ecchymosis on the abdomen, abdominal tenderness, vomiting and, with hemorrhage into the peritoneal cavity, abdominal rigidity. Bowel

sounds are decreased or absent. The patient may have signs of hypovolemic shock, such as hypotension and a rapid, thready pulse.

• *Diet.* Highly acidic foods, such as coffee, chocolate, tomatoes, and citrus products, may cause sharp or gnawing upper quadrant pain.

• *Drugs.* Salicylates and nonsteroidal anti-inflammatory drugs commonly cause burning, gnawing pain in the left upper quadrant or epigastric area and nausea and vomiting.

NURSING CONSIDERATIONS

Help the patient find a comfortable position to ease his distress. A supine position, with his head flat on the table, arms at his sides, and knees slightly flexed, will relax the abdominal muscles. Monitor him closely because abdominal pain can signal a life-threatening disorder.

Alert *Be particularly vigilant for such indications as tachycardia, hypotension, clammy skin, abdominal rigidity, rebound tenderness, a change in the pain's location or intensity, or sudden relief from the pain, which indicate a ruptured abdominal aortic aneurysm. Notify the physician immediately and prepare the patient for emergency surgery. Initiate oxygen therapy, verify that a patent I.V. line is in place, and administer fluids or blood products as ordered.*

Withhold analgesics to avoid masking symptoms that may help to determine the diagnosis; also, withhold food and fluids because the patient may require surgery. Prepare for I.V. infusion and insertion of a nasogastric or other intestinal tube. Peritoneal lavage or abdominal paracentesis may also be required.

PATIENT TEACHING

Inform the patient that pain relief medications may not be ordered immediately because such agents can mask findings that would facilitate diagnosis. Analgesics can also interfere with surgical medications and might therefore be withheld until it's determined whether surgery will be necessary. Teach the patient how to use positioning to help alleviate discomfort. Inform him about what to expect from diagnostic testing, which may include pelvic and rectal examinations, X-rays and computed tomography scans, barium studies, and collection of blood, urine, and stool samples. Ultrasonography, endoscopy, and biopsy may also be performed. If surgery is needed, provide preoperative teaching.

Abdominal rigidity

Abdominal rigidity has been described as abnormal muscle tension or inflexibility of the abdomen, and as an abdominal muscle spasm with involuntary guarding. Rigidity is detected by palpation and may be voluntary or involuntary. Voluntary rigidity reflects the patient's fear or nervousness upon palpation; involuntary rigidity reflects potentially life-threatening peritoneal irritation or inflammation. (See *Recognizing voluntary rigidity*.)

Involuntary rigidity most commonly results from GI disorders, but may also occur in pulmonary and vascular disorders and from the effects of insect toxins. It's typically accompanied by fever, nausea, vomiting, and abdominal tenderness, distention, and pain.

Act now *After palpating abdominal rigidity, quickly take the patient's vital signs. Although he may not appear gravely ill or exhibit markedly abnormal vital signs, abdominal rigidity calls for emergency interventions.*

Prepare to administer oxygen and to insert an I.V. line for fluid and blood replacement. The pa-tient may require vasoactive medications to support blood pressure. He may also need an indwelling urinary catheter with careful monitoring of intake and output. Peritoneal lavage or abdominal para-centesis may be required.

A nasogastric tube may be necessary if abdominal rigidity is accompanied by abdominal distention; the tube relieves this distention. Because emergency surgery may be necessary, the patient should be prepared for laboratory tests and X-rays.

ASSESSMENT
History
If the patient's condition allows further assessment, obtain a brief history; if you're unable to obtain a history from the patient, consult the patient's family. Ask when the abdominal rigidity began and whether it's localized or generalized. Ask him whether the rigidity is accompanied by abdominal pain and, if so, whether the pain and rigidity developed at the same time. Using an established pain scale, ask the patient to rate the pain. Ask about variations. Has the pain increased, decreased, or remained unchanged? Is it constant or intermittent? Is the location of the pain constant, radiating, or has it moved to a completely different location? Next, ask about possible aggravating or alleviating factors, such as position changes, coughing, vomiting, elimination, and walking.

Ask the patient about changes in bowel habits. Has he experienced increased flatulence, constipation, diarrhea, or changes in stool consistency? Note the date of the last bowel movement. Ask about changes in urinary habits. Has he developed urinary frequency, urgency, or pain? Has his urine changed color? Ask the female patient for the date of her last menses and whether changes have occurred in the menstrual cycle.

Physical examination
Inspect the abdomen for peristaltic waves, which may be visible in very thin patients. Check for a visibly distended bowel loop. Next, auscultate bowel sounds. Listen for systolic bruits over the abdominal aorta, renal artery, and iliac artery. Perform light palpation to locate the rigidity and determine its severity. Avoid deep palpation, which may exacerbate abdominal pain. Finally, check for poor skin turgor and dry mucous membranes, which indicate dehydration.

RECOGNIZING VOLUNTARY RIGIDITY

Distinguishing voluntary from involuntary abdominal rigidity is a must for accurate assessment. Review this comparison so that you can quickly tell the two apart.

VOLUNTARY RIGIDITY IS:
◆ usually symmetrical
◆ more rigid on inspiration (expiration causes muscle relaxation)
◆ eased by relaxation techniques, such as positioning the patient comfortably and talking to him in a calm, soothing manner
◆ painless when the patient sits up using his abdominal muscles alone.

INVOLUNTARY RIGIDITY IS:
◆ usually asymmetrical
◆ equally rigid on inspiration and expiration
◆ unaffected by relaxation techniques
◆ painful when the patient sits up using his abdominal muscles alone.

ACCESSORY MUSCLES: LOCATIONS AND FUNCTIONS

The diaphragm and external intercostal muscles are the muscles of normal breathing. When they're taxed by increased work from exercise or disease, accessory muscles provide the extra effort needed to maintain respirations. The upper accessory muscles assist with inspiration, whereas the upper chest, sternum, internal intercostal, and abdominal muscles assist with expiration.

With inspiration, the scalene muscles elevate, fix, and expand the upper chest. The sternocleidomastoid muscles raise the sternum, expanding the chest's anteroposterior and longitudinal dimensions. The pectoralis major elevates the chest, increasing its anteroposterior size, and the trapezius raises the thoracic cage.

With expiration, the internal intercostals depress the ribs, decreasing the chest size. The abdominal muscles pull the lower chest down, depress the lower ribs, and compress the abdominal contents, which exerts pressure on the chest.

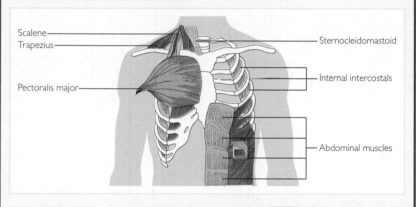

Pediatric pointers

Voluntary rigidity may be difficult to distinguish from involuntary rigidity in a young patient if associated pain makes him restless, tense, or apprehensive. In a child with suspected involuntary rigidity, your priority is early detection of dehydration and shock, which can rapidly become life threatening.

Abdominal rigidity in children can stem from gastric perforation, hypertrophic pyloric stenosis, duodenal obstruction, meconium ileus, intussusception, cystic fibrosis, celiac disease, and appendicitis.

Geriatric pointers

Advanced age and impaired cognition decrease pain perception and intensity in elderly patients. Weakening of abdominal muscles may decrease muscle spasms and rigidity. (See *Accessory muscles: Locations and functions*.) When accessory muscles are used, breathing requires extra effort. The accessory muscles — the sternocleidomastoid, scalene, pectoralis major, trapezius, internal intercostals, and abdominal muscles — stabilize the thorax during respiration. Some accessory muscle use normally takes place during such activities as singing, talking, coughing, defecating, and exercising. However, more pronounced use of these muscles might signal acute respiratory distress, diaphragmatic weakness, or fatigue. It may also result from chronic respiratory disease. Typically, the extent of accessory muscle use reflects the severity of the underlying cause.

MEDICAL CAUSES

● *Abdominal aortic aneurysm (dissecting).* Mild to moderate abdominal rigidity occurs with a dissecting abdominal aortic aneurysm, a life-threatening disorder. The rigidity is typically accompanied by constant upper abdominal pain that may radiate to the lower back or lower abdominal area; it may also manifest as severe chest pain. The pain may worsen when the patient lies down and decrease when he leans forward or sits up. Before rupture, the aneurysm may produce a pulsating mass in the epigastric area, accompanied by a systolic bruit over the aorta. However, the mass stops pulsating after rupture. Associated signs and symptoms include mottled skin below the waist, absence of femoral and pedal pulses, lower blood pressure in the legs than in the arms, and mild to moderate tenderness with guarding. Significant blood loss causes signs of shock, such as tachycardia, tachypnea, and cool, clammy skin.

● *Insect toxins.* Insect stings and bites, especially black widow spider bites, release toxins that can produce abdominal rigidity and generalized, cramping abdominal pain. These toxins may also cause low-grade fever, nausea, vomiting, tremors, and localized pain and swelling. Some patients experience increased salivation, hypertension, paresis, and hyperactive reflexes. Children commonly are restless, have an expiratory grunt, and keep their legs flexed.

● *Mesenteric artery ischemia.* Rigidity occurs in the central or periumbilical region and is accompanied by severe abdominal tenderness, fever, absence of bowel sounds, and signs of shock, including tachycardia, hypotension, and clammy skin. Other findings may include vomiting, anorexia, diarrhea, and constipation. Always suspect mesenteric artery ischemia in patients who are older than age 50 and have a history of heart failure, arrhythmias, cardiovascular infarct, or hypotension if they present with complaints of sudden, severe abdominal pain following 2 to 3 days of colicky periumbilical pain and diarrhea.

● *Peritonitis.* Depending on the cause of peritonitis, abdominal rigidity may be localized (as seen with an acute appendicitis) or generalized (as seen with a perforated ulcer). Peritonitis also causes sudden and severe abdominal pain that can be localized or generalized. The patient with peritonitis generally exhibits abdominal tenderness with distention, rebound tenderness, guarding, hyperalgesia, hypoactive or absent bowel sounds, nausea, and vomiting. He may also experience fever, chills, tachycardia, tachypnea, and hypotension.

● *Pneumonia.* In lower lobe pneumonia, abdominal rigidity is associated with severe referred upper abdominal pain and tenderness. The rigidity diminishes with inspiration. Other findings may include blood-tinged or rusty sputum, a dry and hacking cough, dyspnea, fever, sudden onset of chills, crackles, egophony, decreased breath sounds, and dullness on percussion.

NURSING CONSIDERATIONS

Monitor the patient closely for tachycardia, hypotension, clammy skin, and decreased responsiveness — these signs may indicate the presence of a life-threatening condition. Position him as comfortably as possible, preferably in a supine position, with his head flat on the table, arms at his sides, and knees slightly flexed to relax the abdominal muscles. Withhold analgesics to avoid masking symptoms that may help determine the diagnosis. Monitor for changes in the pain assessment or the development of pain. Withhold food and fluids until surgery has been ruled out. Administer an I.V. antibiotic. Prepare the patient for diagnostic tests, which may include chest and abdominal X-rays, computed tomography scans, magnetic resonance imaging, peritoneal lavage, gastroscopy or colonoscopy, and blood, urine, and stool studies. A pelvic or rectal examination may also be done.

PATIENT TEACHING

Inform the patient that pain medications will be withheld until a definitive diagnosis is made because these agents can mask important symptoms. Reinforce proper positioning to maintain a relaxed abdominal area. Explain the procedures for all tests that are ordered. Prepare the patient for surgery, if indicated.

Analgesia

Analgesia — the absence of sensitivity to pain — can help to identify the type of nervous system lesion and determine its location. For example, thermanesthesia (loss of temperature sensation) without other sensory changes can occur because although all sensory nerve impulses follow the same route, only a few may be blocked when there is an incomplete spinal cord lesion. When all sensory impulses are blocked, the origin of the injury could be in the brain, spinal cord, or peripheral nerves. Examples of other sensory deficits include paresthesia (loss of proprioception and vibratory sense) and tactile anesthesia.

Below the level of the lesion, analgesia can be classified as partial or total and unilateral or bilateral. The onset may be slow and progressive, as seen with a tumor, or abrupt, as seen with trauma. Analgesia may be transient and resolve spontaneously.

Act now *If the patient exhibits unilateral or bilateral analgesia over a large body surface, suspect a spinal cord injury and maintain proper body alignment until the spinal cord is stabilized. A cervical collar and a long backboard are the standards of care. If a collar is unavailable, maintain the patient's head position with sandbags placed around the head and neck. Be prepared for an emergency response if respiratory failure occurs.*

ASSESSMENT
History
After assuring spinal cord stabilization, proceed with assessing the patient. Establish the onset of analgesia (sudden or gradual). Did the patient suffer recent trauma, such as a fall, sports injury, or automobile accident? Obtain a complete medical history, noting incidence of cancer in the patient or his family.

Physical examination
Assess the patient's vital signs, including the pattern of respirations. Determine his level of consciousness. Assist to test pupillary, corneal, cough, and gag reflexes to rule out brain stem and cranial nerve involvement. If the patient is conscious, evaluate his ability to swallow.

Assist to perform a full neurologic assessment, including orientation to person, place, and time. Assess the patient's ability to speak clearly, pupil size and reaction to light, ability to follow commands, ability to wiggle extremities, and awareness of touch. Test for other sensory deficits over all dermatomes (individual skin segments innervated by a specific spinal nerve) by applying light tactile stimulation with a tongue depressor or cotton swab. Perform a more thorough assessment of pain sensitivity, if necessary, using a pin. (See *Testing for analgesia,* pages 18 and 19.) Assess the patient's temperature sensation over all dermatomes, using two test tubes—one filled with warm water, the other with cold water. In each arm and leg, test vibration sense (using a tuning fork), proprioception, and superficial and deep tendon reflexes (DTRs). Check for increased muscle tone by extending and flexing the patient's elbows and knees as he tries to relax.

After a spinal cord injury is ruled out, observe the patient's gait and posture and assess his balance and coordination. Evaluate muscle tone and strength in all extremities.

Pediatric pointers
Because a child may have difficulty describing analgesia, observe him carefully during the assessment for nonverbal clues to pain, such as facial expressions, crying, and retraction from stimuli. Remember that pain thresholds are high in infants, so your assessment findings may not be reliable. Also, remember to test the temperature of bath water carefully for a child who's too young to test it himself.

Geriatric pointers
Pre-existing sensory deficits in elderly patients may make an immediate diagnosis more difficult. Because elderly patients may have some degree of impairment to skin integrity, make sure that the water temperature used for sensory assessment won't burn the skin.

MEDICAL CAUSES
● *Anterior cord syndrome.* Analgesia and thermanesthesia occur bilaterally below the level of the lesion, along with flaccid paralysis and hypoactive DTRs.
● *Central cord syndrome.* Analgesia and thermanesthesia occur bilaterally in several dermatomes, in many cases extending in a capelike fashion over the arms, back, and shoulders. Early weakness in the hands is evident and progresses to weakness and muscle spasms in the arms and shoulder girdle. Hyperactive DTRs and spastic weakness of the legs may develop. (If hypoactive, DTRs and flaccid weakness persist in the legs, a lesion in the lumbar spine may be suspected.)

With brain stem involvement, additional findings include facial analgesia and thermanesthesia, vertigo, nystagmus, atrophy of the tongue, dysarthria, dysphagia, urine retention, anhidrosis, decreased intestinal motility, and hyperkeratosis.

TESTING FOR ANALGESIA

By carefully and systematically testing your patient's sensitivity to pain, you can determine whether his nerve damage has segmental or peripheral distribution and help locate the causative lesion.

Tell the patient to relax, and explain that you're going to lightly touch areas of his skin with a small pin. Have him close his eyes. Apply the pin firmly enough to produce pain without breaking the skin. (Practice on yourself first to learn how to apply the correct pressure.)

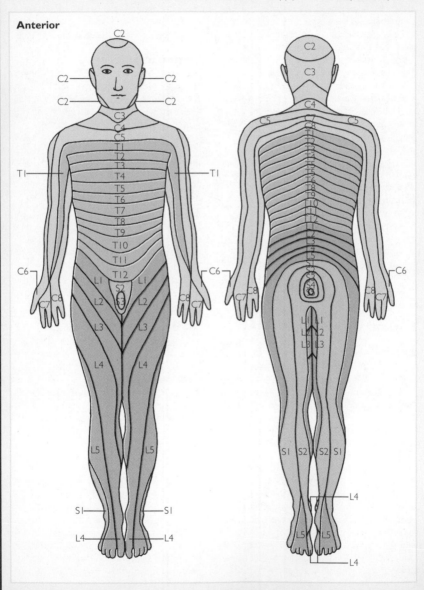

Anterior

Starting with the patient's head and face, move down his body, pricking his skin on alternating sides. Have the patient report when he feels pain. Use the blunt end of the pin occasionally, and vary your test pattern to gauge the accuracy of his response.

Document your findings thoroughly, clearly marking areas of lost pain sensation on a dermatome chart (shown on previous page).

Peripheral nerves

Anterior leg

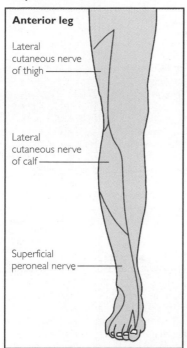

Lateral cutaneous nerve of thigh

Lateral cutaneous nerve of calf

Superficial peroneal nerve

Posterior leg

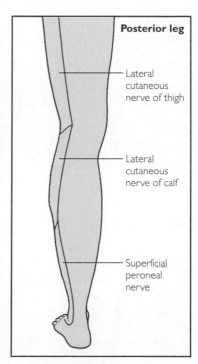

Lateral cutaneous nerve of thigh

Lateral cutaneous nerve of calf

Superficial peroneal nerve

Anterior hand

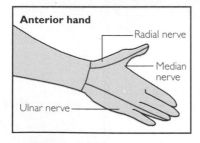

Radial nerve

Median nerve

Ulnar nerve

Posterior hand

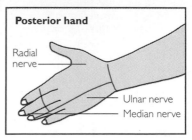

Radial nerve

Ulnar nerve

Median nerve

• **Spinal cord hemisection.** Contralateral analgesia and thermanesthesia occur below the level of the lesion. In addition, loss of proprioception, spastic paralysis, and hyperactive DTRs develop ipsilaterally. Urine retention with overflow incontinence may be present.

OTHER CAUSES
• **Drugs.** Analgesia may occur with the use of a topical or local anesthetic, although numbness and tingling are more common.

NURSING CONSIDERATIONS
Maintain spinal alignment during transport for laboratory or radiologic procedures. Monitor the patient's vital signs and neurologic assessment closely. Provide continuous emotional support to the patient and his family.

Prevent pressure ulcer formation by such measures as meticulous skin care, massage, and frequent repositioning, especially when significant motor deficits hamper the patient's movement. Guard against scalding by testing the water temperature before the patient bathes.

PATIENT TEACHING
Explain all tests and procedures. Advise the patient to test the water at home using a thermometer or a body part with intact sensation before showering or bathing.

Anhidrosis

Anhidrosis is an abnormal deficiency of sweating and can be classified as generalized (complete) or localized (partial). Generalized anhidrosis can lead to life-threatening impairment of thermoregulation and a lack of sweating, eventually leading to retention of excess body heat. Localized anhidrosis rarely interferes with thermoregulation because it affects only a small percentage of the body's sweat glands.

The absence, obstruction, atrophy, or degeneration of sweat glands can produce anhidrosis at the skin surface, even if neurologic stimulation is normal. (See *Eccrine dysfunction in anhidrosis,* pages 22 and 23.)

Other causes of anhidrosis include neurologic disorders that disturb the central or peripheral nervous pathways that normally activate sweating, skin disorders, and congenital, atrophic, or traumatic changes to sweat glands. Use of certain drugs can also lead to anhidrosis.

Anhidrosis may go unrecognized until significant heat or exertion fails to raise sweat. However, localized anhidrosis commonly provokes compensatory hyperhidrosis in the remaining functional sweat glands — which, in many cases, is the patient's chief complaint.

> **Act now** *If the patient's skin feels hot and flushed with an obvious lack of perspiration, ask whether he's experiencing nausea, dizziness, palpitations, and substernal tightness. If these symptoms are present, quickly take the patient's rectal temperature and other vital signs, and assess his level of consciousness (LOC). If a rectal temperature higher than 102.2° F (39° C) is accompanied by tachycardia, tachypnea, altered blood pressure, and decreased LOC, suspect life-threatening heatstroke (anhidrotic asthenia). Start rapid cooling measures, such as swabbing or spraying with very cold water and giving I.V. fluid replacements. Continue these measures and frequently check the patient's vital signs and neurologic status until his temperature drops below 102° F (38.9° C). Then move him to a room with good ventilation, fans, or air conditioning.*

ASSESSMENT
History
Ask the patient to characterize his sweating, especially during heat spells or strenuous activity. Is the sweating slight or profuse? Ask about recent prolonged or extreme exposure to heat and about the onset of anhidrosis or hyperhidrosis. Obtain a complete medical history, focusing on neurologic disorders, skin disorders such as psoriasis, autoimmune disorders such as scleroderma, and systemic diseases such as diabetes mellitus, which can cause peripheral neuropathies. Ask about drug use.

Physical examination
Inspect skin color, texture, and turgor. If you detect skin lesions, document their location, size, color, texture, and pattern. Note the presence of localized sweating and document the area, amount of perspiration, and skin differences in that area.

Pediatric pointers

In infants and children, miliaria rubra and such congenital skin disorders as ichthyosis and anhidrotic ectodermal dysplasia are the most common causes of anhidrosis.

Because delayed development of the thermoregulatory center renders an infant—especially a premature infant—anhidrotic for several weeks after birth, caution parents against overdressing.

Geriatric pointers

Pre-existing disease states and advanced age may place elderly patients at greater risk for anhidrosis. Onset may occur more swiftly in elderly patients.

MEDICAL CAUSES

● *Burns.* Depending on their severity, burns may cause permanent anhidrosis in affected areas as well as blistering, edema, and increased pain or loss of sensation.
● *Cerebral lesions.* Cerebral cortex and brain stem lesions may cause anhidrotic palms and soles, along with various motor and sensory disturbances specific to the site of the lesions.
● *Heatstroke (anhidrotic asthenia).* In the early stages of heatstroke, a life-threatening disorder, the patient may still exhibit signs of sweating and his LOC may be normal, but the rectal temperature may already exceed 102.2° F (39° C). He may experience severe headache and muscle cramps, which later disappear. Associated signs and symptoms include fatigue, nausea and vomiting, dizziness, palpitations, substernal tightness, and elevated blood pressure followed by hypotension. Within minutes, hot, flushed skin will be noted with anhidrosis. Accompanying symptoms include tachycardia, tachypnea, and confusion with a progression to seizures or loss of consciousness.
● *Horner's syndrome.* A supraclavicular spinal cord lesion affecting a cervical nerve produces unilateral facial anhidrosis with compensatory contralateral hyperhidrosis. Other findings include ipsilateral pupillary constriction and ptosis.
● *Miliaria crystallina.* This usually innocuous form of miliaria causes anhidrosis and tiny, clear, fragile blisters, usually under the arms and breasts.
● *Miliaria profunda.* If severe and extensive, this form of miliaria can progress to life-threatening anhidrotic asthenia. Typically, it produces localized anhidrosis with compensatory facial hyperhidrosis. Whitish papules appear mostly on the trunk but also on the extremities. Associated signs and symptoms include inguinal and axillary lymphadenopathy, weakness, shortness of breath, palpitations, and fever.
● *Miliaria rubra (prickly heat).* This common form of miliaria typically produces localized anhidrosis. Small, erythematous papules with centrally placed blisters appear on the trunk and neck and, rarely, on the face, palms, or soles. Pustules may also appear in extensive and chronic miliaria. Related symptoms include paroxysmal itching and paresthesia. In rare instances, severe and extensive miliaria rubra can progress to life-threatening anhidrotic asthenia.
● *Peripheral neuropathy.* Anhidrosis over the legs usually appears with compensatory hyperhidrosis over the head and neck. Associated findings mainly involve extremities and include glossy red skin, diminished or absent deep tendon reflexes, flaccid paralysis and muscle wasting, footdrop, burning pain, and paresthesia, hyperesthesia, or anesthesia in the hands and feet.
● *Shy-Drager syndrome.* Shy-Drager syndrome, a degenerative neurologic syndrome, causes ascending anhidrosis in the legs. Other signs and symptoms include severe orthostatic hypotension, loss of leg hair, impotence, constipation, urine retention or urgency, decreased salivation and tearing, mydriasis, and impaired visual accommodation. Eventually, focal neurologic signs—such as leg tremors, incoordination, and muscle wasting and fasciculation—may appear.
● *Spinal cord lesions.* Anhidrosis may occur symmetrically below the level of the lesion, with compensatory hyperhidrosis in adjacent areas. Other findings vary according to the site and extent of the lesion, but may include partial or total loss of motor and sensory function below the lesion as well as impaired cardiovascular and respiratory function.

OTHER CAUSES

● *Drugs.* Anticholinergics, such as atropine and scopolamine, can cause generalized anhidrosis.

NURSING CONSIDERATIONS

Perform careful monitoring of the patient's vital signs, with particular attention to tem-

Eccrine dysfunction in anhidrosis

Eccrine glands, located over most of the skin, help regulate body temperature by secreting sweat. A change or dysfunction in these glands can result in anhidrosis of varying severity. These illustrations show a normal eccrine gland and some common abnormalities.

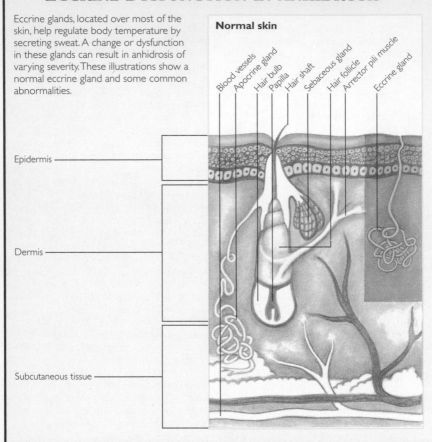

Normal skin

Blood vessels · Apocrine gland · Hair bulb · Papilla · Hair shaft · Sebaceous gland · Hair follicle · Arrector pili muscle · Eccrine gland

Epidermis

Dermis

Subcutaneous tissue

---

perature. Frequently assess the skin and sweating pattern. Assess the patient's LOC.

Because even a careful evaluation can be inconclusive, you may need to administer specific tests to evaluate anhidrosis. These include wrapping the patient in an electric blanket or placing him in a heated box to observe the skin for sweat patterns, applying a topical agent to detect sweat on the skin, and administering a systemic cholinergic drug to stimulate sweating.

PATIENT TEACHING

Review the signs and symptoms of overheating and heatstroke. Inform the patient about measures to prevent dehydration and heatstroke, such as spending time in a cool environment, moving slowly during warm weather, and avoiding strenuous exercise and hot, spicy foods. Tell him to drink about a quart of noncaffeinated, nonalcoholic fluids an hour when in extremely hot environments.

Educate the patient about the anhidrotic effects of certain medications.

Anuria

Anuria is defined as urine output of less than 100 ml in a 24-hour period. Causes include urinary tract obstruction and acute renal fail-

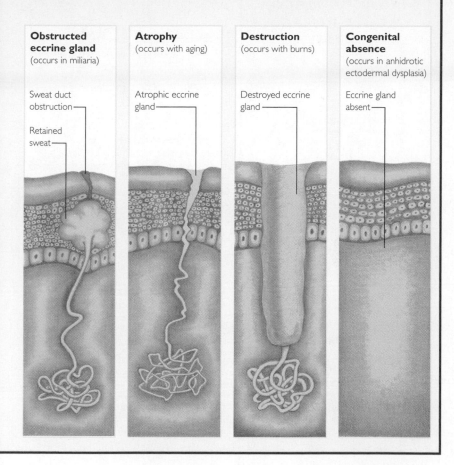

Obstructed eccrine gland (occurs in miliaria)	Atrophy (occurs with aging)	Destruction (occurs with burns)	Congenital absence (occurs in anhidrotic ectodermal dysplasia)
Sweat duct obstruction— Retained sweat—	Atrophic eccrine gland—	Destroyed eccrine gland —	Eccrine gland absent—

ure due to various mechanisms. (See *Major causes of acute renal failure,* page 24.) Anuria is rare; even with renal failure, the kidneys usually produce at least 75 ml of urine daily.

Because urine output is easily measured when the patient is in a controlled setting, anuria rarely goes undetected. However, without immediate treatment, it can rapidly cause uremia and other complications of urine retention.

Act now When anuria is detected, it's essential to determine whether urine formation is present. An indwelling urinary catheter may be inserted to determine the presence of residual urine, mechanical obstruction, or cloudy, foul-smelling urine. Urine output greater than 75 ml/day may indicate a lower urinary tract obstruction. Urine output less than 75 ml/day may indicate renal dysfunction or an obstruction higher in the urinary tract.

ASSESSMENT
History
Obtain a complete history, including changes in voiding pattern or urine characteristics. Ask the patient how much fluid he normally ingests each day, how much he ingested in the past 24 to 48 hours, and the time and amount of his last urination. Note a history of kidney disease, urinary tract obstruction or infection, prostate enlargement, renal calculi, neurogenic bladder, or congenital abnormalities. Ask about abdominal, renal, or urinary tract surgery and about drug use.

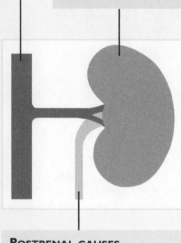
Pediatric pointers

In neonates, anuria is defined as the absence of urine output for 24 hours. It can be classified as primary or secondary. Primary anuria results from bilateral renal agenesis, aplasia, or multicystic dysplasia. Secondary anuria, associated with edema or dehydration, results from renal ischemia, renal vein thrombosis, or congenital anomalies of the genitourinary tract. Anuria in children commonly results from loss of renal function.

Geriatric pointers

In elderly patients, anuria is a gradually occurring sign of underlying pathology. Hospitalized or bedridden elderly patients may be unable to generate the necessary pressure to void if they remain in a supine position. Elderly patients with disease processes; such as Alzheimer's disease or dementia; may be difficult or impossible to evaluate due to urinary incontinence or an inability to record their own urinary output.

MEDICAL CAUSES

● *Acute tubular necrosis (ATN).* Oliguria (occasionally anuria) is a common initial finding with ATN. Associated symptoms may reflect the underlying cause, such as hyperkalemia (muscle weakness, cardiac arrhythmias), uremia (anorexia, nausea, vomiting, confusion, lethargy, twitching, convulsions, pruritus, uremic frost, and Kussmaul's respirations), and heart failure (edema, jugular vein distention, crackles, and dyspnea).

● *Cortical necrosis (bilateral).* Bilateral cortical necrosis is characterized by a sudden change from oliguria to anuria, along with gross hematuria, flank pain, and fever.

● *Glomerulonephritis (acute).* Acute glomerulonephritis produces anuria or oliguria. Related effects include mild fever, malaise, flank pain, gross hematuria, facial and generalized edema, elevated blood pressure, headache, nausea, vomiting, abdominal pain, and signs and symptoms of pulmonary congestion (crackles, dyspnea).

● *Hemolytic-uremic syndrome.* Anuria commonly occurs in the initial stages of hemolytic-uremic syndrome and may last from 1 to 10 days. The patient may experience vomiting, diarrhea, abdominal pain, hematemesis, melena, purpura, fever, elevated blood pressure, hepatomegaly, ecchymosis, edema, hematuria, and pallor. He may also show signs of an upper respiratory tract infection.

Physical examination

Inspect and palpate the abdomen for asymmetry, distention, or bulging. Inspect the flank area for edema or erythema, and percuss and palpate the bladder. Palpate the kidneys anteriorly and posteriorly, and percuss them at the costovertebral angle. Auscultate over the renal arteries, listening for bruits.

- *Papillary necrosis (acute).* Bilateral papillary necrosis produces anuria or oliguria. It also produces flank pain, costovertebral angle tenderness, renal colic, abdominal pain and rigidity, fever, vomiting, decreased bowel sounds, hematuria, and pyuria.
- *Renal artery occlusion (bilateral).* Bilateral renal artery occlusion produces anuria or severe oliguria, commonly accompanied by severe, continuous upper abdominal and flank pain; nausea and vomiting; decreased bowel sounds; fever up to 102° F (38.9° C); and diastolic hypertension.
- *Renal vein occlusion (bilateral).* Bilateral renal vein occlusion occasionally causes anuria; more typical signs and symptoms include acute low back pain, fever, flank tenderness, and hematuria. Development of pulmonary emboli — a common complication — produces sudden dyspnea, pleuritic pain, tachypnea, tachycardia, crackles, pleural friction rub, and possibly hemoptysis.
- *Urinary tract obstruction.* Severe obstruction can produce acute, and sometimes, total anuria, alternating with or preceded by burning and pain on urination, overflow incontinence or dribbling, increased urinary frequency and nocturia, voiding of small amounts, or altered urine stream. Associated findings include bladder distention, pain and a sensation of fullness in the lower abdomen and groin, upper abdominal and flank pain, nausea and vomiting, and signs of secondary infection, such as fever, chills, malaise, and cloudy, foul-smelling urine.
- *Vasculitis.* Vasculitis occasionally produces anuria. More typical findings include malaise, myalgia, polyarthralgia, fever, elevated blood pressure, hematuria, proteinuria, arrhythmias, pallor, and possibly skin lesions, urticaria, and purpura.

OTHER CAUSES

- *Diagnostic tests.* Contrast media used in radiographic studies can cause nephrotoxicity, producing oliguria and, rarely, anuria.
- *Drugs.* Many classes of drugs can cause anuria or, more commonly, oliguria through their nephrotoxic effects. Antibiotics, especially aminoglycosides, are the most typically seen nephrotoxins. Anesthetics, heavy metals, ethyl alcohol, and organic solvents can also be nephrotoxic. Adrenergics and anticholinergics can cause anuria by affecting the nerves and muscles of micturition to produce urine retention.

NURSING CONSIDERATIONS

If catheterization fails to initiate urine flow, prepare the patient for diagnostic studies — such as ultrasonography, cystoscopy, retrograde pyelography, and renal scan — to detect an obstruction higher in the urinary tract. If these tests fail to reveal an obstruction, prepare the patient for further kidney function studies. If these tests reveal an obstruction, immediate surgery may be indicated to remove the obstruction, and a nephrostomy or ureterostomy tube may be inserted to drain urine.

Carefully monitor the patient's vital signs and intake and output, initially saving any urine for inspection. Restrict daily fluid allowance to 600 ml more than the previous day's total urine output. Restrict foods and juices high in potassium and sodium, and make sure that the patient maintains a balanced diet with controlled protein levels. Provide low-sodium hard candy to help decrease thirst. Record fluid intake and output, and weigh the patient daily.

PATIENT TEACHING

Explain all tests and procedures to the patient. Depending on the cause of anuria, review the disorder's early warning signs and symptoms. If the patient requires surgery, withhold food and fluids. Review medications that may worsen renal function.

Aphasia

Aphasia is an impairment in expressing or comprehending written or spoken language. It generally reflects disease or injury to the brain's language centers. (See *Where language originates,* page 26.) Depending on its severity, aphasia may slightly impede communication or may make it impossible. It can be classified as Broca's, Wernicke's, anomic, or global aphasia. Anomic aphasia eventually resolves in more than 50% of patients, but global aphasia is usually irreversible. (See *Identifying types of aphasia,* page 27.)

Act now *Quickly look for signs and symptoms of increased intracranial pressure (ICP), such as pupillary changes, decreased level of consciousness (LOC), vomiting, seizures, bradycardia, widening pulse pressure, and irregular respirations. If you detect signs of increased ICP, insert a*

WHERE LANGUAGE ORIGINATES

Aphasia reflects damage to one or more of the brain's primary language centers, which, in most people, are located in the left hemisphere. *Broca's area* lies next to the region of the motor cortex that controls the muscles necessary for speech. *Wernicke's area* is the center of auditory, visual, and language comprehension. It lies between *Heschl's gyrus*, the primary receiver of auditory stimuli, and the *angular gyrus*, a "way station" between the brain's auditory and visual regions. Connecting Wernicke's and Broca's areas is a large nerve bundle, the *arcuate fasciculus*, which enables speech repetition.

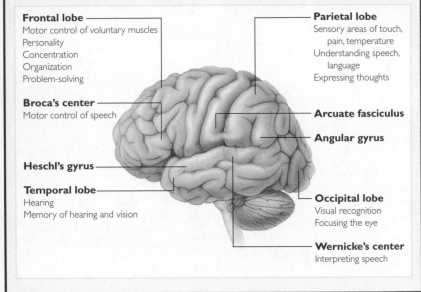

Frontal lobe
Motor control of voluntary muscles
Personality
Concentration
Organization
Problem-solving

Broca's center
Motor control of speech

Heschl's gyrus

Temporal lobe
Hearing
Memory of hearing and vision

Parietal lobe
Sensory areas of touch,
pain, temperature
Understanding speech,
language
Expressing thoughts

Arcuate fasciculus

Angular gyrus

Occipital lobe
Visual recognition
Focusing the eye

Wernicke's center
Interpreting speech

---

urinary catheter to prevent bladder rupture and then administer mannitol I.V. to decrease cerebral edema. In addition, make sure that emergency resuscitation equipment is readily available to support respiratory and cardiac function, if necessary. You may have to prepare the patient for emergency surgery.

ASSESSMENT
History

A history will probably need to be obtained from the patient's family or companion because of the patient's impairment. Determine if the aphasia is new or when it began. Determine if the patient has a history of headaches, hypertension, seizure disorders, or drug use.

Physical examination

Perform a complete neurologic examination. Take the patient's vital signs and assess his LOC. Be aware, though, that assessing LOC is commonly difficult because the patient's verbal responses may be unreliable. Assess the patient's pupillary response, eye movements, and motor function, especially his mouth and tongue movement, swallowing ability, and spontaneous movements and gestures. To best assess motor function, first demonstrate the motions and then have the patient imitate them. Don't give liquids to drink until ordered due to the risk of aspiration.

Also, recognize that dysarthria (impaired articulation due to weakness or paralysis of the muscles necessary for speech) or speech apraxia (inability to voluntarily control the muscles of speech) may accompany aphasia; therefore, speak slowly and distinctly, and allow the patient ample time to respond. Check for obvious signs of neurologic

IDENTIFYING TYPES OF APHASIA

TYPE	LOCATION OF LESION	SIGNS AND SYMPTOMS
Anomic aphasia	Temporal-parietal area; may extend to angular gyrus, but sometimes poorly localized	Patient's understanding of written and spoken language is relatively unimpaired. His speech, although fluent, lacks meaningful content. Word-finding difficulty and circumlocution are characteristic. Rarely, the patient also displays paraphasia.
Broca's aphasia (expressive aphasia)	Broca's area; usually in third frontal convolution of the left hemisphere	Patient's understanding of written and spoken language is relatively spared, but speech is nonfluent, evidencing word-finding difficulty, jargon, paraphasia, limited vocabulary, and simple sentence construction. He can't repeat words and phrases. If Wernicke's area is intact, he recognizes speech errors and shows frustration. He's commonly hemiparetic.
Global aphasia	Broca's and Wernicke's areas	Patient has profoundly impaired receptive and expressive ability. He can't repeat words or phrases and can't follow directions. His occasional speech is marked by paraphasia or jargon.
Wernicke's aphasia (receptive aphasia)	Wernicke's area; usually in posterior or superior temporal lobe	Patient has difficulty understanding written and spoken language. He can't repeat words or phrases or can't follow directions. His speech is fluent but may be rapid and rambling, with paraphasia. He has difficulty naming objects (anomia) and is unaware of speech errors.

deficit, such as ptosis or fluid leakage from the nose and ears.

Pediatric pointers

Recognize that the term *childhood aphasia* is sometimes mistakenly applied to children who fail to develop normal language skills but who aren't considered mentally retarded or developmentally delayed. *Aphasia* refers solely to the loss of previously developed communication skills.

Brain damage associated with aphasia in children most commonly follows anoxia — the result of near-drowning or airway obstruction.

Geriatric pointers

Pre-existing diseases, such as dementia (Alzheimer's type, vascular, or others) or previous stroke may make it more difficult to assess the patient for aphasia.

MEDICAL CAUSES

- *Alzheimer's disease.* With Alzheimer's disease, a degenerative disease, anomic aphasia may begin insidiously and then progress to severe global aphasia. Associated signs and symptoms include behavioral changes, memory loss, poor judgment, restlessness, myoclonus, and muscle rigidity. Incontinence is usually a late sign.
- *Brain abscess.* Any type of aphasia may occur with brain abscess. Usually, aphasia develops insidiously and may be accompanied by hemiparesis, ataxia, facial weakness, and signs of increased ICP.
- *Brain tumor.* A brain tumor may cause any type of aphasia. As the tumor enlarges, other aphasias may occur along with behavioral changes, memory loss, motor weakness, seizures, auditory hallucinations, visual field deficits, and increased ICP.

- *Creutzfeldt-Jakob disease.* Creutzfeldt-Jacob disease is a rapidly progressive dementia accompanied by neurologic signs and symptoms, such as myoclonic jerking, ataxia, aphasia, vision disturbances, and paralysis. It generally affects adults ages 40 to 65.
- *Encephalitis.* Encephalitis usually produces transient aphasia. Its early signs and symptoms include fever, headache, and vomiting. Seizures, confusion, stupor or coma, hemiparesis, asymmetrical deep tendon reflexes, positive Babinski's reflex, ataxia, myoclonus, nystagmus, ocular palsies, and facial weakness may accompany aphasia.
- *Head trauma.* Any type of aphasia may accompany severe head trauma, which occurs suddenly and may be transient or permanent, depending on the extent of brain damage. Associated signs and symptoms include blurred or double vision, headache, pallor, diaphoresis, numbness and paresis, cerebrospinal otorrhea or rhinorrhea, altered respirations, tachycardia, disorientation, behavioral changes, and signs of increased ICP.
- *Seizures.* Seizures and the postictal state may cause transient aphasia if the seizures involve the language centers.
- *Stroke.* The most common cause of aphasia, stroke may produce Wernicke's, Broca's, or global aphasia. Associated findings include decreased LOC, right-sided hemiparesis, homonymous hemianopia, paresthesia, and loss of sensation. (These signs and symptoms may appear on the left side if the right hemisphere contains the language centers.)
- *Transient ischemic attack (TIA).* A TIA can produce any type of aphasia, which occurs suddenly and resolves within 24 hours of the TIA. Associated signs and symptoms include transient hemiparesis, hemianopia, and paresthesia (all usually right-sided), dizziness, and confusion.

NURSING CONSIDERATIONS

Maintain reality by frequently explaining what has happened, where the patient is located and why, and what the date is. Later, expect periods of depression as the patient recognizes his disability. Facilitate communication by providing a relaxed, accepting environment with a minimum of distracting stimuli. Prepare the patient for a psychiatric consultation if the depression becomes debilitating or is demonstrated by personality changes.

When you speak to the patient, don't assume that he understands you. He may simply be interpreting subtle clues to meaning, such as social context, facial expressions, and gestures. To help avoid misunderstanding, use nonverbal techniques, speak to him in simple phrases, and use demonstration to clarify your verbal directions.

Remember that aphasia is a language disorder, not an emotional or auditory one, so speak to the patient in a normal tone of voice. Make sure that he has necessary aids, such as eyeglasses or dentures, to facilitate communication. Refer the patient to a speech pathologist early to help him cope with his aphasia.

PATIENT TEACHING

Carefully explain diagnostic tests, such as skull X-rays, computed tomography or magnetic resonance imaging, angiography, and electroencephalography. Explain the related effects of aphasia to the patient and his family, such as possible depression or the use of profanity.

Apnea

Apnea is the cessation of spontaneous respiration and is usually a life-threatening emergency that requires immediate intervention to prevent death. It may occur as a temporary and self-limiting event, such as Cheyne-Stokes and Biot's respirations.

Apnea usually results from one or more of six pathophysiologic mechanisms, each of which has numerous causes. Its most common causes include trauma, cardiac arrest, neurologic disease, aspiration of foreign objects, bronchospasm, and drug overdose. (See *Causes of apnea.*)

Act now Upon discovering a patient with apnea, immediately begin resuscitative measures. Place the patient in a supine position. Open the airway using the head tilt/chin lift technique, and look, listen, and feel for spontaneous respirations. (If there's suspected head, neck, or spine trauma, use the jaw thrust maneuver to open the airway). If breaths are absent, begin artificial ventilation. If apnea was prolonged, full cardiac ar-

Causes of apnea

AIRWAY OBSTRUCTION
- Asthma
- Bronchospasm
- Chronic bronchitis
- Chronic obstructive pulmonary disease
- Foreign body aspiration
- Hemothorax or pneumothorax
- Mucus plug
- Obstruction by tongue or tumor
- Obstructive sleep apnea
- Secretion retention
- Tracheal or bronchial rupture

BRAIN STEM DYSFUNCTION
- Brain abscess
- Brain stem injury
- Brain tumor
- Central nervous system depressants
- Central sleep apnea

- Cerebral hemorrhage
- Cerebral infarction
- Encephalitis
- Head trauma
- Increased intracranial pressure
- Medullary or pontine hemorrhage or infarction
- Meningitis
- Transtentorial herniation

NEUROMUSCULAR FAILURE
- Amyotrophic lateral sclerosis
- Botulism
- Diphtheria
- Guillain-Barré syndrome
- Myasthenia gravis
- Phrenic nerve paralysis
- Rupture of the diaphragm
- Spinal cord injury

PARENCHYMATOUS DISEASE
- Acute respiratory distress syndrome
- Diffuse pneumonia
- Emphysema
- Near drowning
- Pulmonary edema
- Pulmonary fibrosis
- Secretion retention

PLEURAL PRESSURE GRADIENT DISRUPTION
- Flail chest
- Open chest wounds

PULMONARY CAPILLARY PERFUSION DECREASE
- Arrhythmias
- Cardiac arrest
- Myocardial infarction
- Pulmonary embolism
- Pulmonary hypertension
- Shock

---

rest may be present. Palpate the patient's carotid pulse, and if absent, begin chest compressions.

For an infant or a child, the airway is opened in the same manner as an adult. For a child, a carotid pulse is palpated, and for an infant, a brachial pulse is palpated.

ASSESSMENT
History
When the patient is stabilized, obtain a history from the family. Determine the onset and events immediately preceding the event. Determine if there were related events, such as headache, chest pain, muscle weakness, sore throat, or dyspnea. Ask about a history of respiratory, cardiac, or neurologic disease and about allergies and drug use.

Physical examination
Inspect the head, face, neck, and trunk for soft-tissue injury, hemorrhage, or skeletal deformity. Don't overlook obvious clues, such as oral and nasal secretions reflecting fluid-filled airways and alveoli, or facial soot and

singed nasal hair suggesting thermal injury to the tracheobronchial tree.

Auscultate over all lung lobes for adventitious breath sounds, particularly crackles and rhonchi. Percuss the lung fields for increased dullness or hyperresonance. Auscultate the heart for murmurs, pericardial friction rub, and arrhythmias. Assess for cyanosis, pallor, jugular vein distention, and edema. If appropriate, perform a neurologic assessment. Evaluate the patient's level of consciousness (LOC), orientation, and mental status; test cranial nerve function and motor function, sensation, and reflexes in all extremities.

Pediatric pointers
Premature infants are especially susceptible to periodic apneic episodes because of central nervous system (CNS) immaturity. Other common causes of apnea in infants include sepsis, intraventricular and subarachnoid hemorrhage, seizures, bronchiolitis, and sudden infant death syndrome.

In toddlers and older children, the primary cause of apnea is acute airway obstruction from aspiration of foreign objects. Other causes include acute epiglottiditis, enlarged tonsils and adenoids, croup, asthma, and systemic disorders, such as muscular dystrophy and cystic fibrosis. Therefore, in children and infants who have been ill with fever and develop signs of respiratory impairment, immediate access to the health care system is of primary importance. Emergency intubation may be required.

Geriatric pointers
In elderly patients, increased sensitivity to analgesics, sedative-hypnotics, or any combination of these drugs may produce apnea, even with normal dosage ranges.

MEDICAL CAUSES
● *Airway obstruction.* Occlusion or compression of the trachea, central airways, or smaller airways can cause sudden apnea by blocking the patient's airflow and producing acute respiratory failure.
● *Brain stem dysfunction.* Primary or secondary brain stem dysfunction can cause apnea by destroying the brain stem's ability to initiate respirations. Apnea may arise suddenly (as in trauma, hemorrhage, or infarction) or gradually (as in degenerative disease or a tumor). Apnea may be preceded by a decreased LOC and by various motor and sensory deficits.
● *Neuromuscular failure.* Trauma or disease can disrupt the mechanics of respiration, causing sudden or gradual apnea. Associated findings include diaphragmatic or intercostal muscle paralysis from injury, or respiratory weakness or paralysis from acute or degenerative disease.
● *Parenchymatous lung disease.* An accumulation of fluid within the alveoli produces apnea by interfering with pulmonary gas exchange and producing acute respiratory failure. Apnea may arise suddenly, as in near drowning and acute pulmonary edema, or gradually, as in emphysema. Apnea also may be preceded by crackles and labored respirations with accessory muscle use.
● *Pleural pressure gradient disruption.* Conversion of normal negative pleural air pressure to positive pressure by chest wall injuries, such as flail chest, causes lung collapse, producing respiratory distress and, if untreated, apnea. Associated signs include an asymmetrical chest wall and asymmetrical or paradoxical respirations.

● *Pulmonary capillary perfusion decrease.* Apnea can stem from obstructed pulmonary circulation, most commonly due to heart failure or lack of circulatory patency. It occurs suddenly in cardiac arrest, massive pulmonary embolism, and most cases of severe shock. In contrast, it occurs progressively in septic shock and pulmonary hypertension. Related findings include hypotension, tachycardia, and edema.

OTHER CAUSES
● *Drugs.* CNS depressants may cause hypoventilation and apnea. Benzodiazepines may cause respiratory depression and apnea when given I.V. along with other CNS depressants to elderly or acutely ill patients.
● *Neuromuscular blockers.* These medications, such as curariform drugs and anticholinesterases, may produce sudden apnea because of respiratory muscle paralysis.
● *Sleep-related apnea.* These repetitive apneas occur during sleep from airflow obstruction or brain stem dysfunction.

NURSING CONSIDERATIONS
Perform continuous assessment of the patient's respiratory and cardiac systems until he's stable. Obtain his vital signs, and perform a full neurologic examination.

PATIENT TEACHING
If the cause of the apnea was preventable, review the standards with the patient, if applicable, and his family. Educate the patient about safety measures related to aspiration of medications. Encourage cardiopulmonary resuscitation training for all adolescents and adults.

Apraxia

Apraxia is the inability to perform purposeful movements in the absence of significant weakness, sensory loss, poor coordination, or lack of comprehension or motivation. Apraxia usually indicates a lesion in the cerebral hemisphere. Its onset, severity, and duration vary.

Apraxia is classified as ideational, ideomotor, or kinetic, depending on the stage at which voluntary movement is impaired. It can also be classified by type of motor or

HOW APRAXIA INTERFERES WITH PURPOSEFUL MOVEMENT

TYPE OF APRAXIA	DESCRIPTION	EXAMINATION TECHNIQUE
Ideational apraxia	The patient can physically perform the steps required to complete a task but fails to remember the sequence in which they're performed.	Ask the patient to tie his shoelace. Typically, he can grasp the shoelace, loop it, and pull on it. However, he can't remember the sequence of steps needed to tie a knot.
Ideomotor apraxia	The patient understands and can physically perform the steps required to complete the task but can't formulate a plan to carry them out.	Ask the patient to wave or cross his arms. Typically, he won't respond, but he may be able to spontaneously perform the gesture.
Kinetic apraxia	The patient understands the task and formulates a plan but fails to set the proper muscles in motion.	Ask the patient to comb his hair. Typically, he can't move his arm and hand correctly to do so. However, he can state that he needs to pick up the comb and draw it through his hair.

skill impairment. For example, *facial* and *gait apraxia* involve specific motor groups and are easily perceived. *Constructional apraxia* refers to the inability to copy simple drawings or patterns. *Dressing apraxia* refers to the inability to correctly dress oneself. *Callosal apraxia* refers to normal motor function on one side of the body accompanied by the inability to reproduce movements on the other side. (See *How apraxia interferes with purposeful movement*.)

ASSESSMENT
History
Obtain the patient's history. Ask whether he has a previous history of neurologic disease. Does he have a history of headaches or dizziness?

Ask about previous cerebrovascular disease, atherosclerosis, neoplastic disease, infection, or hepatic disease.

Physical examination
First, obtain the patient's vital signs and assess his level of consciousness. Perform a neurologic assessment, staying alert for evidence of aphasia or dysarthria. Assess motor function, observing for weakness and tremors. Assist with testing sensory function, deep tendon reflexes, and visual field deficits.

Stay alert for signs and symptoms of increased intracranial pressure (ICP), such as headache and vomiting. If present, elevate the head of the bed 30 degrees and monitor the patient closely for altered pupil size and reactivity, bradycardia, widened pulse pressure, and irregular respirations. Have emergency resuscitation equipment nearby, and be prepared to give mannitol I.V. to decrease cerebral edema after inserting a urinary catheter to avoid bladder rupture.

If the patient is experiencing seizures, stay with him and have another nurse notify the physician immediately. Avoid restraining the patient. Assist him into a supine position, loosen tight clothing, and place a pillow or other soft object beneath his head. Don't place anything into his mouth. Turn the patient's head to the side to provide an open airway.

Pediatric pointers
Detecting apraxia in children can be difficult. However, a sudden inability to perform a previously accomplished movement warrants prompt neurologic evaluation because a brain tumor — the most common cause of apraxia in children — can be treated effectively if detected early.

Brain damage in a young child may cause developmental apraxia, which interferes with

APRAXIA:
CAUSES AND ASSOCIATED FINDINGS

MAJOR ASSOCIATED SIGNS AND SYMPTOMS

COMMON CAUSES	Amnesia	Aphasia	Decreased level of consciousness	Decreased mental acuity	Dysarthria	Fetor hepaticus	Headache	Hyperreflexia	Incontinence	Seizures	Tremors	Visual field deficits
Alzheimer's disease	●	●							●		●	
Brain abscess		●		●	●		●	●	●	●		●
Brain tumor		●		●	●		●	●	●	●		●
Hepatic encephalopathy		●		●		●	●		●			●
Stroke		●	●						●			●

the ability to learn activities that require sequential movement, such as hopping, jumping, hitting or kicking a ball, or dancing. When caring for a child with apraxia, be aware of his limitations and provide an environment conducive to rehabilitation. Provide emotional support because playmates will usually tease a child who can't perform normal physical activities.

Geriatric pointers

Pre-existing diseases, such as dementia (Alzheimer's type, vascular, or others), previous stroke, or dehydration, may interfere with assessing the patient for apraxia.

MEDICAL CAUSES

See *Apraxia: Causes and associated findings*.
- *Alzheimer's disease.* Alzheimer's disease sometimes causes gradual and irreversible ideomotor apraxia. It can also cause amnesia, anomia, decreased attention span, apathy, aphasia, restlessness, agitation, paranoid delusions, incontinence, social withdrawal, ataxia, and tremors.
- *Brain abscess.* Apraxia occasionally results from a large brain abscess; it typically resolves spontaneously after the infection subsides. Depending on the location of the abscess, apraxia may be accompanied by

headache, fever, drowsiness, decreased mental acuity, aphasia, dysarthria, hemiparesis, hyperreflexia, incontinence, focal or generalized seizures, and ocular disturbances, such as nystagmus, visual field deficits, and unequal pupils.
- *Brain tumor.* With a brain tumor, progressive apraxia may be preceded by decreased mental acuity, headache, dizziness, and seizures. It may occur with or directly after pupil changes or other early signs of increased ICP. Apraxia may also accompany other localizing signs and symptoms of the tumor, such as aphasia, dysarthria, visual field deficits, weakness, stiffness, and hyperreflexia in the extremities.
- *Hepatic encephalopathy.* Hepatic encephalopathy may cause a gradual onset of constructional apraxia, which may be reversible with treatment. Early associated signs and symptoms include disorientation, amnesia, slurred speech, dysarthria, asterixis, and lethargy. Later signs include hyperreflexia, positive Babinski's reflex, agitation, seizures, fetor hepaticus, stupor, and coma.
- *Stroke.* The onset of apraxia is typically sudden in stroke; it commonly resolves spontaneously, but may persist in some patients. Associated signs and symptoms vary according to the affected artery, but can in-

clude headache, confusion, stupor or coma, hemiplegia, unilateral or bilateral visual field deficits, aphasia, agnosia, dysarthria, and urinary incontinence.

NURSING CONSIDERATIONS

Prepare the patient for diagnostic studies, which may include computed tomography and radionuclide brain scans. Because weakness, sensory deficits, confusion, and seizures may accompany apraxia, take measures to ensure the patient's safety. For example, assist him with gait apraxia in walking.

PATIENT TEACHING

Explain the disorder to the patient. Encourage him to participate in his normal activities as tolerated. Help him overcome frustration arising from the inability to perform routine tasks by breaking each task down into separate steps, demonstrating these steps, and having the patient repeat the actions you demonstrated as taught by the physical and occupational therapists. Allow him sufficient time to perform each step. Avoid giving complex directions. Encourage family members to assist in the patient's rehabilitation.

Ataxia

Ataxia is defined as an incoordination and irregularity of voluntary, purposeful movements. Ataxia can be classified as cerebellar or sensory. Cerebellar ataxia is caused by disease of the cerebellum and its pathways between the cerebral cortex, the brain stem, and the spinal cord. Gait, trunk, limb and, possibly, speech abnormalities may occur in cerebellar ataxia. In sensory ataxia, position sense (proprioception) is impaired due to interruption of afferent nerve fibers in the peripheral nerves, posterior roots, posterior columns of the spinal cord, or medial lemnisci. Although uncommon, sensory ataxia may also be caused by a lesion in both parietal lobes. Sensory ataxia results in gait abnormalities. (See *Identifying ataxia,* page 34.)

Ataxia can be acute or chronic. Acute ataxia occurs with stroke, hemorrhage, or a large tumor in the posterior fossa. A large tumor in the posterior fossa is a life-threatening condition in which the cerebellum may herniate downward through the foramen magnum behind the cervical spinal cord, or upward through the tentorium of the cerebral hemispheres. Herniation may lead to compression of the brain stem. Acute ataxia may also result from drug toxicity or poisoning. Chronic ataxia can be progressive and may be seen with acute disease such as metabolic imbalances and with chronic degenerative neurologic disease.

Act now *If ataxic movements develop abruptly, assess the patient for signs of increased intracranial pressure and impending herniation. Elevate the head of the bed. Determine the patient's level of consciousness (LOC) and stay alert for pupillary changes, motor weakness or paralysis, neck stiffness, pain, and vomiting. Check the patient's vital signs, noting rate and pattern of respirations. Have emergency resuscitation equipment readily available. Prepare the patient for a computed tomography scan or surgery.*

ASSESSMENT
History

If the patient's condition permits, obtain his history. Ask about the onset and initial presentation of ataxia, noting whether it developed suddenly or gradually. Note a history of multiple sclerosis, diabetes, central nervous system infection, neoplastic disease, previous stroke, or a family history of ataxia. Inquire about chronic alcohol abuse or prolonged exposure to industrial toxins such as mercury.

Physical examination

If the patient is able to stand, perform Romberg's test to help distinguish between cerebellar and sensory ataxia. Instruct the patient to stand with his feet together and his arms at his sides. Note his posture and balance, first with his eyes open, and then closed. Minimal swaying indicates normal posture and balance, swaying and an inability to maintain balance with eyes open or closed suggests cerebellar ataxia, and increased swaying and an inability to maintain balance with eyes closed indicates sensory ataxia. Stand close to the patient during this test to provide support if he falls.

Evaluate motor strength when testing for gait and limb ataxia because motor weakness may mimic ataxic movements. Gait ataxia may be severe even when limb ataxia is minimal. Ask the patient with gait ataxia whether he tends to fall to one side and whether falls typically occur at night. With

Ataxia may be observed in the patient's speech, in the movements of his trunk and limbs, or in his gait.

◆ With speech ataxia, a form of dysarthria, the patient typically speaks slowly and stresses usually unstressed words and syllables. Speech content is unaffected.

◆ With truncal ataxia, a disturbance in equilibrium, the patient can't sit or stand without falling. Also, his head and trunk may bob and sway (titubation). If he can walk, his gait is reeling.

◆ With limb ataxia, the patient loses the ability to gauge distance, speed, and power of movement, resulting in poorly controlled, variable, and inaccurate voluntary movements. He may move too quickly or too slowly, or his movements may break down into component parts, giving him the appearance of a puppet or robot. Other effects include a coarse, irregular tremor in purposeful movement (but not at rest) and reduced muscle tone.

◆ With gait ataxia, the patient's gait is wide based, unsteady, and irregular.

◆ With cerebellar ataxia, the patient may stagger or lurch in zigzag fashion, turn with extreme difficulty, and lose his balance when his feet are together.

◆ With sensory ataxia, the patient moves abruptly and stomps or taps his feet. This occurs because he throws his feet forward and outward, and then brings them down first on the heels and then on the toes. The patient also fixes his eyes on the ground, watching his steps. However, if he can't watch them, staggering worsens. When he stands with his feet together, he sways or loses his balance.

◆ With limb ataxia, the patient loses the ability to gauge distance, speed, and power of movement, resulting in poorly controlled, variable, and inaccurate voluntary movements. He may move too quickly or too slowly, or his movements may break down into component parts, giving him the appearance of a puppet or robot. Other effects include a coarse, irregular tremor in purposeful movement (but not at rest) and reduced muscle tone.

◆ With gait ataxia, the patient's gait is wide based, unsteady, and irregular.

◆ With cerebellar ataxia, the patient may stagger or lurch in zigzag fashion, turn with extreme difficulty, and lose his balance when his feet are together.

◆ With sensory ataxia, the patient moves abruptly and stomps or taps his feet. This occurs because he throws his feet forward and outward, and then brings them down first on the heels and then on the toes. The patient also fixes his eyes on the ground, watching his steps. However, if he can't watch them, staggering worsens. When he stands with his feet together, he sways or loses his balance.

---

truncal ataxia, remember that the patient who has no symptoms while lying down but can't walk or stand may appear to be experiencing hysteria or drug or alcohol intoxication.

Pediatric pointers

Ataxia occurs in acute and chronic forms in children. It can result from congenital or acquired disease. Acute ataxia may arise from febrile infection, brain tumors, mumps, and other disorders. Chronic ataxia may occur due to Gaucher's disease, Refsum's disease, and other inborn errors of metabolism.

When assessing a child for ataxia, consider his level of motor skills and his emotional state. Your examination may be limited to observing the child in spontaneous activity and carefully questioning his parents about such changes in motor activity as increased unsteadiness or falling. If you suspect ataxia, refer the child for a neurologic evaluation to rule out a brain tumor.

Geriatric pointers

Pre-existing diseases, such as dementia (Alzheimer's type, vascular, or others) or previous stroke, may hamper an ataxia assessment. Functional problems may also impede the assessment of new symptoms.

MEDICAL CAUSES

● *Cerebellar abscess.* Cerebellar abscess commonly causes limb ataxia on the same side as the lesion as well as gait and truncal ataxia. Typically, the initial symptom is headache localized behind the ear or in the occipital region, followed by oculomotor palsy, fever, vomiting, altered LOC, and coma.

- *Cerebellar hemorrhage.* With cerebellar hemorrhage, a life-threatening disorder, ataxia is usually acute but transient. Unilateral or bilateral ataxia affects the trunk, gait, or limbs. The patient initially experiences repeated vomiting, occipital headache, vertigo, oculomotor palsy, dysphagia, and dysarthria. Later signs, such as decreased LOC or coma, signal impending herniation.
- *Cranial trauma.* Ataxia is rare with cranial trauma; if it occurs, it's typically unilateral. Bilateral ataxia suggests traumatic hemorrhage. Associated signs and symptoms include vomiting, headache, decreased LOC, irritability, and focal neurologic defects. If the cerebral hemispheres are also affected, focal or generalized seizures may occur.
- *Creutzfeldt-Jakob disease.* Creutzfeldt-Jacob disease is a rapidly progressive dementia accompanied by neurologic signs and symptoms, such as myoclonic jerking, ataxia, aphasia, vision disturbances, and paralysis.
- *Diabetic neuropathy.* Peripheral nerve damage due to diabetes mellitus may cause sensory ataxia, extremity pain, slight leg weakness, skin changes, and bowel and bladder dysfunction.
- *Diphtheria.* Within 4 to 8 weeks of the onset of diphtheria symptoms, a life-threatening neuropathy develops, possibly producing sensory ataxia and paralysis of respiratory muscles. Diphtheria can be accompanied by fever, paresthesia, and limb paralysis and, sometimes, respiratory muscle paralysis.
- *Encephalomyelitis.* Encephalomyelitis can, rarely, be accompanied by cerebellar ataxia. Encephalomyelitis, which may lead to damage of the cerebrospinal white matter, is a complication associated with measles, smallpox, chickenpox, or rubella. It may also occur due to rabies or smallpox vaccinations. Signs and symptoms of encephalomyelitis include headache, fever, vomiting, altered LOC, paralysis, seizures, oculomotor palsy, and pupillary changes.
- *Friedreich's ataxia.* Friedreich's ataxia, a progressive familial disorder, affects the spinal cord and cerebellum. It causes gait ataxia initially, followed by truncal, limb, and speech ataxia. Other signs and symptoms include pes cavus, kyphoscoliosis, cranial nerve palsy, and motor and sensory deficits. A positive Babinski's response may appear.
- *Guillain-Barré syndrome.* Peripheral nerve involvement usually follows a mild viral infection and may, rarely, lead to sensory ataxia. Guillain-Barré syndrome also causes ascending paralysis and may lead to respiratory distress.
- *Hepatocerebral degeneration.* Residual neurologic defects, including mild cerebellar ataxia with a wide-based, unsteady gait, occasionally remain following recovery from hepatic coma. Ataxia may be accompanied by altered LOC, dysarthria, rhythmic arm tremors, and choreoathetosis of the face, neck, and shoulders.
- *Hyperthermia.* Cerebellar ataxia can occur in patients who survive the coma and seizures characteristic of the acute phase of hyperthermia. Subsequent findings include spastic paralysis, dementia, and slowly resolving confusion.
- *Metastatic cancer.* Cancer that metastasizes to the cerebellum may cause gait ataxia accompanied by headache, dizziness, nystagmus, decreased LOC, nausea, and vomiting.
- *Multiple sclerosis (MS).* Nystagmus and cerebellar ataxia commonly occur in MS; limb weakness and spasticity may occur as well. Speech ataxia (especially scanning) may occur, and spinal cord involvement may result in sensory ataxia. During remissions, ataxia may subside or even disappear. During exacerbations, it may reappear, worsen, or become permanent. MS also causes optic neuritis, optic atrophy, numbness and weakness, diplopia, dizziness, and bladder dysfunction.
- *Olivopontocerebellar atrophy.* Olivopontocerebellar atrophy produces gait ataxia and, later, limb and speech ataxia. In rare instances, it produces an intention tremor. It's accompanied by choreiform movements, dysphagia, and loss of sphincter tone.
- *Poisoning.* Chronic arsenic poisoning may cause sensory ataxia, along with headache, seizures, altered LOC, motor deficits, and muscle aching. Chronic mercury poisoning causes gait and limb ataxia, principally of the arms. It also causes mental confusion, mood changes, dysarthria, and tremors of the extremities, tongue, and lips.
- *Polyarteritis nodosa.* Acute or subacute polyarteritis may cause sensory ataxia, abdominal and limb pain, hematuria, fever, and elevated blood pressure.
- *Polyneuropathy.* Carcinomatous and myelomatous polyneuropathy may occur before detection of the primary tumor in cancer, multiple myeloma, or Hodgkin's dis-

ease. Signs and symptoms include ataxia, severe motor weakness, muscle atrophy, and sensory loss in the limbs. Pain and skin changes may also occur.

- *Porphyria.* Porphyria affects the sensory and, more commonly, the motor nerves, possibly leading to ataxia. It also causes abdominal pain, mental disturbances, vomiting, headache, focal neurologic defects, altered LOC, generalized seizures, and skin lesions.
- *Posterior fossa tumor.* Gait, truncal, or limb ataxia may occur early and worsen as the tumor enlarges. Other signs and symptoms include vomiting, headache, papilledema, vertigo, oculomotor palsy, decreased LOC, and motor and sensory impairments on the same side as the lesion.
- *Spinocerebellar ataxia.* With spinocerebellar ataxia, the patient may initially experience fatigue, followed by stiff-legged gait ataxia. Eventually, limb ataxia, dysarthria, static tremor, nystagmus, cramps, paresthesia, and sensory deficits occur.
- *Stroke.* Occlusions in the vertebrobasilar arteries halt blood flow, leading to infarction in the medulla, pons, or cerebellum. Ataxia may occur at the onset of stroke and remain as a residual deficit. Worsening ataxia during the acute phase may indicate extension of the stroke or severe swelling. Ataxia may be accompanied by unilateral or bilateral motor weakness, possible altered LOC, sensory loss, vertigo, nausea, vomiting, oculomotor palsy, and dysphagia.
- *Syringomyelia.* Syringomyelia, a chronic, degenerative disorder, may cause a mixed spastic-ataxic gait. It's associated with loss of pain and temperature sensations (but preservation of touch sensation), skin changes, amyotrophy, and thoracic scoliosis.
- *Wernicke's disease.* The result of thiamine deficiency, Wernicke's disease produces gait ataxia and, rarely, intention tremor or speech ataxia. With severe ataxia, the patient may be unable to stand or walk. Ataxia decreases with thiamine therapy. Associated signs and symptoms include nystagmus, diplopia, ocular palsies, confusion, tachycardia, exertional dyspnea, and orthostatic hypotension.

OTHER CAUSES

- *Drugs.* Toxic levels of anticonvulsants, especially phenytoin, may result in gait ataxia. Toxic levels of anticholinergics and tricyclic antidepressants may also result in ataxia. Aminoglutethimide causes ataxia in

about 10% of patients; however, this effect usually disappears 4 to 6 weeks after drug therapy is discontinued.

NURSING CONSIDERATIONS

Assess the patient's neurologic status frequently. Prepare the patient for laboratory studies, such as blood tests for toxic drug levels and radiologic tests. Then focus on helping the patient adapt to his condition; refer him to psychiatric consultation if ordered. Promote rehabilitation goals set forth by the physical, occupational, and speech therapists, and implement safety measures. Refer the patient with progressive disease for counseling, if appropriate.

PATIENT TEACHING

Instruct the patient with sensory ataxia to move slowly, especially when turning or rising from a chair. Provide a cane or walker for extra support. Ask the patient's family to assess his home for safety hazards, such as uneven surfaces or the absence of handrails on stairs. Refer the patient for home care follow-up nursing and rehabilitative services as ordered.

B

Back pain

Back pain affects an estimated 80% of the population and is the second leading cause of absence from work. Although this symptom may indicate a spondylogenic disorder, it may also result from a genitourinary, GI, cardiovascular, or neoplastic disorder. Postural imbalance associated with pregnancy may also cause back pain.

The onset, location, and distribution of back pain and its responses to activity and rest provide important clues about the cause. Back pain may be acute or chronic, constant or intermittent. It may remain localized in the back or radiate along the spine or down one or both legs. Back pain may be exacerbated by activity — typically by bending, stooping, or lifting — and alleviated by rest, or it may be unaffected by either.

Intrinsic back pain results from muscle spasm, nerve root irritation, fracture, or a combination of these mechanisms. It usually occurs in the lower back or lumbosacral area. Back pain may also be referred from the abdomen or flank; such referred pain can signal such life-threatening conditions as a perforated ulcer, acute pancreatitis, or a dissecting abdominal aortic aneurysm. Back pain in the scapular area may reflect referred cardiac pain, such as that seen in myocardial infarction, another life-threatening condition.

ASSESSMENT
History

Ask the patient where the pain is located; back pain in some areas can signal the presence of a life-threatening condition.

Act now *If the patient reports acute, severe back pain, quickly obtain his vital signs and perform a rapid evaluation to rule out life-threatening causes. If he describes deep lumbar pain unaffected by activity, observe for a pulsating epigastric mass. Presence of this sign may indicate a dissecting abdominal aortic aneurysm. Withhold food and fluids because the patient may require emergency surgery. Prepare for I.V. fluid replacement and oxygen administration.*

If he reports severe epigastric pain that radiates through the abdomen to the back, assess for absent bowel sounds and abdominal rigidity and tenderness. These symptoms may indicate a perforated ulcer or acute pancreatitis. Start an I.V. line for fluids and medications, administer oxygen, insert a nasogastric tube, and withhold food.

If the patient complains of scapular area back pain, especially if accompanied by shortness of breath or diaphoresis, give oxygen via a nasal cannula or mask and obtain a 12-lead electrocardiogram to rule out myocardial infarction.

After you have ruled out potential life-threatening causes of back pain, continue to obtain the patient's history. Observe him for expressions of pain while gathering information. Ask about previous injuries and illnesses, dietary habits, alcohol intake, and cigarette smoking. Inquire about medications, including past and present prescriptions, use of over-the-counter drugs, and disease processes or pain control regimens.

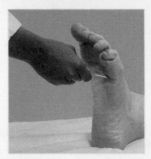
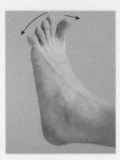
Ask the patient about the onset of his back pain. Were there precipitating factors? Ask the patient to rate the pain on a standardized pain scale. Ask him for details about the pain — is it burning, stabbing, throbbing, or aching? Constant or intermittent? If it's intermittent, does it occur at a specific time of day? Does the pain radiate? Is there associated weakness? Does he experience repetitive pain or different types of pain? What, if anything, lessens the pain? What aggravates it? The patient's answers will help identify the cause of his back pain. For example, visceral referred back pain is indicated if the patient states that the pain isn't affected by activity and rest. In contrast, spondylogenic-referred back pain is likely if the pain increases with activity and decreases with rest. Pain of neoplastic origin is indicated if the patient reports that he can obtain relief by walking and that the pain increases at night.

Physical examination

Perform a thorough physical examination. Observe skin color, especially in the patient's legs, and palpate skin temperature. Palpate femoral, popliteal, posterior tibial, and pedal pulses. Ask the patient about unusual sensations in the legs, such as numbness and tingling. If pain doesn't prevent standing, observe the patient's posture — does he stand erect or lean toward one side? Observe the level of the shoulders and pelvis and the curvature of the back. Ask the patient to bend forward, backward, and from side to side while you palpate for paravertebral muscle spasms. Note rotation of the spine on the trunk. Palpate the dorsolumbar spine for point tenderness. Then ask the patient to walk — first on his heels, then on his toes (stand close by during these tests so that you can assist the patient if he falls). Weakness may reflect a muscular disorder or spinal nerve root irritation.

Place the patient in a sitting position to evaluate and compare patellar tendon (knee), Achilles tendon, and Babinski's reflexes. (See *How to elicit Babinski's reflex.*) Evaluate the strength of the extensor hallucis longus by asking the patient to keep his great toe firmly in place against resistance. Measure leg length and hamstring and quadriceps muscles bilaterally. Note a difference of more than ⅜″ (1 cm) in muscle size, especially in the calf.

To reproduce leg and back pain, assist the patient into a supine position on the examining table. Grasp his heel and slowly lift his leg. If he feels pain, note its exact location and the angle between the table and his leg when it occurs. Repeat this maneuver with the opposite leg. Pain along the sciatic nerve may indicate disk herniation or sciatica.

Note the range of motion of the hip and knee. Palpate the flanks and percuss with your fingertips or fist to reveal the presence of costovertebral angle (CVA) tenderness.

Pediatric pointers

Because a child may have difficulty describing back pain, stay alert for nonverbal clues, such as wincing or a refusal to walk.

Back pain in children may stem from intervertebral disk inflammation (diskitis), neoplasms, idiopathic juvenile osteoporosis, and spondylolisthesis. Disk herniation typically doesn't cause back pain. Scoliosis, a common disorder in adolescents, rarely causes back pain.

While obtaining the child's history, pay close attention to family dynamics, noting factors that suggest child abuse.

Geriatric pointers

Suspect metastatic cancer—especially of the prostate, colon, or breast—in elderly patients with recent onset of back pain that worsens at night and isn't usually relieved by rest. Remember that assessing back pain may be hampered in elderly patients with functional disabilities.

MEDICAL CAUSES

- *Abdominal aortic aneurysm (dissecting).* Life-threatening dissection of an abdominal aortic aneurysm may initially cause low back pain or dull abdominal pain. More commonly, it produces constant upper abdominal pain. A pulsating abdominal mass may be palpated in the epigastrium; pulsation ceases if rupture occurs. Aneurysmal dissection can also cause mottled skin below the waist, absence of femoral and pedal pulses, mild to moderate tenderness with guarding, and abdominal rigidity. Blood pressure in the patient's legs may be lower than blood pressure in his arms. Signs of shock, such as cool, clammy skin, occur with significant blood loss.

- *Ankylosing spondylitis.* Ankylosing spondylitis is a chronic, progressive disorder that causes sacroiliac pain that radiates up the spine and is aggravated by lateral pressure on the pelvis. The pain is usually most severe in the morning or after a period of inactivity; it isn't relieved by rest. Abnormal rigidity of the lumbar spine with forward flexion is also characteristic. Ankylosing spondylitis can cause local tenderness, fatigue, fever, anorexia, weight loss, and occasional iritis.

- *Appendicitis.* Appendicitis is a life-threatening disorder in which vague and dull discomfort in the epigastric or umbilical region gradually localizes in McBurney's point in the right lower quadrant. With retrocecal appendicitis, pain may also radiate to the back. The localization of the pain is preceded by anorexia and nausea and is accompanied by fever, occasional vomiting, abdominal tenderness (especially over McBurney's point), and rebound tenderness. Some patients also report painful, urgent urination.

- *Cholecystitis.* Cholecystitis produces severe pain that occurs in the right upper quadrant of the abdomen and may radiate to the right shoulder, chest, or back. The pain may occur abruptly or gradually, increasing over several hours. Patients typically report a history of similar pain after consuming high-fat meals. Accompanying signs and symptoms include anorexia, fever, nausea, vomiting, right upper quadrant tenderness, abdominal rigidity, pallor, and sweating.

- *Chordoma.* A slow-developing malignant tumor, chordoma causes persistent pain in the lower back, sacrum, and coccyx. As the tumor expands, pain may be accompanied by constipation and bowel or bladder incontinence.

- *Endometriosis.* Endometriosis causes deep sacral pain and severe, cramping pain in the lower abdomen. The pain worsens just before or during menstruation and may be aggravated by defecation. It's accompanied by constipation, abdominal tenderness, dysmenorrhea, and dyspareunia.

- *Intervertebral disk rupture.* Disk rupture produces gradual or abrupt lower back pain with or without leg pain (sciatica). It rarely produces leg pain alone. Pain usually begins in the back and radiates to the buttocks and leg. It's exacerbated by activity, coughing, and sneezing and lessened by rest. Accompanying symptoms include paresthesia (most commonly, numbness or tingling in the lower leg and foot), paravertebral muscle spasm, and decreased reflexes on the affected side. This disorder also affects posture and gait. The patient's spine is slightly flexed and he leans toward the painful side. He walks slowly and rises from a sitting to a standing position with extreme difficulty.

- *Lumbosacral sprain.* Aching, localized pain and tenderness due to muscle spasm on lateral motion is the primary symptom of a lumbosacral sprain. The recumbent patient typically flexes his knees and hips to ease pain. Flexion of the spine intensifies pain, whereas rest facilitates relief.

- *Metastatic tumors.* The spread of metastatic tumors to the spine — a common occurrence — leads to low back pain in approximately 25% of patients. It typically begins abruptly and is accompanied by cramping muscular pain. This pain is usually worse at night and isn't relieved by rest.
- *Myeloma.* Back pain caused by myeloma — a primary malignant tumor — usually begins abruptly and worsens with exercise. It may be accompanied by arthritic signs and symptoms, such as achiness, joint swelling, and tenderness. Other signs and symptoms include fever, malaise, peripheral paresthesia, and weight loss.
- *Pancreatitis (acute).* Acute pancreatitis is a life-threatening disorder that typically produces fulminating, continuous upper abdominal pain that may radiate to both flanks and the back. To relieve this pain, the patient may bend forward, draw his knees to his chest, or move restlessly.

   Early associated signs and symptoms include abdominal tenderness, nausea, vomiting, fever, pallor, tachycardia and, in some patients, abdominal guarding, rigidity, rebound tenderness, and hypoactive bowel sounds. Jaundice may be a late sign. Occurring as inflammation subsides, Turner's sign (ecchymosis of the abdomen or flank) or Cullen's sign (bluish discoloration of skin around the umbilicus and in both flanks) signals hemorrhagic pancreatitis.
- *Perforated ulcer.* In some patients, perforation of a duodenal or gastric ulcer causes sudden, prostrating epigastric pain that may radiate throughout the abdomen and to the back. This life-threatening disorder also causes boardlike abdominal rigidity, tenderness with guarding, generalized rebound tenderness, absent bowel sounds, and grunting, shallow respirations. Associated signs include fever, tachycardia, and hypotension.
- *Prostate cancer.* Chronic, aching back pain may be the only symptom of prostate cancer, although hematuria and decreased urine stream may also occur.
- *Pyelonephritis (acute).* Acute pyelonephritis produces back pain or tenderness (especially over the CVA) as well as progressive pain in the flank and lower abdomen. Other signs and symptoms include high fever and chills, nausea and vomiting, flank and abdominal tenderness, and urinary frequency and urgency.

- *Reiter's syndrome.* In some patients, sacroiliac pain is the first sign of Reiter's syndrome. Pain is accompanied by the classic triad of conjunctivitis, urethritis, and arthritis.
- *Renal calculi.* The colicky pain of renal calculi usually results from irritation of the ureteral lining, which increases the frequency and force of peristaltic contractions. The pain travels from the CVA to the flank, suprapubic region, and external genitalia. Its intensity varies; it may become excruciating if calculi travel down a ureter. Calculi in the renal pelvis and calyces result in dull and constant flank pain. Renal calculi also cause nausea, vomiting, urinary urgency (if a calculus lodges near the bladder), hematuria, and agitation due to pain. Pain resolves or significantly decreases after calculi move to the bladder. Encourage the patient to recover the calculi for analysis.
- *Rift Valley fever.* Typical signs and symptoms of Rift Valley fever — a viral disease — include back pain, fever, myalgia, weakness, and dizziness. It may present as several different clinical syndromes. A small percentage of patients may develop encephalitis or hemorrhagic fever leading to shock and hemorrhage. Inflammation of the retina may result in some permanent vision loss. Although Rift Valley fever is typically found in Africa, outbreaks have also occurred in Saudi Arabia and Yemen. The disease is transmitted to humans through the bite of an infected mosquito or exposure to infected animals.
- *Sacroiliac strain.* Sacroiliac strain causes pain that may radiate to the buttock, hip, and lateral aspect of the thigh. The pain is aggravated by weight bearing on the affected extremity and by abduction with resistance of the leg. Associated signs and symptoms include tenderness of the symphysis pubis and a limp or a gluteus medius or abductor lurch.
- *Smallpox (variola major).* Worldwide eradication of smallpox was achieved in 1977. The United States and Russia have the only documented storage sites of the virus, which is considered a potential agent for biological warfare. Initial signs and symptoms of smallpox include back pain, high fever, malaise, prostration, severe headache, and abdominal pain. A maculopapular rash develops on the mucosa of the mouth, pharynx, face, and forearms and spreads to the trunk and legs. Within 2 days, the rash becomes vesicular and, later, pustular. The le-

EXERCISES FOR CHRONIC LOW BACK PAIN

Dear Patient,
If you have chronic low back pain, the exercises illlustrated here may help relieve your discomfort and prevent further lumbar deterioriation. When you perform these exercises, keep in mind the following points:
◆ Breathe slowly, inhaling through your nose and exhaling completely through pursed lips.
◆ Begin gradually, performing each exercsie only once per day and progressing to 10 repetitions.
◆ Exercise moderately; expect mild discomfort, but stop if you experience severe pain.

BACK PRESS

Lie on your back, with your arms on your chest or abdomen and your knees bent. Press the small (lower portion) of your back to the floor while tightening your abdominal muscles and buttocks. Count to 10, and then slowly relax.

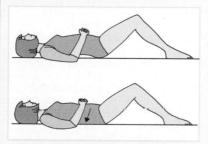

KNEE GRASP

Lie on your back, with your knees bent. Bring one knee to your chest, grasping it firmly with both hands, and lower your knee. Repeat with the other knee — then with *both* knees, as shown here.

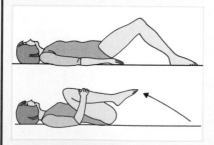

KNEE BEND

Stand with your hands on the back of a chair for support. Keeping your back straight, slowly bend your knees until you're in a squatting position. Return to your starting position.

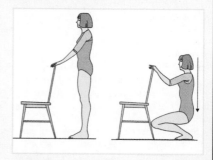

TRUNK CURL

Lie on your back, with your knees bent and feet flat. Cross your arms on your chest. Lift your head and shoulders off of the floor, and hold for a count of 2. Repeat 10 times. Work up to at least 30, taking brief rests as needed.

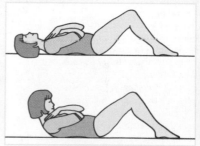

sions, which develop simultaneously rather than gradually increasing in number, occur more frequently on the face and extremities. The pustules are round, firm, and embedded in the skin. After 8 to 9 days, the pustules form a crust. Later, the scab separates from the skin, leaving a pitted scar. In fatal cases, death results from encephalitis, extensive bleeding, or secondary infection.

- *Spinal neoplasm (benign)*. This neoplasm typically causes severe, localized back pain and scoliosis.
- *Spinal stenosis.* Resembling a ruptured intervertebral disk, spinal stenosis produces back pain that may be accompanied by sciatica, commonly affecting both legs. The pain may radiate to the toes and may progress to numbness or weakness unless the patient rests.
- *Spondylolisthesis.* A major structural disorder characterized by forward slippage of one vertebra onto another, spondylolisthesis may be asymptomatic or may cause low back pain, with or without nerve root involvement. Associated symptoms of nerve root involvement include paresthesia, buttock pain, and pain radiating down the leg. Palpation of the lumbar spine may reveal a "step-off" of the spinous process. Flexion of the spine may be limited.
- *Transverse process fracture.* This injury causes severe, localized back pain with muscle spasm and hematoma.
- *Vertebral compression fracture.* Initially, a vertebral compression fracture may be painless. Several weeks later, it causes back pain aggravated by weight bearing and local tenderness. Fracture of a thoracic vertebra may cause referred pain in the lumbar area.
- *Vertebral osteomyelitis.* Initially, vertebral osteomyelitis causes insidious back pain. As it progresses, the pain may become constant, more pronounced at night, and aggravated by spinal movement. Accompanying signs and symptoms include vertebral and hamstring spasms, tenderness of the spinous processes, fever, and malaise.
- *Vertebral osteoporosis.* Vertebral osteoporosis causes chronic, aching back pain that's aggravated by activity and somewhat relieved by rest. Tenderness may also occur.

OTHER CAUSES
- *Neurologic tests.* Lumbar puncture and myelography can produce transient back pain.

NURSING CONSIDERATIONS
Monitor the patient closely if the type and location of back pain suggest a life-threatening cause. Stay alert for increasing pain, altered neurovascular status in the legs, loss of bowel or bladder control, altered vital signs, sweating, and cyanosis.

Until a tentative diagnosis is made, withhold analgesics to avoid masking symptoms. Withhold food and fluids until it's determined whether the patient requires surgery. Once a medical emergency is ruled out, make him as comfortable as possible by elevating the head of the bed, placing a pillow under his knees, and administering pain medications. Prepare the patient for a rectal or pelvic examination, routine blood tests, urinalysis, computed tomography scan, biopsies, and X-rays of the chest, abdomen, and spine.

Fit the patient for a corset or lumbosacral support. Refer him to a physical therapist, occupational therapist, massage therapist, or psychologist, as indicated.

PATIENT TEACHING
Explain all tests and procedures. Instruct the patient not to wear a lumbosacral support in bed. Describe such pain-relief measures as cold therapy, warm baths, mattress choices, and backboards. Instruct the patient and his family about relaxation techniques, such as deep breathing, biofeedback, and transcutaneous electrical nerve stimulation.

If the patient has chronic back pain, reinforce instructions about bed rest, analgesics, anti-inflammatory medications, and exercise. (See *Exercises for chronic low back pain,* page 41.) Help him recognize the need to make lifestyle changes, such as losing weight or correcting poor posture. Advise the patient with acute back pain secondary to a musculoskeletal problem to continue his daily activities as tolerated rather than staying on total bed rest.

Battle's sign

Battle's sign—ecchymosis over the mastoid process of the temporal bone—is typically the only outward sign of a basilar skull fracture. In fact, this type of fracture may go undetected even by skull X-rays. If left untreated, it can cause death due to involvement of nearby cranial nerves, brain stem, blood vessels, or meninges.

Appearing behind one or both ears, Battle's sign is easily overlooked or hidden by the patient's hair. During emergency care of a trauma victim, it may be overshadowed by more visible or imminently life-threatening injuries.

A force strong enough to fracture the base of the skull causes Battle's sign by damaging supporting tissues of the mastoid area and causing seepage of blood from the fracture site to the mastoid. Battle's sign usually develops 24 to 36 hours after the fracture and may persist for weeks.

Act now *If you observe Battle's sign, keep the patient flat and monitor neurologic signs closely. Prepare him for skull X-rays and a computed tomography (CT) scan.*

ASSESSMENT
History

Obtain the patient's history, noting recent trauma to the head such as involvement in a motor vehicle accident. Assess his level of consciousness and the appropriateness of his responses to your questions.

Physical examination

Perform a complete neurologic assessment. Check the patient's vital signs; stay alert for widening pulse pressure and bradycardia — these are signs of increased intracranial pressure. Assess cranial nerve (CN) function in CN II, III, IV, VI, VII, and VIII. Evaluate pupillary size and response to light as well as motor and verbal responses. Relate these data to the Glasgow Coma Scale. Assess for cerebrospinal fluid (CSF) leakage from the nose or ears. Ask about postnasal drip, which may reflect CSF drainage down the throat. Look for the halo sign — a bloodstain encircled by a yellowish ring — on bed linens or dressings. Test drainage to determine the presence of CSF. Follow the neurologic examination with a complete physical examination to detect other injuries associated with a basilar skull fracture.

Pediatric pointers

Children who are victims of abuse frequently sustain basilar skull fractures from severe blows to the head. As in adults, Battle's sign may be the only outward sign of fracture and, perhaps, the only clue to child abuse. If

you suspect child abuse, follow facility protocol for reporting the incident.

Geriatric pointers

Many elderly people experience some degree of functional loss with serious effects (such as falling) that can precipitate a basilar skull fracture. Elder neglect and abuse is also on the rise and should be considered when examining older patients.

MEDICAL CAUSES

- *Basilar skull fracture.* Battle's sign may be the only outward sign of a basilar skull fracture or it may be accompanied by periorbital ecchymosis (raccoon eyes), conjunctival hemorrhage, nystagmus, ocular deviation, epistaxis, anosmia, a bulging tympanic membrane (from CSF or blood accumulation), visible fracture lines on the external auditory canal, tinnitus, difficulty hearing, facial paralysis, or vertigo.

NURSING CONSIDERATIONS

Assess the patient's neurologic function frequently. Keep him in a supine position to decrease pressure on dural tears and to minimize CSF leakage. Avoid nasogastric intubation and nasopharyngeal suction, which may cause cerebral infection. Also, caution the patient against blowing his nose, which may worsen a dural tear.

The patient may need skull X-rays and a CT scan to help confirm a basilar skull fracture and to evaluate the severity of the head injury. Typically, a basilar skull fracture and associated dural tears heal spontaneously within several days to weeks. However, if the patient has a large dural tear, a craniotomy may be necessary to repair the tear with a graft patch. If the injury was due to abuse, notify the appropriate authority in the facility.

PATIENT TEACHING

Explain all procedures and tests. Inform the patient with a basilar skull fracture that he'll require bed rest for several days to weeks. Explain the need to avoid placing pressure on the brain tissue, and advise him on proper positioning. Also tell him to refrain from blowing his nose.

If the injury was due to an accidental fall, advise the patient's family to assess the household for safety hazards and remove precipitating factors such as throw rugs.

Bladder distention

Bladder distention is an abnormal enlargement of the bladder due to the accumulation of urine arising from an inability to excrete urine. Distention can be caused by a mechanical or anatomic obstruction, neuromuscular disorder, or the use of certain drugs. Although it's relatively common in all ages and both sexes, it's most common in older men with prostate disorders that cause urine retention.

Distention usually develops gradually, but the onset can also be sudden. Gradual distention usually remains asymptomatic until stretching of the bladder produces discomfort. Acute distention produces suprapubic fullness, pressure, and pain. If severe distention isn't corrected promptly by catheterization or massage, the bladder rises within the abdomen, its walls become thin, and renal function can be impaired.

Bladder distention is aggravated by the intake of caffeine, alcohol, large quantities of fluid, and diuretics.

Act now If the patient has severe distention, insert an indwelling urinary catheter to help relieve discomfort and prevent bladder rupture. If greater than 700 ml is emptied from the bladder, compressed blood vessels dilate and may make the patient feel faint. Typically, the indwelling catheter is clamped for 30 to 60 minutes to permit vessel compensation.

ASSESSMENT
History
Ask the patient about voiding patterns, the time and amount of the last voiding, and the amount of fluid he consumed since the last voiding. Does he have a history of difficulty when urinating? Ask whether Valsalva's maneuver or Credé's maneuver is required to initiate urination. Does he experience an urgent need to urinate? Does the urge to urinate arise without warning? Is urination painful or irritating? Ask about the force and continuity of the urine stream and whether the bladder is empty after voiding.

Assess the patient's history for the presence of a urinary tract obstruction or infections, venereal disease, lower abdominal or urinary tract trauma, systemic or neurologic disorders, and neurologic, intestinal, or pelvic surgery. Note medication history, including the use of over-the-counter or recreational drugs.

Physical examination
Take the patient's vital signs, and percuss and palpate the bladder. (Remember that if the bladder is empty, it can't be palpated through the abdominal wall.) Inspect the urethral meatus. Document the appearance and amount of any discharge. Finally, test for perineal sensation and anal sphincter tone; in male patients, digitally examine the prostate gland.

Pediatric pointers
Look for urine retention and bladder distention in an infant who fails to void normal amounts. (In the first 48 hours of life, an infant excretes about 60 ml of urine; during the following week, he excretes about 300 ml of urine daily.) In males, posterior urethral valves, meatal stenosis, phimosis, spinal cord anomalies, bladder diverticula, and other congenital defects may cause urinary obstruction and resultant bladder distention.

Geriatric pointers
Pre-existing disease states may hamper adequate assessment of bladder distention in elderly patients.

MEDICAL CAUSES
See *Bladder distention: Causes and associated findings,* pages 46 and 47.
- **Benign prostatic hyperplasia (BPH).** With BPH, bladder distention gradually develops as the prostate enlarges. Occasionally, its onset is acute. Initially, the patient experiences urinary hesitancy, straining, and frequency; reduced force of and the inability to stop the urine stream; nocturia; and postvoiding dribbling. As the disorder progresses, it produces prostate enlargement, sensations of suprapubic fullness and incomplete bladder emptying, perineal pain, constipation, and hematuria.
- **Bladder calculi.** Bladder calculi may produce bladder distention, but more commonly it produces pain as its only symptom. The pain is usually referred to the tip of the penis, the vulvar area, the lower back, or the heel. It worsens during walking or exercise and abates when the patient lies down. It can be accompanied by urinary frequency and urgency, terminal hematuria, and dysuria. Pain

is usually most severe when micturition ceases.

- *Bladder cancer.* By blocking the urethral orifice, neoplasms can cause bladder distention. Associated signs and symptoms include hematuria (most common sign); urinary frequency and urgency; nocturia; dysuria; pyuria; pain in the bladder, rectum, pelvis, flank, back, or legs; vomiting; diarrhea; and sleeplessness. A mass may be palpable on bimanual examination.

- *Multiple sclerosis (MS).* With MS, urine retention and bladder distention result from interruption of upper motor neuron control of the bladder. Associated signs and symptoms include optic neuritis, paresthesia, impaired position and vibratory senses, diplopia, nystagmus, dizziness, abnormal reflexes, dysarthria, muscle weakness, emotional lability, Lhermitte's sign (transient, electric-like shocks that spread down the body when the head is flexed), Babinski's sign, and ataxia.

- *Prostate cancer.* Prostate cancer eventually causes bladder distention in about 25% of patients. Usual signs and symptoms include dysuria, urinary frequency and urgency, nocturia, weight loss, fatigue, perineal pain, constipation, and induration of the prostate or a rigid, irregular prostate on digital rectal examination. For some patients, urine retention and bladder distention are the only signs.

- *Prostatitis.* With acute prostatitis, bladder distention occurs rapidly along with perineal discomfort and suprapubic fullness. Other signs and symptoms include perineal pain; tense, a boggy, tender, and warm enlarged prostate; decreased libido; impotence; decreased force of the urine stream; dysuria; hematuria; and urinary frequency and urgency. Additional signs and symptoms include fatigue, malaise, myalgia, fever, chills, nausea, and vomiting.

  With chronic prostatitis, bladder distention is rare. However, it may be accompanied by sensations of perineal discomfort and suprapubic fullness, prostatic tenderness, decreased libido, urinary frequency and urgency, dysuria, pyuria, hematuria, persistent urethral discharge, ejaculatory pain, and dull pain radiating to the lower back, buttocks, penis, or perineum.

- *Spinal neoplasms.* Disrupting upper neuron control of the bladder, spinal neoplasms cause neurogenic bladder and resultant distention. Associated signs and symptoms include a sense of pelvic fullness, continuous overflow dribbling, back pain that usually mimics sciatica pain, constipation, tender vertebral processes, sensory deficits, and muscle weakness, flaccidity, and atrophy. Signs and symptoms of urinary tract infection (dysuria, urinary frequency and urgency, nocturia, tenesmus, hematuria, and weakness) may also occur.

- *Urethral calculi.* With urethral calculi, urethral obstruction leads to bladder distention. The patient experiences interrupted urine flow. The obstruction causes pain radiating to the penis or vulva and referred to the perineum or rectum. It may also produce a palpable stone and urethral discharge.

- *Urethral stricture.* Urethral stricture results in urine retention and bladder distention with chronic urethral discharge (most common sign), urinary frequency (also common), dysuria, urgency, decreased force and diameter of the urine stream, and pyuria. Urinoma and urosepsis may also develop.

OTHER CAUSES

- *Catheterization.* Using an indwelling urinary catheter can result in urine retention and bladder distention. While the catheter is in place, inadequate drainage due to kinked tubing or an occluded lumen may lead to urine retention. In addition, a misplaced urinary catheter or irritation with catheter removal may cause edema, thereby blocking urine outflow.

- *Drugs.* Parasympatholytics, anticholinergics, ganglionic blockers, sedatives, anesthetics, and opiates can produce urine retention and bladder distention.

NURSING CONSIDERATIONS

Monitor the patient's vital signs and the extent of bladder distention. Obtain bladder urinary volume with a bladder scanner. Encourage the patient to change positions to alleviate discomfort. Administer medications for pain relief.

Prepare the patient for diagnostic tests, such as endoscopy and radiologic studies, to determine the cause of bladder distention. Withhold fluids and food if surgery is indicated.

PATIENT TEACHING

If the patient doesn't require immediate urinary catheterization, provide privacy and suggest that a normal voiding position be assumed. Teach Valsalva's maneuver, or gently

BLADDER DISTENTION: CAUSES AND ASSOCIATED FINDINGS

MAJOR ASSOCIATED SIGNS AND SYMPTOMS

COMMON CAUSES	Ataxia	Constipation	Dysuria	Fatigue	Fever	Hematuria	Muscle weakness	Myalgia	Nausea	Nocturia	Pain, buttock and sacral	
Benign prostatic hyperplasia		●				●				●		
Bladder calculi			●			●						
Bladder cancer			●			●				●	●	
Multiple sclerosis	●						●					
Prostate cancer		●	●	●						●		
Prostatitis (acute)			●	●	●	●		●	●			
Prostatitis (chronic)			●			●					●	
Spinal neoplasms		●	●			●	●			●		
Urethral calculi											●	
Urethral strictures			●									

perform Credé's maneuver. Use the power of suggestion to stimulate voiding. For example, run water in the sink, pour warm water over his perineum, place his hands in warm water, or play tapes of aquatic sounds.

Blood pressure decrease

Low blood pressure or hypotension refers to inadequate intravascular pressure to maintain the oxygen requirements of the body's tissues. Although commonly linked to shock, this sign may also result from a cardiovascular, respiratory, neurologic, or metabolic disorder. Hypoperfusion states especially affect the kidneys, brain, and heart, and may lead to renal failure, change in the patient's level of consciousness (LOC), or myocardial ischemia. Low blood pressure may be drug-induced or may accompany diagnostic tests — most commonly those using contrast media.

Hypotension may be due to stress or change of position — specifically, rising abruptly from a supine or sitting position to a standing position (orthostatic hypotension).

Normal blood pressure varies considerably; what qualifies as low blood pressure for one person may be normal for another. Consequently, every blood pressure reading must be compared against the patient's baseline and clinical status. Typically, a reading below 90/60 mm Hg, or a drop of 30 mm Hg from the baseline, is considered low blood pressure.

Pain, flank	Pain, lower back	Pain, pelvic	Pain, penile	Pain, perineal	Pain, vulvar	Prostatic enlargement	Prostatic rigidity	Pyuria	Suprapubic fullness	Urethral discharge	Urinary frequency	Urinary stream changes	Urinary urgency	Vomiting
			●			●			●		●	●		
			●	●							●		●	
●	●	●						●			●		●	●
				●			●				●			
				●		●			●		●		●	●
		●				●		●	●	●	●			
		●		●	●						●			
				●	●	●				●				
								●		●	●		●	●

Low blood pressure can reflect an expanded intravascular space (as in severe infections, allergic reactions, or adrenal insufficiency), reduced intravascular volume (as in dehydration and hemorrhage), or decreased cardiac output (as in impaired cardiac muscle contractility). Because the body's pressure-regulating mechanisms are complex and interrelated, a combination of these factors usually contributes to low blood pressure.

Act now *If the patient's systolic pressure is less than 80 mm Hg, or 30 mm Hg below his baseline, suspect shock immediately. Quickly evaluate the patient for a decreased LOC. Check his apical pulse for tachycardia and respirations for tachypnea. Also, inspect him for cool, clammy skin. Elevate the patient's legs above the level of his heart, or place him in Trendelenburg's position if the bed can be adjusted. Then start an I.V. line using a large-bore needle to replace fluids and blood or to administer drugs. Prepare to administer oxygen with mechanical ventilation, if necessary. Monitor the patient's intake and output and insert an indwelling urinary catheter to accurately measure urine output. The patient may also need a central venous line or a pulmonary artery catheter to facilitate monitoring of fluid status. Prepare the patient for cardiac monitoring to evaluate cardiac rhythm. Be ready to insert a nasogastric tube to prevent aspiration in the comatose patient. Throughout emergency interventions, keep the patient's spinal column immobile until spinal cord trauma is ruled out.*

ASSESSMENT
History

Obtain the patient's history from the patient or his family, paying particular attention to associated symptoms, such as weakness, fatigue, dizziness, fainting, blurred vision, nausea or vomiting, blood in stool, unsteady gait, palpitations, chest or abdominal pain, difficulty breathing, or generalized pain. De-

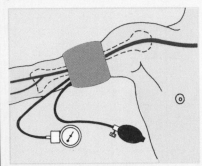
termine if symptoms appear when the patient changes positions suddenly.

Physical examination

Obtain blood pressure measurements with the patient lying down, sitting, and then standing, and compare readings. A drop in systolic or diastolic pressure of 10 mm Hg or more and an increase in heart rate of more than 15 beats/minute between position changes suggest orthostatic hypotension.

(See *Ensuring accurate blood pressure measurement.*)

Obtain the patient's other vital signs. Inspect the skin for pallor, sweating, and clamminess. Palpate peripheral pulses. Note paradoxical pulse — an accentuated fall in systolic pressure during inspiration — which suggests pericardial tamponade. Then auscultate for abnormal heart sounds (gallops, murmurs), rate (bradycardia, tachycardia), or rhythm. Auscultate the lungs for abnormal breath sounds (diminished sounds, crackles,

NORMAL PEDIATRIC BLOOD PRESSURE

AGE	NORMAL SYSTOLIC PRESSURE	NORMAL DIASTOLIC PRESSURE
Birth to 3 months	40 to 80 mm Hg	Not detectable
3 months to 1 year	80 to 100 mm Hg	Not detectable
1 to 4 years	100 to 108 mm Hg	60 mm Hg
4 to 12 years	108 to 124 mm Hg	60 to 70 mm Hg

wheezing), rate (bradypnea, tachypnea), or rhythm (agonal or Cheyne-Stokes respirations). Look for signs of hemorrhage, including visible bleeding and palpable masses, bruising, tenderness, or a positive stool occult blood test. Assess the patient for abdominal rigidity and rebound tenderness; auscultate for abnormal bowel sounds. Also, carefully assess the patient for possible sources of infection such as open wounds.

Pediatric pointers

Normal blood pressure in children is lower than that of adults. (See *Normal pediatric blood pressure.*)

Because accidents occur frequently in children, suspect trauma or shock first as a possible cause of low blood pressure. Remember that even though low blood pressure typically doesn't accompany head injury in adults (because intracranial hemorrhage is insufficient to cause hypovolemia), it does accompany head injury in infants and young children; their expandable cranial vaults allow significant blood loss into the cranial space, resulting in hypovolemia.

Another common cause of low blood pressure in children is dehydration, which results from failure to thrive or from persistent diarrhea and vomiting for as little as 24 hours.

Geriatric pointers

In elderly patients, low blood pressure commonly results from the use of multiple drugs that potentiate this adverse effect. Orthostatic hypotension due to autonomic dysfunction is another common cause of low blood pressure.

MEDICAL CAUSES

- *Acute adrenal insufficiency.* Orthostatic hypotension is characteristic with acute adrenal insufficiency, accompanied by fatigue, weakness, nausea, vomiting, abdominal discomfort, weight loss, fever, and tachycardia. The patient may also have hyperpigmentation of fingers, nails, nipples, scars, and body folds; pale, cool, clammy skin; restlessness; decreased urine output; tachypnea; and coma.
- *Alcohol toxicity.* Low blood pressure occurs infrequently; more commonly, alcohol toxicity produces distinct alcohol breath odor, tachycardia, bradypnea, hypothermia, decreased LOC, seizures, staggering gait, nausea, vomiting, diuresis, and slow, stertorous breathing.
- *Anaphylactic shock.* Following exposure to an allergen, such as penicillin or insect venom, a dramatic fall in blood pressure and narrowed pulse pressure signal anaphylactic shock, a severe allergic reaction. Initially, it causes anxiety, restlessness, a feeling of doom, intense itching (especially of the hands and feet), and pounding headache. Later, it may also produce weakness, sweating, nasal congestion, coughing, difficulty breathing, nausea, abdominal cramps, involuntary defecation, seizures, flushing, change or loss of voice due to laryngeal edema, urinary incontinence, and tachycardia.
- *Anthrax (inhalation).* Anthrax is an acute infectious disease that's caused by the gram-positive, spore-forming bacterium *Bacillus anthracis.* Although the disease most commonly occurs in wild and domestic grazing animals, such as cattle, sheep, and goats, the spores can live in the soil for many years. The disease can occur in humans exposed to infected animals, tissue from infected animals, or

biological warfare. Most natural cases occur in agricultural regions worldwide. Anthrax may occur in cutaneous, inhalation, or GI form.

Inhalation anthrax is caused by inhaling aerosolized spores. Initial signs and symptoms are flulike and include fever, chills, weakness, cough, and chest pain. The disease generally occurs in two stages with a period of recovery after the initial signs and symptoms. The second stage develops abruptly with rapid deterioration marked by fever, dyspnea, stridor, and hypotension generally leading to death within 24 hours. Radiologic findings include mediastinitis and symmetric mediastinal widening.

- *Cardiac arrhythmias.* With an arrhythmia, blood pressure may fluctuate between normal and low readings. Dizziness, chest pain, difficulty breathing, light-headedness, weakness, fatigue, and palpitations may also occur. Auscultation typically reveals an irregular rhythm and a pulse rate greater than 100 beats/minute or less than 60 beats/minute.

- *Cardiac contusion.* With cardiac contusion, low blood pressure occurs along with tachycardia and, at times, anginal pain and dyspnea.

- *Cardiac tamponade.* An accentuated fall in systolic pressure (more than 10 mm Hg) during inspiration, known as *paradoxical pulse,* is characteristic in patients with cardiac tamponade. This disorder also causes restlessness, cyanosis, tachycardia, jugular vein distention, muffled heart sounds, dyspnea, and Kussmaul's sign (increased venous distention with inspiration).

- *Cardiogenic shock.* A fall in systolic pressure to less than 80 mm Hg or to 30 mm Hg less than the patient's baseline, because of decreased cardiac contractility, is characteristic in patients with cardiogenic shock. Accompanying low blood pressure are tachycardia, narrowed pulse pressure, diminished Korotkoff sounds, peripheral cyanosis, and pale, cool, clammy skin. Cardiogenic shock also causes restlessness and anxiety, which may progress to disorientation and confusion. Associated signs and symptoms include angina, dyspnea, jugular vein distention, oliguria, ventricular gallop, tachypnea, and weak, rapid pulse.

- *Cholera.* Cholera is an acute infection caused by the bacterium *Vibrio cholerae* that may be mild with uncomplicated diarrhea or severe and life threatening. Cholera is spread by ingestion of contaminated water or food, especially shellfish. Signs include abrupt watery diarrhea and vomiting. Severe water and electrolyte loss leads to thirst, weakness, muscle cramps, decreased skin turgor, oliguria, tachycardia, and hypotension. Without treatment, death can occur within hours.

- *Diabetic ketoacidosis (DKA).* Hypovolemia triggered by osmotic diuresis in hyperglycemia is responsible for the low blood pressure associated with DKA, which is usually present in patients with type 1 diabetes mellitus. It also commonly produces polydipsia, polyuria, polyphagia, dehydration, weight loss, abdominal pain, nausea, vomiting, fruity breath odor, Kussmaul's respirations, tachycardia, seizures, confusion, and stupor that may progress to coma.

- *Heart failure.* With heart failure, blood pressure may fluctuate between normal and low readings. However, a precipitous drop in blood pressure may signal cardiogenic shock. Other signs and symptoms of heart failure include exertional dyspnea, dyspnea of abrupt or gradual onset, paroxysmal nocturnal dyspnea or difficulty breathing in the supine position (orthopnea), fatigue, weight gain, pallor or cyanosis, sweating, and anxiety. Auscultation reveals ventricular gallop, tachycardia, bilateral crackles, and tachypnea. Dependent edema, jugular vein distention, increased capillary refill time, and hepatomegaly may also occur.

- *Hyperosmolar hyperglycemic nonketotic syndrome (HHNS).* HHNS, which is common in people with type 2 diabetes mellitus, decreases blood pressure — at times dramatically, if the patient loses significant fluid from diuresis due to severe hyperglycemia and hyperosmolarity. It also produces dry mouth, poor skin turgor, tachycardia, confusion progressing to coma and, occasionally, generalized tonic-clonic seizure.

- *Hypovolemic shock.* A fall in systolic pressure to less than 80 mm Hg or 30 mm Hg less than the patient's baseline, secondary to acute blood loss or dehydration, is characteristic in patients with hypovolemic shock. Accompanying it are diminished Korotkoff sounds, narrowed pulse pressure, and rapid, weak, and irregular pulse. Peripheral vasoconstriction causes cyanosis of the extremities and pale, cool, clammy skin. Other signs and symptoms include oliguria, confusion, disorientation, restlessness, and anxiety.

- **Hypoxemia.** Initially, blood pressure may be normal or slightly elevated, but as hypoxemia becomes more pronounced, blood pressure drops. The patient may also display tachycardia, tachypnea, dyspnea, and confusion, and may progress from stupor to coma.
- **Myocardial infarction (MI).** With MI — a life-threatening disorder — blood pressure may be low or high. However, a precipitous drop in blood pressure may signal cardiogenic shock. Associated signs and symptoms include chest pain that may radiate to the jaw, shoulder, arm, back, or epigastrium; dyspnea; anxiety; nausea or vomiting; sweating; and cool, pale, or cyanotic skin. Auscultation may reveal an atrial gallop, a murmur and, occasionally, an irregular pulse.
- **Neurogenic shock.** The result of sympathetic denervation due to cervical injury or anesthesia, neurogenic shock produces low blood pressure and bradycardia. However, the patient's skin remains warm and dry because of cutaneous vasodilation and sweat gland denervation. Depending on the cause of shock, there may also be motor weakness of the limbs or diaphragm.
- **Pulmonary embolism.** Pulmonary embolism causes sudden, sharp chest pain and dyspnea accompanied by cough and, occasionally, low-grade fever. Low blood pressure occurs with narrowed pulse pressure and diminished Korotkoff sounds. Associated signs include tachycardia, tachypnea, paradoxical pulse, jugular vein distention, and hemoptysis.
- **Septic shock.** Initially, septic shock produces fever and chills. Low blood pressure, tachycardia, and tachypnea may also develop early, but the patient's skin remains warm. Later, low blood pressure becomes increasingly severe — less than 80 mm Hg, or 30 mm Hg less than the patient's baseline — and is accompanied by narrowed pulse pressure. Other late signs and symptoms include pale skin, cyanotic extremities, apprehension, thirst, oliguria, and coma.
- **Vasovagal syncope.** Vasovagal syncope is a transient attack of loss or near-loss of consciousness that's characterized by low blood pressure, pallor, cold sweats, nausea, palpitations or slowed heart rate, and weakness following stressful, painful, or claustrophobic experiences.

OTHER CAUSES

- **Diagnostic tests.** These include the gastric acid stimulation test using histamine and X-ray studies using contrast media. The latter may trigger an allergic reaction, which causes low blood pressure.
- **Drugs.** Calcium channel blockers, diuretics, vasodilators, alpha- and beta-adrenergic blockers, general anesthetics, opioid analgesics, monoamine oxidase inhibitors, anxiolytics (such as benzodiazepines), tranquilizers, and most I.V. antiarrhythmics can cause low blood pressure.

NURSING CONSIDERATIONS

Check the patient's vital signs frequently to determine if low blood pressure is constant or intermittent. If blood pressure is extremely low, an arterial catheter may be inserted to allow close monitoring of pressures. Alternatively, a Doppler flowmeter may be used.

Place the patient on bed rest. Keep the side rails of the bed up. If the patient is ambulatory, assist him as necessary. To avoid falls, don't leave a dizzy patient unattended when he's sitting or walking.

Prepare the patient for laboratory tests, which may include bedside glucose check, urinalysis, routine blood studies, an electrocardiogram, and chest, cervical, and abdominal X-rays.

PATIENT TEACHING

If the patient has orthostatic hypotension, instruct him to stand up slowly. Advise the patient with vasovagal syncope to avoid situations that trigger the episodes. Evaluate the patient's need for a cane or walker. Explain all procedures and tests.

Blood pressure increase

Elevated blood pressure (hypertension) is defined as an intermittent or sustained increase in blood pressure exceeding 140/90 mm Hg. Hypertension strikes more men than women and twice as many blacks as whites. Its causes can be life threatening; however, patients are usually unaware that it exists.

Elevated blood pressure may develop suddenly or gradually. A sudden, severe rise

PATHOPHYSIOLOGY OF ELEVATED BLOOD PRESSURE

Blood pressure—the force blood exerts on vessels as it flows through them—depends on cardiac output, peripheral resistance, and blood volume. A brief review of its regulating mechanisms—nervous system control, capillary fluid shifts, kidney excretion, and hormonal changes—will help you understand how elevated blood pressure develops.

◆ *Nervous system control* involves the sympathetic system, chiefly baroreceptors and chemoreceptors, which promotes moderate vasoconstriction to maintain normal blood pressure. When this system responds inappropriately, increased vasoconstriction enhances peripheral resistance, resulting in elevated blood pressure.

◆ *Capillary fluid shifts* regulate blood volume by responding to arterial pressure. Increased pressure forces fluid into the interstitial space; decreased pressure allows it to be drawn back into the arteries by osmosis. However, this fluid shift may take several hours to adjust blood pressure.

◆ *Kidney excretion* also helps regulate blood volume by increasing or decreasing urine formation. Normally an arterial pressure of about 60 mm Hg maintains urine output. When pressure drops below this reading, urine formation ceases, thus increasing blood volume. Like capillary fluid shifts, this mechanism may take several hours to adjust blood pressure.

◆ *Hormonal changes* reflect stimulation of the kidney's renin-angiotension-aldosterone system in response to low arterial pressure. This system affects vasoconstriction, which increases arterial pressure, and stimulates aldosterone release, which regulates sodium retention—a key determinant of blood volume.

Elevated blood pressure signals the breakdown or inappropriate response of these pressure-regulating mechanisms. Its associated signs and symptoms concentrate in the target organs and tissues illustrated here.

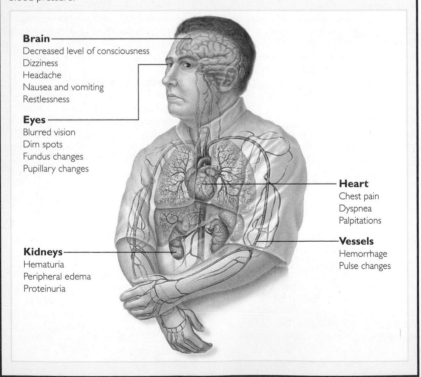

Brain
Decreased level of consciousness
Dizziness
Headache
Nausea and vomiting
Restlessness

Eyes
Blurred vision
Dim spots
Fundus changes
Pupillary changes

Kidneys
Hematuria
Peripheral edema
Proteinuria

Heart
Chest pain
Dyspnea
Palpitations

Vessels
Hemorrhage
Pulse changes

MANAGING ELEVATED BLOOD PRESSURE

Blood pressure exceeding 180/110 mm Hg may indicate hypertensive crisis — a life-threatening condition requiring prompt treatment. Maintain a patent airway and institute seizure precautions. Prepare to administer an I.V. antihypertensive and diuretic. You'll also need to insert an indwelling urinary catheter to accurately monitor urine output.

If blood pressure is less severely elevated, continue to rule out other life-threatening causes. If the patient is pregnant, suspect preeclampsia or eclampsia. Place her on bed rest, and insert an I.V. line. Administer magnesium sulfate (to decrease neuromuscular irritability) and an antihypertensive. Monitor her vital signs closely for the next 24 hours. If diastolic blood pressure continues to exceed 100 mm Hg despite drug therapy, you may need to prepare the patient for induced labor and delivery or for cesarean birth. Offer emotional support if she must face delivery of a premature neonate.

If the patient isn't pregnant, quickly observe for equally obvious clues. Assess the patient for exophthalmos and an enlarged thyroid gland. If these signs are present, ask about a history of hyperthyroidism. Then look for other associated signs and symptoms, including tachycardia, widened pulse pressure, palpi-

tations, severe weakness, diarrhea, fever exceeding 100° F (37.8° C), and nervousness. Prepare to administer an antithyroid drug orally or by nasogastric tube, if necessary. Also, evaluate fluid status; look for signs of dehydration such as poor skin turgor. Prepare for I.V. fluid replacement and temperature control using a cooling blanket, if necessary.

If the patient shows signs of increased intracranial pressure (such as decreased level of consciousness and fixed or dilated pupils), ask him or a family member if he has recently experienced head trauma. Then check for an increased respiratory rate and bradycardia. You'll need to maintain a patent airway in case the patient vomits. In addition, institute seizure precautions, and prepare to give an I.V. diuretic. Insert an indwelling urinary catheter, and monitor intake and output. Check the patient's vital signs every 15 minutes until he's stable.

If the patient has absent or weak peripheral pulses, ask about chest pressure or pain, which suggests a dissecting aortic aneurysm. Enforce bed rest until a diagnosis has been established. As appropriate, give the patient an I.V. antihypertensive or prepare him for surgery.

---

in pressure (exceeding 180/110 mm Hg) may indicate life-threatening hypertensive crisis. However, even a less dramatic rise may be equally significant if it heralds a dissecting aortic aneurysm, increased intracranial pressure (ICP), myocardial infarction (MI), eclampsia, or thyrotoxicosis.

Usually associated with essential hypertension, elevated blood pressure may also result from a renal or endocrine disorder, a treatment that affects fluid status such as dialysis, or a drug's adverse effect. Ingestion of large amounts of certain foods, such as black licorice and cheddar cheese, may temporarily elevate blood pressure. (See *Pathophysiology of elevated blood pressure*.) Sometimes, elevated blood pressure may simply reflect inaccurate blood pressure measurement. (See *Ensuring accurate blood pressure measurement,* page 48.) However, careful measurement alone doesn't ensure a clinical-

ly useful reading. To be useful, each blood pressure reading must be compared with the patient's baseline. Also, serial readings may be necessary to establish elevated blood pressure.

Act now   *If you detect sharply elevated blood pressure, quickly rule out possible life-threatening causes. (See* Managing elevated blood pressure.*)*

ASSESSMENT
History
Determine if the patient has a history of cardiovascular or cerebrovascular disease, diabetes, or renal disease. Ask about a family history of high blood pressure — a likely finding with essential hypertension, pheochromocytoma, or polycystic kidney disease. If hypertension was a pre-existing disease, determine its onset, age at onset, medical treatment regimen, and associated symp-

toms. Pheochromocytoma and primary aldosteronism usually occur between ages 40 and 60. If you suspect either, check for orthostatic hypotension.

Note headache, palpitations, blurred vision, and sweating. Ask about wine-colored urine and decreased urine output; these signs suggest glomerulonephritis, which can cause elevated blood pressure.

Obtain a medication history, including past and present prescriptions, herbal preparations, and over-the-counter (OTC) drugs (especially decongestants). Determine if the patient takes prescribed antihypertensives as recommended.

✸ **Alert** *A sudden onset of high blood pressure in middle-age or elderly patients suggests renovascular stenosis. Although essential hypertension may begin in childhood, it typically isn't diagnosed until around age 35.*

Hypertension has been reported to be two to three times more common in women taking hormonal contraceptives than those not taking them. Women age 35 and older who smoke cigarettes should be strongly encouraged to stop; if they continue to smoke, they should be discouraged from using hormonal contraceptives.

Physical examination
Take the patient's blood pressure with him lying down, sitting, and then standing. Normally, systolic pressure falls and diastolic pressure rises on standing. With orthostatic hypotension, both pressures fall.

Using a funduscope, check for intraocular hemorrhage, exudate, and papilledema, which characterize severe hypertension. Perform a thorough cardiovascular assessment. Check for carotid bruits and jugular vein distention. (See *Preventing false bruits.*) Assess skin color, temperature, and turgor. Palpate peripheral pulses. Auscultate for abnormal heart sounds (gallops, louder second sound, murmurs), rate (bradycardia, tachycardia), or rhythm. Then auscultate for abnormal breath sounds (crackles, wheezing), rate (bradypnea, tachypnea), or rhythm.

Palpate the abdomen for tenderness, masses, or liver enlargement. Auscultate for abdominal bruits. Renal artery stenosis produces bruits over the upper abdomen or in the costovertebral angles (CVAs). Easily palpable, enlarged kidneys and a large, tender liver suggest polycystic kidney disease. Obtain a urine sample to check for microscopic hematuria.

Pediatric pointers
Normally, blood pressure in children is lower than in adults—an essential point to recognize when assessing a patient for elevated blood pressure. (See *Normal pediatric blood pressure,* page 49.)

Elevated blood pressure in children may result from lead or mercury poisoning, essential hypertension, renovascular stenosis, chronic pyelonephritis, coarctation of the aorta, patent ductus arteriosus, glomerulonephritis, adrenogenital syndrome, or neuroblastoma. Treatment typically begins with drug therapy. Surgery may then follow in patients with patent ductus arteriosus, coarctation of the aorta, neuroblastoma, and some cases of renovascular stenosis. Diuretics and antibiotics are used to treat glomerulonephritis and chronic pyelonephritis; hormonal therapy, to treat adrenogenital syndrome.

Geriatric pointers
Atherosclerosis commonly produces isolated systolic hypertension in elderly patients. Treatment is warranted to prevent long-term complications.

MEDICAL CAUSES
● *Aldosteronism (primary).* With aldosteronism, elevated diastolic pressure may be accompanied by orthostatic hypotension. Other findings include constipation, muscle weakness, polyuria, polydipsia, and personality changes.
● *Anemia.* Accompanying elevated systolic pressure in anemia are pulsations in the capillary beds, bounding pulse, tachycardia, systolic ejection murmur, pale mucous membranes and, in patients with sickle cell anemia, ventricular gallop and crackles.
● *Aortic aneurysm (dissecting).* Initially, aortic aneurysm—a life-threatening disorder—causes a sudden rise in systolic pressure (which may be the precipitating event), but no change in diastolic pressure. However, this increase is brief. The body's ability to compensate fails, resulting in hypotension.

Other signs and symptoms vary, depending on the type of aortic aneurysm. An abdominal aneurysm may cause persistent abdominal and back pain, weakness, sweating, tachycardia, dyspnea, a pulsating abdominal mass, restlessness, confusion, and cool,

PREVENTING FALSE BRUITS

Auscultating bruits accurately requires practice and skill. These sounds typically stem from arterial luminal narrowing or arterial dilation, but they can also result from excessive pressure applied to the stethoscope's bell during auscultation. This pressure compresses the artery, creating turbulent blood flow and a false bruit.

To prevent false bruits, place the bell lightly on the patient's skin. Also, if you're auscultating for a popliteal bruit, help the patient to a supine position, place your hand behind his ankle, and lift his leg slightly before placing the bell behind the knee.

Normal blood flow, no bruit

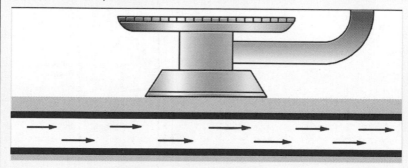

Turbulent blood flow and resultant bruit caused by aneurysm

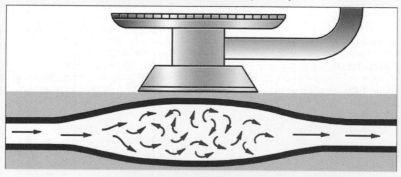

Turbulent blood flow and false bruit caused by compression of artery

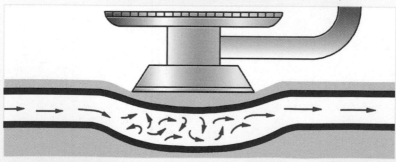

clammy skin. A thoracic aneurysm may cause a ripping or tearing sensation in the chest, which may radiate to the neck, shoulders, lower back, or abdomen; pallor; syncope; blindness; loss of consciousness; sweating; dyspnea; tachycardia; cyanosis; leg weakness; murmur; and absent radial and femoral pulses.

● *Atherosclerosis.* With atherosclerosis, systolic pressure rises while diastolic pressure commonly remains normal or slightly elevated. The patient may show no other signs, or he may have a weak pulse, flushed skin, tachycardia, angina, and claudication.

● *Cushing's syndrome.* Twice as common in females as in males, Cushing's syndrome causes elevated blood pressure and widened pulse pressure as well as truncal obesity, moon face, and other cushingoid signs. It's usually caused by corticosteroid use.

● *Hypertension.* Essential hypertension develops insidiously and is characterized by a gradual increase in blood pressure from decade to decade. Except for this high blood pressure, the patient may be asymptomatic or (rarely) may complain of suboccipital headache, light-headedness, tinnitus, and fatigue.

With malignant hypertension, diastolic pressure abruptly rises above 120 mm Hg, and systolic pressure may exceed 200 mm Hg. Typically, the patient has pulmonary edema marked by jugular vein distention, dyspnea, tachypnea, tachycardia, and coughing up pink, frothy sputum. Other characteristic signs and symptoms include severe headache, confusion, blurred vision, tinnitus, epistaxis, muscle twitching, chest pain, nausea, and vomiting.

● *Increased ICP.* Increased ICP causes an increased respiratory rate initially, followed by increased systolic pressure and widened pulse pressure. Increased ICP affects heart rate last, causing bradycardia (Cushing's reflex). Associated signs and symptoms include headache, projectile vomiting, decreased level of consciousness, and fixed or dilated pupils.

● *Myocardial infarction (MI).* MI — a life-threatening disorder — may cause high or low blood pressure. Common findings include crushing chest pain that may radiate to the jaw, shoulder, arm, back, or epigastrium. Other findings include dyspnea, anxiety, nausea, vomiting, weakness, diaphoresis, atrial gallop, and murmurs.

● *Pheochromocytoma.* Paroxysmal or sustained elevated blood pressure characterizes pheochromocytoma and may be accompanied by orthostatic hypotension. Associated signs and symptoms include anxiety, diaphoresis, palpitations, tremors, pallor, nausea, weight loss, and headache.

● *Polycystic kidney disease.* Elevated blood pressure is typically preceded by flank pain. Other signs and symptoms include enlarged kidneys; enlarged, tender liver; and intermittent gross hematuria.

● *Preeclampsia and eclampsia.* Potentially life threatening to the mother and fetus, preeclampsia and eclampsia characteristically increase blood pressure. They're defined as a reading of 140/90 mm Hg or more in the first trimester, a reading of 130/80 mm Hg or more in the second or third trimester, an increase of 30 mm Hg above the patient's baseline systolic pressure, or an increase of 15 mm Hg above the patient's baseline diastolic pressure. Accompanying elevated blood pressure are generalized edema, sudden weight gain of 3 lb (1.4 kg) or more per week during the second or third trimester, severe frontal headache, blurred or double vision, decreased urine output, proteinuria, midabdominal pain, neuromuscular irritability, nausea, and possibly seizures (eclampsia).

● *Renovascular stenosis.* Renovascular stenosis produces abruptly elevated systolic and diastolic pressures. Other characteristic signs and symptoms include bruits over the upper abdomen or in the CVAs, hematuria, and acute flank pain.

● *Thyrotoxicosis.* Accompanying the elevated systolic pressure associated with thyrotoxicosis — a potentially life-threatening disorder — are widened pulse pressure, tachycardia, bounding pulse, pulsations in the capillary nail beds, palpitations, weight loss, exophthalmos, an enlarged thyroid gland, weakness, diarrhea, fever over 100° F (37.8° C), and warm, moist skin. The patient may appear nervous and emotionally unstable, displaying occasional outbursts or even psychotic behavior. Heat intolerance, exertional dyspnea and, in females, decreased or absent menses may also occur.

OTHER CAUSES

● *Drugs.* Central nervous system stimulants (such as amphetamines), sympathomimetics, corticosteroids, nonsteroidal anti-inflammatory drugs, hormonal contraceptives, monoamine oxidase inhibitors, and OTC cold remedies can increase blood pressure, as can cocaine abuse.

- *Herbal supplements.* Ephedra (ma huang), ginseng, and licorice may cause high blood pressure or an irregular heartbeat. St. John's wort can also raise blood pressure, especially when taken with substances that antagonize hypericin, such as amphetamines, cold and hay fever medications, nasal decongestants, pickled foods, beer, coffee, wine, and chocolate.
- *Treatments.* Kidney dialysis and transplantation cause transient elevation of blood pressure.

NURSING CONSIDERATIONS

Prepare the patient for routine blood tests and urinalysis. Depending on the suspected cause of the increased blood pressure, radiographic studies, especially of the kidneys, may be necessary, as well as cardiac monitoring.

Obtain the patient's vital signs frequently. Monitor the effects of treatment. Perform neurologic and respiratory assessments frequently.

PATIENT TEACHING

If the patient has essential hypertension, explain the importance of long-term control of elevated blood pressure and the purpose, dosage, schedule, route, and adverse effects of prescribed antihypertensives. Encourage him to report adverse reactions; the drug dosage or schedule may simply need adjustment. Then teach the patient and his family how to monitor his blood pressure so that he can evaluate the effectiveness of drug therapy and lifestyle changes. Have him record blood pressure readings and symptoms, and ask him to share this information on his return visits.

Bowel sounds, absent

Absent bowel sounds refers to an inability to hear bowel sounds through a stethoscope after listening for at least 5 minutes in each abdominal quadrant. Bowel sounds cease when mechanical or vascular obstruction or neurogenic inhibition halts peristalsis. When peristalsis stops, gas from bowel contents

and fluid secreted from the intestinal walls accumulate and distend the lumen, leading to life-threatening complications, such as perforation, peritonitis, and sepsis, or hypovolemic shock.

Simple mechanical obstruction, resulting from adhesions, hernia, or tumor, causes loss of fluids and electrolytes and induces dehydration. Vascular obstruction cuts off circulation to the intestinal walls, leading to ischemia, necrosis, and shock. Neurogenic inhibition, affecting innervation of the intestinal wall, may result from infection, bowel distention, or trauma. It may also follow mechanical or vascular obstruction or metabolic derangement such as hypokalemia.

Abrupt cessation of bowel sounds, when accompanied by abdominal pain, rigidity, and distention, signals a life-threatening crisis requiring immediate intervention. Absent bowel sounds following a period of hyperactive sounds are equally ominous and may indicate strangulation of a mechanically obstructed bowel. (See *Are bowel sounds really absent?* page 58.)

Act now *If you fail to detect bowel sounds and the patient reports sudden, severe abdominal pain and cramping or exhibits severe abdominal distention, prepare to insert a nasogastric (NG) or intestinal tube to suction lumen contents and decompress the bowel. Administer I.V. fluids and electrolytes to offset dehydration and imbalances caused by the dysfunctional bowel.*

Because the patient may require surgery to relieve an obstruction, withhold oral intake. Take the patient's vital signs, and stay alert for signs of shock, such as hypotension, tachycardia, and cool, clammy skin. Measure his abdominal girth as a baseline for gauging subsequent changes.

ASSESSMENT
History

If the patient's condition permits, proceed with a brief history. Determine if abdominal pain is present, and if so, the time of its onset, precipitating or aggravating factors, location and radiation, sensation of bloating, presence or absence of flatulence, changes in bowel habits or characteristics, or absence of bowel movements (a possible sign of complete obstruction or paralytic ileus).

Determine conditions that commonly lead to mechanical obstruction, such as abdominal tumors, hernias, and adhesions from past surgery. Determine if the patient was involved in an accident — even a seemingly minor one, such as falling off a stepladder — that may have caused vascular clots. Check for a history of acute pancreatitis, diverticulitis, or gynecologic infection, which may have led to intra-abdominal infection and bowel dysfunction. Be sure to ask about previous toxic conditions, such as uremia, and about spinal cord injury, which can lead to paralytic ileus.

Physical examination

Complete a full GI assessment by inspecting abdominal contour. Stoop at the recumbent patient's side and then at the foot of his bed to detect localized or generalized distention. Auscultate for dullness over fluid-filled areas and tympany over pockets of gas. Percuss and palpate the abdomen gently, examining the area of pain last. Palpate for abdominal rigidity and guarding, which suggest peritoneal irritation that can lead to paralytic ileus.

Pediatric pointers

Absent bowel sounds in children may result from Hirschsprung's disease, volvulus, or in-

tussusception, both of which can lead to life-threatening obstruction.

Geriatric pointers

Older patients with a bowel obstruction that doesn't respond to decompression should be considered for early surgical intervention to avoid the risk of bowel infarct.

MEDICAL CAUSES

● *Complete mechanical intestinal obstruction.* Absent bowel sounds follow a period of hyperactive bowel sounds with complete mechanical intestinal obstruction — a potentially life-threatening disorder. This silence accompanies acute, colicky abdominal pain that arises in the quadrant of obstruction and may radiate to the flank or lumbar regions. Associated signs and symptoms include abdominal distention, bloating, constipation, and nausea and vomiting (the higher the blockage, the earlier and more severe the vomiting). In late stages, signs of shock may occur with fever, rebound tenderness, and abdominal rigidity.

● *Mesenteric artery occlusion.* With mesenteric artery occlusion — a life-threatening disorder — bowel sounds disappear after a brief period of hyperactive sounds. Sudden, severe midepigastric or periumbilical pain occurs next, followed by abdominal distention, bruits, vomiting, constipation, and signs of shock. Fever is common. Abdominal rigidity may appear later.

● *Paralytic (adynamic) ileus.* The cardinal sign of paralytic ileus is absent bowel sounds. In addition to abdominal distention, associated signs and symptoms include generalized discomfort and constipation or passage of small, liquid stools. If paralytic ileus follows acute abdominal infection, the patient may also experience fever and abdominal pain.

OTHER CAUSES

● *Abdominal surgery.* Bowel sounds are normally absent after abdominal surgery — the result of anesthetic use and surgical manipulation.

NURSING CONSIDERATIONS

After you've inserted an NG tube or an intestinal tube, elevate the head of the patient's bed at least 30 degrees, and turn the patient to facilitate passage of the tube through the GI tract. (Remember not to tape an intestinal tube to the patient's face.) Ensure tube patency by checking for drainage and properly functioning suction devices, and irrigate accordingly. Withhold food and fluids until it's determined whether the patient needs surgery.

Continue to administer I.V. fluids and electrolytes, and make sure that you send a serum specimen to the laboratory for electrolyte analysis at least once per day. The patient may need X-ray studies and further blood work to determine the cause of absent bowel sounds.

After mechanical obstruction and intra-abdominal sepsis have been ruled out as the cause of absent bowel sounds, give the patient drugs to control pain and stimulate peristalsis.

PATIENT TEACHING

Explain all procedures and tests to the patient.

Bowel sounds, hyperactive

Sometimes audible without a stethoscope, hyperactive bowel sounds reflect increased intestinal motility (peristalsis). They're commonly characterized as rapid, rushing, gurgling waves of sound. (See *Characteristics of bowel sounds.*) They may stem from life-threatening bowel obstruction or GI hemorrhage, or from GI infection, inflammatory bowel disease (IBD), which usually follows a chronic course; food allergies; or stress.

Act now *After detecting hyperactive bowel sounds, quickly check the patient's vital signs and ask him about associated symptoms, such as abdominal pain, vomiting, and diarrhea. If cramping abdominal pain or vomiting is present, continue to auscultate for bowel sounds. If bowel sounds stop abruptly, suspect complete bowel obstruction. Prepare to assist with GI suction and decompression, give I.V. fluids and electrolytes, and prepare the patient for surgery.*

ASSESSMENT
History

Determine if there's a history of hernia or abdominal surgery because these may cause mechanical intestinal obstruction. Determine if there's a history of IBD, eruptions of gastroenteritis among family members, friends, or coworkers. Ask if the patient has traveled recently, even within the United States.

In addition, determine whether stress may have contributed to the patient's problem. Ask about food allergies and recent ingestion of unusual foods or fluids. Obtain a full medication history, including over-the-counter medications.

Alert *Homosexual males who report acute diarrhea and exhibit negative fecal ova and parasite cultures may be infected with chlamydial proctitis not associated with lymphogranuloma venereum. Because rectal cultures will probably be negative, treatment with tetracycline is appropriate.*

Physical examination

Check for fever, which suggests infection. Complete a full GI assessment by inspecting abdominal contour. Stoop at the recumbent patient's side and then at the foot of his bed to detect localized or generalized distention. Auscultate the abdomen and note bowel sounds. Percuss and palpate the abdomen gently. Palpate for abdominal rigidity and guarding, which suggest peritoneal irritation that can lead to paralytic ileus.

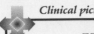

HYPERACTIVE BOWEL SOUNDS: CAUSES AND ASSOCIATED FINDINGS

MAJOR ASSOCIATED SIGNS AND SYMPTOMS

COMMON CAUSES	Abdominal distention	Abdominal pain	Anorexia	Constipation	Diarrhea	Fever	Nausea	Perianal lesions	Rectal bleeding	Tenesmus	Vomiting	Weight loss
Crohn's disease	●	●	●		●	●		●				●
Food hypersensitivity					●		●				●	
Gastroenteritis		●			●	●	●				●	
GI hemorrhage	●	●			●				●			
Mechanical intestinal obstruction	●	●		●			●				●	
Ulcerative colitis (acute)			●		●	●				●		●

Pediatric pointers

Hyperactive bowel sounds in children usually result from gastroenteritis, erratic eating habits, excessive ingestion of certain foods (such as unripened fruit), or food allergy.

Geriatric pointers

Medication interactions and pre-existing diseases may produce pronounced symptoms in the elderly. Dehydration and fluid and electrolyte imbalances can quickly develop if there's fluid loss present.

MEDICAL CAUSES

See *Hyperactive bowel sounds: Causes and associated findings.*

● *Crohn's disease.* Hyperactive bowel sounds usually arise insidiously. Associated signs and symptoms of Crohn's disease include diarrhea, cramping abdominal pain that may be relieved by defecation, anorexia, low-grade fever, abdominal distention and tenderness and, in many cases, a fixed mass in the right lower quadrant. Perianal and vaginal lesions are common. Muscle wasting, weight loss, and signs of dehydration may occur as the disease progresses.

● *Food hypersensitivity.* Malabsorption—typically lactose intolerance—may cause hyperactive bowel sounds. Associated signs and symptoms of food hypersensitivity include diarrhea and, possibly, nausea and vomiting, angioedema, and urticaria.

● *Gastroenteritis.* Hyperactive bowel sounds follow sudden nausea and vomiting and accompany "explosive" diarrhea. Abdominal cramping or pain is common, typically after a peristaltic wave. Fever may occur, depending on the causative organism.

● *GI hemorrhage.* Hyperactive bowel sounds provide the most immediate indication of persistent upper GI bleeding. Other findings include hematemesis, coffee-ground vomitus, abdominal distention, bloody diarrhea, rectal passage of bright red clots and jellylike material or melena, and pain during bleeding. Decreased urine output, tachycardia, and hypotension accompany blood loss.

● *Mechanical intestinal obstruction.* Hyperactive bowel sounds occur simultaneously with cramping abdominal pain every few minutes in patients with intestinal obstruction, a potentially life-threatening disorder. Bowel sounds may later become hypoactive and then disappear. With small-bowel obstruction, nausea and vomiting occur earlier and with greater severity than in large-bowel obstruction. With complete bowel obstruction, hyperactive sounds are also accompanied by abdominal distention and constipation, although the part of the bowel distal to the obstruction may continue to empty for up to 3 days.

● *Ulcerative colitis (acute).* Hyperactive bowel sounds arise abruptly in patients with ulcerative colitis and are accompanied by bloody diarrhea, anorexia, abdominal pain, nausea and vomiting, fever, and tenesmus. Weight loss, arthralgia, and arthritis may occur.

NURSING CONSIDERATIONS

Obtain the patient's vital signs. Prepare him for diagnostic tests. These may include endoscopy to view a suspected lesion, barium X-rays, computed tomography scan, or stool analysis.

Monitor intake and output closely. If diarrhea is present, monitor for signs and symptoms of dehydration.

PATIENT TEACHING

Explain prescribed dietary changes to the patient. These may range from complete food and fluid restrictions to a liquid or bland diet. Because stress commonly precipitates or aggravates bowel hyperactivity, teach the patient relaxation techniques such as deep breathing. Encourage rest and restrict the patient's physical activity.

Bradycardia

Bradycardia refers to a heart rate of less than 60 beats/minute. It occurs normally in young adults, trained athletes, and elderly people as well as during sleep. It's also a normal response to vagal stimulation caused by coughing, vomiting, or straining during defecation. When bradycardia results from these causes, the heart rate rarely drops below 40 beats/minute. However, when it results from pathologic causes, such as cardiovascular disorders, the heart rate may be slower.

By itself, bradycardia is a nonspecific sign. However, in conjunction with such symptoms as chest pain, dizziness, syncope, arrhythmias, and shortness of breath, it can signal a life-threatening disorder.

Act now Depending on the accompanying signs and symptoms, the patient with bradycardia may require immediate emergency care. For symptomatic bradycardia, atropine I.V. may be ordered, a transcutaneous pacemaker may be required, and full cardiorespiratory arrest may occur.

ASSESSMENT
History

After detecting bradycardia, check for related signs of life-threatening disorders before proceeding with a history. (See *Managing severe bradycardia,* page 62.) Determine if the patient or a family member has a history of a slow pulse rate. Check for underlying metabolic disorders, such as hypothyroidism, which can precipitate bradycardia. Obtain a medication history and make sure that the prescribed schedule and dosage is followed.

Physical examination

Monitor the patient's vital signs, temperature, pulse, respirations, blood pressure, and oxygen saturation. If he's on a cardiac monitor, frequently assess cardiac rhythm and note changes.

Assess for changes in the patient's level of consciousness (LOC) or respiratory status.

Pediatric pointers

Heart rates are normally higher in children than in adults. Fetal bradycardia — a heart rate of less than 120 beats/minute — may occur during prolonged labor or complications of delivery, such as compression of the umbilical cord, partial abruptio placentae, and placenta previa. Intermittent bradycardia, sometimes accompanied by apnea, commonly occurs in premature neonates. Bradycardia rarely occurs in full-term neonates or children. However, it can result from congenital heart defects, acute glomerulonephritis, and transient or complete heart block associated with cardiac catheterization or cardiac surgery.

Geriatric pointers

Sinus node dysfunction is the most common bradyarrhythmia encountered among the elderly. A patient with this disorder may have as his chief complaint fatigue, exercise intolerance, dizziness, or syncope. If the patient is asymptomatic, no intervention is nec-

MANAGING SEVERE BRADYCARDIA

Bradycardia can signal a life-threatening disorder when accompanied by pain, shortness of breath, dizziness, or syncope or in a patient with prolonged exposure to cold or head or neck trauma. Take the patient's vital signs immediately, connect him to a cardiac monitor, and insert an I.V. line. Depending on the cause of bradycardia, you'll need to administer fluids, atropine, steroids, or thyroid medication. If indicated, insert an indwelling urinary catheter. Intubation, mechanical ventilation, or pacemaker placement may be necessary if the patient's respiratory rate falls.

If appropriate, perform a focused evaluation to help locate the cause of bradycardia. For example, ask about pain. Viselike pressure or crushing or burning chest pain that radiates to the arms, back, or jaw may indicate an acute myocardial infarction (MI); a severe headache, increased intracranial pressure. Also, ask about nausea, vomiting, or shortness of breath — signs and symptoms associated with an acute MI and cardiomyopathy. Observe the patient for peripheral cyanosis, edema, or jugular vein distention, which may indicate cardiomyopathy. Look for a thyroidectomy scar because severe bradycardia may result from hypothyroidism caused by failure to take thyroid hormone replacements.

If the cause of bradycardia is evident, provide supportive care. For example, keep the hypothermic patient warm by applying blankets, and monitor his core temperature until it reaches 99° F (37.2° C); stabilize the head and neck of a trauma patient until cervical spinal injury is ruled out.

essary. A symptomatic patient, however, requires careful scrutiny of his drug therapy. Beta-adrenergic blockers, verapamil, diazepam, sympatholytics, antihypertensives, and some antiarrhythmics have been implicated; symptoms may clear when these drugs are discontinued. Pacing is usually indicated in the patient with symptomatic bradycardia lacking a correctable cause.

MEDICAL CAUSES

● *Cardiac arrhythmias.* Depending on the type of arrhythmia and the patient's tolerance of it, bradycardia may be transient or sustained, benign or life threatening. Related findings include hypotension, palpitations, dizziness, weakness, syncope, and fatigue.

● *Cardiomyopathy.* Cardiomyopathy is a potentially life-threatening disorder that may cause transient or sustained bradycardia. Other findings include dizziness, syncope, edema, fatigue, jugular vein distention, orthopnea, dyspnea, and peripheral cyanosis.

● *Cervical spinal injury.* Bradycardia may be transient or sustained, depending on the severity of the injury. Its onset coincides with sympathetic denervation. Associated signs and symptoms include hypotension, decreased body temperature, slowed peristalsis, leg paralysis, and partial arm and respiratory muscle paralysis.

● *Hypothermia.* Bradycardia usually appears when the core temperature drops below 89.6° F (32° C). It's accompanied by shivering, peripheral cyanosis, muscle rigidity, bradypnea, and confusion leading to stupor.

● *Hypothyroidism.* Hypothyroidism causes severe bradycardia in addition to fatigue, constipation, unexplained weight gain, and sensitivity to cold. Related signs include cool, dry, thick skin; sparse, dry hair; facial swelling; periorbital edema; thick, brittle nails; and confusion leading to stupor.

● *Increased intracranial pressure (ICP).* Bradycardia occurs as a late sign of increased ICP along with rapid respiratory rate, elevated systolic pressure, decreased diastolic pressure, and widened pulse pressure. Associated signs and symptoms include persistent headache, projectile vomiting, decreased LOC, and fixed, unequal and, possibly, dilated pupils.

● *Myocardial infarction (MI).* Sinus bradycardia is the most common arrhythmia associated with an acute MI. Accompanying signs and symptoms of an MI include an aching, burning, or viselike pressure in the chest that may radiate to the jaw, shoulder, arm, back, or epigastric area; nausea and vomiting; cool, clammy, and pale or cyanotic skin; anxiety; and dyspnea. Blood pressure may be elevated or depressed. Auscultation may reveal abnormal heart sounds.

OTHER CAUSES
- *Diagnostic tests.* Cardiac catheterization and electrophysiologic studies can induce temporary bradycardia.
- *Drugs.* Beta-adrenergic blockers and some calcium channel blockers, cardiac glycosides, topical miotics (such as pilocarpine), protamine, quinidine and other antiarrhythmics, and sympatholytics may cause transient bradycardia. Failure to take thyroid replacements may also cause bradycardia.
- *Invasive treatments.* Suctioning can induce hypoxia and vagal stimulation, causing bradycardia. Cardiac surgery can cause edema or damage to conduction tissues, causing bradycardia.

NURSING CONSIDERATIONS
Continue to monitor the patient's vital signs frequently. Stay especially alert for changes in his cardiac rhythm, respiratory rate, and LOC.

Prepare the patient for laboratory tests, which can include complete blood count; cardiac enzyme, serum electrolyte, blood glucose, blood urea nitrogen, arterial blood gas, and blood drug levels; thyroid function tests; and a 12-lead electrocardiogram. If appropriate, prepare the patient for 24-hour Holter monitoring.

PATIENT TEACHING
Explain all tests and procedures to the patient and his family. Explain the need for cardiac monitoring and common alarms that may be heard. Teach the patient and his family how to take a radial pulse.

Bradypnea

Commonly preceding life-threatening apnea or respiratory arrest, bradypnea is a pattern of regular respirations with a rate of less than 10 breaths/minute. This sign results from neurologic and metabolic disorders and drug overdose, which depress the brain's respiratory control centers. (See *Understanding how the nervous system controls breathing,* page 64.)

Act now Depending on the degree of central nervous system (CNS) depression, the patient with severe bradypnea may require constant stimulation to breathe. If the patient seems excessively sleepy, try to arouse him by shaking and instructing him to breathe. Quickly take his vital signs. Assess his neurologic status by checking pupil size and reactions and by evaluating his level of consciousness (LOC) and his ability to move his extremities.

Place the patient on an apnea monitor, keep emergency airway equipment available, and be prepared to assist with intubation and mechanical ventilation if spontaneous respirations cease. To prevent aspiration, position the patient on his side or keep the head elevated 30 degrees higher than the rest of the body, and clear his airway with suction or finger sweeps, if necessary.

ASSESSMENT
History
Obtain a brief history from the patient or his family. Determine if the patient may be experiencing a drug overdose and, if so, try to determine what drugs were ingested, the amount, time, and by what route. Checking extremities for needle marks may indicate possible drug abuse.

After drug overdose is ruled out, determine any chronic illnesses, such as diabetes and renal failure. Check for a medical identification bracelet or an I.D. card that identifies an underlying condition. Also, ask whether the patient has a history of head trauma, brain tumor, neurologic infection, or stroke.

Physical examination
Perform a full respiratory and neurologic assessment, noting respiratory rate and pattern.

Pediatric pointers
Because respiratory rates are higher in children than in adults, bradypnea in children is defined according to age. (See *Respiratory rates in children,* page 65.)

Geriatric pointers
When drugs are prescribed for older patients, keep in mind that they are at higher risk for developing bradypnea secondary to drug toxicity because many of these patients take several drugs that can potentiate this effect and typically have other conditions that predispose them to it. Warn older patients about this potentially life-threatening complication.

UNDERSTANDING HOW THE NERVOUS SYSTEM CONTROLS BREATHING

Stimulation from external sources and from higher brain centers acts on respiratory centers in the pons and medulla. These centers, in turn, send impulses to various parts of the respiratory system to alter respiration patterns.

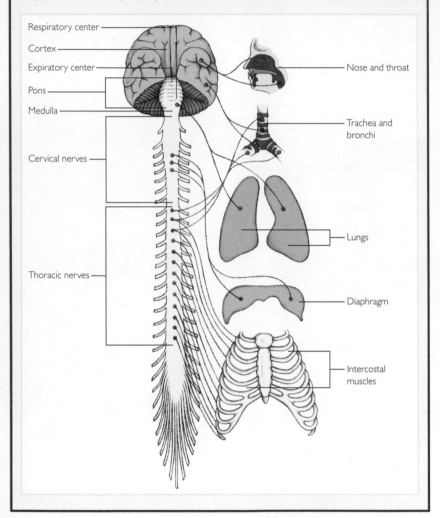

MEDICAL CAUSES

● *Diabetic ketoacidosis.* Bradypnea occurs late in patients with severe, uncontrolled diabetes. Patients with severe ketoacidosis may experience Kussmaul's respirations. Associated signs and symptoms include decreased LOC, fatigue, weakness, fruity breath odor, and oliguria.

● *Hepatic failure.* Occurring with end-stage hepatic failure, bradypnea may be accompanied by coma, hyperactive reflexes, asterixis, a positive Babinski's sign, fetor hepaticus, and other signs.

- *Increased intracranial pressure (ICP).* A late sign of increased ICP—a life-threatening condition—bradypnea is preceded by decreased LOC, deteriorating motor function, and fixed, dilated pupils. The triad of bradypnea, bradycardia, and hypertension is a classic sign of late medullary strangulation.
- *Renal failure.* Occurring with end-stage renal failure, bradypnea may be accompanied by convulsions, decreased LOC, GI bleeding, hypotension or hypertension, uremic frost, and diverse other signs.
- *Respiratory failure.* Bradypnea occurs with end-stage respiratory failure along with cyanosis, diminished breath sounds, tachycardia, mildly increased blood pressure, and decreased LOC.

OTHER CAUSES
- *Drugs.* Overdose with an opioid analgesic or, less commonly, a sedative, barbiturate, phenothiazine, or other CNS depressant can cause bradypnea. Use of any of these drugs with alcohol can also cause bradypnea.

NURSING CONSIDERATIONS
Because a patient with bradypnea may develop apnea, check his respiratory status frequently and be prepared to give ventilatory support if necessary. Don't leave the patient unattended, especially if his LOC is decreased. Obtain blood for arterial blood gas analysis, electrolyte studies, and a possible drug screen. Ready the patient for chest X-rays and possibly a computed tomography scan of the head.

Administer prescribed drugs and oxygen. Administration of I.V. nalozone, an opioid antagonist, may be required depending on the cause of the respiratory depression. Avoid giving the patient a CNS depressant because it can exacerbate bradypnea. Similarly, give oxygen judiciously to a patient with chronic carbon dioxide retention, which may occur with chronic obstructive pulmonary disease, because excess oxygen therapy can have a negative effect.

When dealing with slow breathing in hospitalized patients, always review all drugs and dosages given during the last 24 hours.

PATIENT TEACHING
Inform the patient who regularly takes an opioid—for example, a patient with advanced cancer or sickle cell anemia—that bradypnea is a serious complication. Teach him the early signs of toxicity, such as nausea and vomiting. It's also important to identify the patient who may be abusing these drugs.

Encourage the family to take a cardiopulmonary resuscitation class.

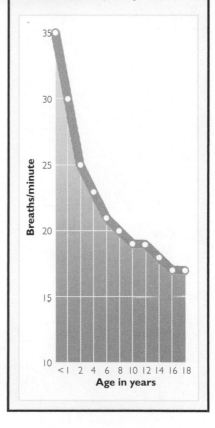

RESPIRATORY RATES IN CHILDREN

This graph shows normal respiratory rates in children, which are higher than normal rates in adults. Accordingly, bradypnea in children is defined by the age of the child.

Breaths/minute (y-axis: 10, 15, 20, 25, 30, 35)

Age in years (x-axis: <1, 2, 4, 6, 8, 10, 12, 14, 16, 18)

Breath odor, fecal

Fecal breath odor typically accompanies fecal vomiting associated with a long-standing intestinal obstruction or gastrojejunocolic fistula. It represents an important late diagnostic clue to a potentially life-threatening GI disorder because complete obstruction of any part of the bowel, if untreated, can cause death within hours from vascular collapse and shock.

When the obstructed or adynamic intestine attempts self-decompression by regurgitating its contents, vigorous peristaltic waves propel bowel contents backward into the stomach. When the stomach fills with intestinal fluid, further reverse peristalsis results in vomiting. The odor of feculent vomitus lingers in the mouth.

Fecal breath odor may also occur in patients with a nasogastric (NG) or intestinal tube. The odor is detected only while the underlying disorder persists and abates soon after its resolution.

Act now Because fecal breath odor signals a potentially life-threatening intestinal obstruction, you'll need to quickly evaluate your patient's condition. Monitor his vital signs, and stay alert for signs of shock, such as hypotension, tachycardia, narrowed pulse pressure, and cool, clammy skin. Determine if the patient has experienced nausea or has vomited. Find out the frequency of vomiting as well as the color, odor, amount, and consistency of the vomitus. Have an emesis basin nearby to collect and accurately measure the vomitus.

Anticipate emergency surgery to relieve an obstruction or repair a fistula, and withhold all food and fluids. Be prepared to insert an NG or intestinal tube for GI tract decompression. Insert a peripheral I.V. line for vascular access, or assist with central line insertion for large-bore access and central venous pressure monitoring. Obtain a blood sample and send it to the laboratory for complete blood count and electrolyte analysis because large fluid losses and shifts can produce electrolyte imbalances. Maintain adequate hydration and support circulatory status with additional fluids.

ASSESSMENT
History
Determine if the patient has had previous abdominal surgery because adhesions can develop and cause an obstruction. Ask if there has been a loss of appetite; abdominal pain with a description of its onset, duration, and intensity; and normal bowel habits, noting constipation, diarrhea, date of last bowel movement, color and consistency of stool, and leakage of stool.

Physical examination
Perform a full GI assessment. Auscultate for bowel sounds — hyperactive, high-pitched sounds may indicate *impending* bowel obstruction, whereas hypoactive or absent sounds occur *late* in obstruction and paralytic ileus. Inspect the abdomen, noting its contour and any surgical scars. Measure the patient's abdominal girth to provide baseline data for subsequent assessment of distention. Percuss for tympany, indicating a gas-filled bowel, and dullness, indicating fluid. Palpate for tenderness, distention, and rigidity.

Rectal and pelvic examinations should be performed. All patients with a suspected bowel obstruction should have a flat and upright abdominal X-ray; some will also need a chest X-ray, sigmoidoscopy, and barium enema.

Pediatric pointers
Carefully monitor the child's fluid and electrolyte status because dehydration can occur rapidly from persistent vomiting. The absence of tears and dry or parched mucous membranes are important clinical signs of dehydration.

Geriatric pointers
Elderly patients may require early surgical intervention for a bowel obstruction that doesn't respond to decompression because of the high risk of bowel infarct.

MEDICAL CAUSES
● *Distal small-bowel obstruction.* With late obstruction, nausea is present although vomiting may be delayed. Vomitus initially consists of gastric contents, then changes to bilious contents, followed by fecal contents with resultant fecal breath odor. Accompanying symptoms include achiness, malaise, drowsiness, and polydipsia. Bowel changes (ranging from diarrhea to constipation) are accompanied by abdominal distention, persistent epigastric or periumbilical colicky pain, and hyperactive bowel sounds and borborygmi. As the obstruction becomes complete, bowel sounds become hypoactive or

absent. Fever, hypotension, tachycardia, and rebound tenderness may indicate strangulation or perforation.

● **Gastrojejunocolic fistula.** With gastrojejunocolic fistula, symptoms may be variable and intermittent because of temporary plugging of the fistula. Fecal vomiting with resulting fecal breath odor may occur, but the most common chief complaint is diarrhea, accompanied by abdominal pain. Related GI findings include anorexia, weight loss, abdominal distention, and possibly marked malabsorption.

● **Large-bowel obstruction.** Vomiting is usually absent at first, but fecal vomiting with resultant fecal breath odor occurs as a late sign. Typically, symptoms develop more slowly than in small-bowel obstruction. Colicky abdominal pain appears suddenly, followed by continuous hypogastric pain. Marked abdominal distention and tenderness occur, and loops of large bowel may be visible through the abdominal wall. Although constipation develops, defecation may continue for up to 3 days after complete obstruction because of stool remaining in the bowel below the obstruction. Leakage of stool is common with partial obstruction.

NURSING CONSIDERATIONS

After an NG or intestinal tube has been inserted, keep the head of the bed elevated at least 30 degrees and turn the patient to facilitate passage of the intestinal tube through the GI tract. Don't tape the intestinal tube to the patient's face. Ensure tube patency by monitoring drainage and watching that suction devices function properly. Irrigate as required and monitor GI drainage. Provide meticulous oral care. Send serum samples to the laboratory for electrolyte analysis at least once per day. Prepare the patient for diagnostic tests, such as abdominal X-rays, barium enema, and proctoscopy.

PATIENT TEACHING

Explain all procedures and tests. Preoperative teaching is needed if the patient requires surgery. Encourage the patient to brush his teeth and gargle with a flavored mouthwash or half-strength hydrogen peroxide mixture to minimize offensive breath odor. Assure him that the fecal odor is temporary and will abate after treatment of the underlying cause.

Breath odor, fruity

Fruity breath odor results from respiratory elimination of excess acetone. This sign characteristically occurs with ketoacidosis — a potentially life-threatening condition that requires immediate treatment to prevent severe dehydration, irreversible coma, and death.

Ketoacidosis results from the excessive catabolism of fats for cellular energy in the absence of usable carbohydrates. This process begins when insulin levels are insufficient to transport glucose into the cells, as in diabetes mellitus, or when glucose is unavailable and hepatic glycogen stores are depleted, as in low-carbohydrate diets and malnutrition. Lacking glucose, the cells burn fat faster than enzymes can handle the ketones, the acidic end products. As a result, the ketones (acetone, beta-hydroxybutyric acid, and acetoacetic acid) accumulate in the blood and urine. To compensate for increased acidity, Kussmaul's respirations expel carbon dioxide with enough acetone to flavor the breath. Eventually, this compensatory mechanism fails, producing ketoacidosis.

Act now *When you detect fruity breath odor, check for Kussmaul's respirations and examine the patient's level of consciousness (LOC). Take his vital signs and check skin turgor. Stay alert for fruity breath odor that accompanies rapid, deep respirations; stupor; and poor skin turgor. Try to obtain a brief history, noting if the patient has type 1 diabetes mellitus, nutritional problems such as anorexia nervosa, and fad diets with little or no carbohydrates. Obtain venous and arterial blood samples for complete blood count and glucose, electrolyte, acetone, and arterial blood gas (ABG) levels. Also obtain a urine specimen to test for glucose and acetone. Administer I.V. fluids to maintain hydration and electrolyte balance; dehydration may be profound at the initial diagnosis. In the patient with diabetic ketoacidosis (DKA), give regular insulin to reduce blood glucose levels.*

If the patient is obtunded, you'll need to insert endotracheal and nasogastric (NG) tubes. Suction as needed. Insert an indwelling urinary catheter, and monitor intake and output. Insert central venous pressure and arterial lines to monitor the patient's fluid status and blood pressure. Place the patient on a cardiac monitor, monitor his vital signs and neurologic status, and draw blood hourly to check glucose, electrolyte, acetone, and ABG levels.

ASSESSMENT
History

If the patient isn't in severe distress, obtain a thorough history. Ask about the onset and duration of fruity breath odor. Find out about changes in breathing pattern. Ask about increased thirst, frequent urination, weight loss, fatigue, and abdominal pain. Ask the female patient if she has had candidal vaginitis or vaginal secretions with itching. If the patient has a history of diabetes mellitus, ask about stress, infections, and adherence to the treatment regimen. If you suspect that the patient has anorexia nervosa, obtain a dietary and weight history.

Physical examination

Perform a full neurologic examination, noting the patient's LOC. Assess him for signs of dehydration and shock. Assess the patient's GI system.

Pediatric pointers

Fruity breath odor in an infant or child usually stems from uncontrolled diabetes mellitus. Ketoacidosis develops rapidly in this age-group because of low glycogen reserves. As a result, prompt administration of insulin and correction of fluid and electrolyte imbalance are necessary to prevent shock and death.

Geriatric pointers

Elderly patients may have poor oral hygiene, increased dental caries, decreased salivary function with dryness, and poor dietary intake. In addition, many take multiple drugs. Consider all of these factors when evaluating an elderly patient with mouth odor.

MEDICAL CAUSES

● *Anorexia nervosa*. Severe weight loss associated with anorexia nervosa may produce fruity breath, usually with nausea, constipation, and cold intolerance as well as dental enamel erosion and scars or calluses in the dorsum of the hand, related to induced vomiting.
● *Ketoacidosis.* Fruity breath odor accompanies alcoholic ketoacidosis, which is usually seen in poorly nourished alcoholics with vomiting, abdominal pain, and only minimal food intake over several days. Kussmaul's respirations begin abruptly and accompany dehydration, abdominal pain and distention, and absent bowel sounds. Blood glucose levels are normal or slightly decreased.

With DKA, fruity breath odor commonly occurs as ketoacidosis develops over 1 to 2 days. Other findings include polydipsia, polyuria, nocturia, weak and rapid pulse, hunger, weight loss, weakness, fatigue, nausea, vomiting, and abdominal pain. Eventually, Kussmaul's respirations, orthostatic hypotension, dehydration, tachycardia, confusion, and stupor occur. Signs and symptoms may lead to coma.

Starvation ketoacidosis is a potentially life-threatening disorder that has a gradual onset. Besides fruity breath odor, typical findings include signs of cachexia and dehydration, decreased LOC, bradycardia, and a history of severely limited food intake (anorexia nervosa).

OTHER CAUSES

● *Drugs.* Any drug known to cause metabolic acidosis, such as nitroprusside and salicylates, can result in fruity breath odor.
● *Low-carbohydrate diets.* Low-carbohydrate diets, which encourage little or no carbohydrate intake, may cause ketoacidosis and the resulting fruity breath odor.

NURSING CONSIDERATIONS

Monitor fluid status. Perform neurologic and respiratory assessments. Provide emotional support for the patient and his family. Explain tests and treatments clearly. When the patient is more alert and his condition stabilizes, remove the NG tube and start him on an appropriate diet. Switch his insulin from the I.V. to the subcutaneous route.

PATIENT TEACHING

Teach the patient and provide appropriate referrals. For example, teach the patient with uncontrolled diabetes mellitus to recognize the signs of hyperglycemia and to wear a medical identification bracelet. Refer the patient with anorexia nervosa to a psychologist or a support group, and recognize the need for possible long-term follow-up.

Carpopedal spasm

Carpopedal spasm is the violent, painful contraction of the muscles in the hands and feet. (See *Recognizing carpopedal spasm,* page 70.) It's an important sign of tetany, a potentially life-threatening condition characterized by increased neuromuscular excitation and sustained muscle contraction. Carpopedal spasm is commonly associated with hypocalcemia.

Carpopedal spasm requires prompt evaluation and intervention. If the causative factor isn't identified and treated promptly, the patient can also develop laryngospasm, seizures, cardiac arrhythmias, and cardiac and respiratory arrest.

🐾 ***Act now*** *If you detect carpopedal spasm, quickly examine the patient for signs of respiratory distress (laryngospasm, stridor, loud crowing noises, cyanosis) or cardiac arrhythmias, which indicate hypocalcemia. Obtain blood specimens for electrolyte analysis (especially calcium) and perform an electrocardiogram. Connect the patient to a monitor to watch for the appearance of arrhythmias. Administer an I.V. calcium preparation and provide emergency respiratory and cardiac support, as ordered. If calcium infusion doesn't control the spasms, administer a sedative, as ordered.*

ASSESSMENT
History
Ask the patient about the onset and duration of the spasms and the degree of pain they produce. Assess him for related signs and symptoms of hypocalcemia, such as numbness and tingling of the hands and feet, other muscle cramps or spasms, and nausea, vomiting, and abdominal pain. Determine whether the patient's history includes previous neck surgery, calcium or magnesium deficiency, tetanus exposure, or hypoparathyroidism.

Ask the patient's family members whether they noticed changes in his behavior. Mental confusion — even personality changes — may occur with hypocalcemia.

Physical examination
Inspect the patient's skin and fingernails, noting dryness or scaling and ridged, brittle nails. Obtain his vital signs. Perform a head-to-toe assessment with a complete respiratory assessment. Check Chvostek's sign (tapping of the facial nerve, which results in facial nerve spasm).

Pediatric pointers
Idiopathic hypoparathyroidism is a common cause of hypocalcemia in children. Carefully monitor children with this condition because carpopedal spasm may herald the onset of epileptiform seizures or generalized tetany followed by prolonged tonic spasms.

Geriatric pointers
Always ask elderly patients about their immunization record. Suspect tetanus in anyone who comes into your facility with carpopedal spasm, difficulty swallowing, and seizures. Such patients may have incomplete immunizations or may not have had a recent booster shot. Always ask about a recent wound, no matter how inconsequential it may seem.

RECOGNIZING CARPOPEDAL SPASM

In the hand, carpopedal spasm involves adduction of the thumb over the palm, followed by flexion of the metacarpophalangeal joints, extension of the interphalangeal joints (fingers together), adduction of the hyperextended fingers, and flexion of the wrist and elbow joints. Similar effects occur in the joints of the feet.

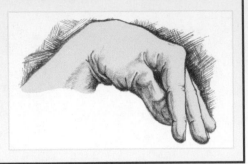

MEDICAL CAUSES

● *Hypocalcemia.* Carpopedal spasm is an early sign of hypocalcemia. It's usually accompanied by paresthesia of the fingers, toes, and perioral area; muscle weakness, twitching, and cramping; hyperreflexia; chorea; fatigue; and palpitations. Positive Chvostek's and Trousseau's signs can be elicited. Laryngospasm, stridor, and seizures may appear in severe hypocalcemia.

Chronic hypocalcemia may be accompanied by mental status changes; cramps; dry, scaly skin; brittle nails; and thin, patchy hair and eyebrows.

● *Tetanus.* Tetanus is an infectious disease that develops when *Clostridium tetani* enters a wound in a nonimmunized individual. The patient develops muscle spasms and painful seizures. Difficulty swallowing and low-grade fever are also present. If the patient isn't treated or treatment is delayed, the mortality rate is very high.

OTHER CAUSES

● *Medical treatments.* Multiple blood transfusions and parathyroidectomy may cause hypocalcemia, resulting in carpopedal spasm. Surgical procedures that impair calcium absorption, such as ileostomy formation and gastric resection with gastrojejunostomy, may also cause hypocalcemia.

NURSING CONSIDERATIONS

Prepare the patient for laboratory tests, such as complete blood count and serum calcium, phosphorus, and parathyroid hormone studies.

Carpopedal spasm can cause severe pain and anxiety; provide a quiet, dark environment to help the patient remain calm. Observe him closely for other signs of hypocalcemia until laboratory results rule out the disorder.

PATIENT TEACHING

Advise the patient to report numbness, tingling, or pain during hospitalization. If he has a disease that increases his risk of low serum calcium level, emphasize the need for dietary calcium replacement upon discharge from the hospital. Teach the patient the importance of receiving immunization against tetanus and keeping a vaccination record. If his immunization status is uncertain, he must receive the vaccine. Tetanus toxoid booster shots must be given every 10 years after the initial immunization.

Chest expansion, asymmetrical

Asymmetrical chest expansion is the uneven extension of portions of the chest wall during inspiration. During normal respiration, the thorax uniformly expands upward and outward, and then contracts downward and inward. When this process is disrupted, breathing becomes uncoordinated, resulting in asymmetrical chest expansion.

The onset may be sudden or gradual and may affect one or both sides of the chest wall. It may occur as delayed expiration (chest lag), abnormal movement during inspiration (for example, intercostal retractions,

Recognizing life-threatening causes of asymmetrical chest expansion

Asymmetrical chest expansion can result from several life-threatening disorders. Two common causes — bronchial obstruction and flail chest — produce distinctive chest wall movements that provide important clues about the underlying disorder.

With *bronchial obstruction*, only the unaffected portion of the chest wall expands during inspiration. Intercostal bulging during expiration may indicate that the air is trapped in the chest.

INSPIRATION

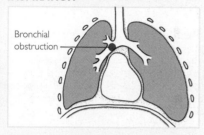

EXPIRATION

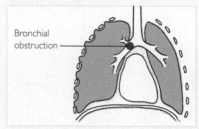

With *flail chest* — a disruption of the thorax due to multiple rib fractures — the unstable portion of the chest wall collapses inward at

inspiration and balloons outward at expiration.

INSPIRATION

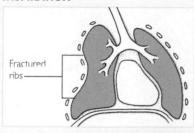

EXPIRATION

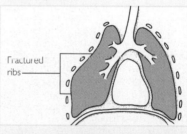

paradoxical movement, or chest-abdomen asynchrony), or unilateral absence of movement. Asymmetrical chest expansion usually results from pleural disorders, such as life-threatening hemothorax or tension pneumothorax. (See *Recognizing life-threatening causes of asymmetrical chest expansion.*) It can also result from a musculoskeletal or urologic disorder, airway obstruction, or trauma. Regardless of its underlying cause, asymmetrical chest expansion produces rapid and shallow or deep respirations that increase the work of breathing.

Act now *If you detect asymmetrical chest expansion, first consider traumatic injury to the patient's ribs or sternum, which can cause flail*

chest, a life-threatening emergency characterized by paradoxical chest movement. Quickly take the patient's vital signs and look for signs of acute respiratory distress — rapid and shallow respirations, tachycardia, and cyanosis. Provide pain management and pulmonary toilet. Don't tape or use sandbags to temporarily splint the unstable flair segment because these actions will impede chest expansion and decrease oxygenation and clearance of secretions.

Depending on the severity of respiratory distress, administer oxygen by nasal cannula, mask, or mechanical ventilator. Prepare the patient for emergency intubation, if indicated. Insert an I.V. line to allow fluid replacement and administration of pain medication.

Obtain a blood sample for arterial blood gas analysis, and connect the patient to a cardiac monitor.

Although asymmetrical chest expansion may result from hemothorax, tension pneumothorax, bronchial obstruction, and other life-threatening causes, it isn't a cardinal sign of these disorders. Because any form of asymmetrical chest expansion can compromise the patient's respiratory status, don't leave the patient unattended, and stay alert for signs of respiratory distress.

ASSESSMENT
History
Ask the patient whether he experiences dyspnea or pain during breathing. If he reports shortness of breath, ask whether it's constant or intermittent. If the patient reports that the pain worsens with inspiration or expiration, ask him if there are precipitating or aggravating factors or factors that alleviate the pain.

Ask the patient whether he has a history of pulmonary or systemic illness, such as frequent upper respiratory tract infections, asthma, tuberculosis, pneumonia, or cancer, or if he has had thoracic surgery. Any of these findings can produce asymmetrical chest expansion on the affected side. Ask about a history of blunt or penetrating chest trauma, which may have caused pulmonary injury. Ask the patient whether he may have inhaled toxic fumes or aspirated a toxic substance, perhaps at his place of employment.

Physical examination
Examine the posterior chest wall for areas of tenderness or deformity. To evaluate the extent of asymmetrical chest expansion, place your hands — fingers together and thumbs abducted toward the spine — flat on both sections of the lower posterior chest wall. Position your thumbs at the 10th rib, and grasp the lateral rib cage with your hands. As the patient inhales, note the uneven separation of your thumbs, and gauge the distance between them. Then repeat this technique on the upper posterior chest wall. Next, use the ulnar surface of your hand to palpate for vocal or tactile fremitus on both sides of the chest. To check for vocal fremitus, ask the patient to repeat "99" as you proceed. Note asymmetrical vibrations and areas of enhanced, diminished, or absent fremitus. Gently palpate the trachea for midline posi-

tioning. Then percuss and auscultate to detect air and fluid in the lungs and pleural spaces. Finally, auscultate all lung fields for normal and adventitious breath sounds. Examine the patient's anterior chest wall, using the same assessment techniques.

Alert *Be prepared for immediate intervention if your examination of the patient reveals deviation of the trachea, which typically indicates an acute problem. Prepare the patient for emergency intubation and possible mechanical ventilation. Plan for emergency X-rays or a computed tomography scan to identify the problem.*

Pediatric pointers
Children have a greater risk than adults of mainstem bronchi (especially left bronchus) intubation. However, because children's breath sounds are usually referred from one lung to the other because of the small size of the thoracic cage, use chest wall expansion as an indicator of correct tube position. Children also develop asymmetrical chest expansion, paradoxical breathing, and retractions with acute respiratory illnesses, such as bronchiolitis, asthma, and croup.

Congenital abnormalities, such as cerebral palsy and diaphragmatic hernia, can also cause asymmetrical chest expansion. With cerebral palsy, asymmetrical facial muscles usually accompany chest-abdomen asynchrony. With a life-threatening diaphragmatic hernia, asymmetrical expansion usually occurs on the left side of the chest.

Geriatric pointers
Asymmetrical chest expansion may be more difficult to identify in elderly patients due to the structural changes associated with aging.

MEDICAL CAUSES
● *Bronchial obstruction.* With bronchial obstruction, life-threatening loss of airway patency may occur gradually or suddenly. Typically, lack of chest movement indicates complete obstruction; chest lag signals partial obstruction. If air is trapped in the chest, you may detect intercostal bulging during expiration and hyperresonance on percussion. You may also note dyspnea, accessory muscle use, decreased or absent breath sounds, and suprasternal, substernal, or intercostal retractions.
● *Flail chest.* With flail chest — a life-threatening injury to the ribs or sternum — the unstable portion of the chest

wall collapses inward during inspiration and balloons outward during expiration (paradoxical movement). The patient may have ecchymoses, severe localized pain, or other signs of traumatic injury to the chest wall. He may also exhibit rapid, shallow respirations, tachycardia, and cyanosis.

● *Hemothorax.* Bleeding into the pleural space causes chest lag during inspiration in hemothorax, a life-threatening condition. Other findings include signs of traumatic chest injury, stabbing pain at the injury site, anxiety, dullness on percussion, tachypnea, tachycardia, and hypoxemia. If hypovolemia occurs, you'll note signs of shock, such as hypotension and a rapid, weak pulse.

● *Kyphoscoliosis.* Abnormal curvature of the thoracic spine in the anteroposterior direction (kyphosis) and the lateral direction (scoliosis) gradually compresses one lung and distends the other. This produces decreased chest wall movement on the compressed-lung side and expands the intercostal muscles during inspiration on the opposite side. It can also produce ineffective coughing, dyspnea, back pain, and fatigue.

● *Myasthenia gravis.* Progressive loss of ventilatory muscle function produces asynchrony of the chest and abdomen during inspiration ("abdominal paradox"), which can lead to the onset of acute respiratory distress. Typically, the patient's shallow respirations and increased muscle weakness cause severe dyspnea, tachypnea and, possibly, apnea.

● *Phrenic nerve dysfunction.* With phrenic nerve dysfunction, the paralyzed hemidiaphragm fails to contract downward, causing asynchrony of the thorax and upper abdomen on the affected side during inspiration ("abdominal paradox"). Its onset may be sudden, as in trauma, or gradual, as in infection or spinal cord disease. If the patient has underlying pulmonary dysfunction that contributes to hyperventilation, his inability to breathe deeply or to cough effectively may cause atelectasis of the affected lung.

● *Pleural effusion.* Chest lag at end-inspiration occurs gradually in pleural effusion — a life-threatening accumulation of fluid, blood, or pus in the pleural space. Usually, some combination of dyspnea, tachypnea, and tachycardia precedes chest lag; the patient may also have pleuritic pain that worsens with coughing or deep breathing. The area of the effusion is delineated by dullness on percussion and by egophony, bronchophony, whispered pectoriloquy, decreased or absent breath sounds, and decreased tactile fremitus. Fever appears if infection causes the effusion.

● *Pneumonia.* Depending on whether fluid consolidation in the lungs develops unilaterally or bilaterally, asymmetrical chest expansion occurs as inspiratory chest lag or as chest-abdomen asynchrony. The patient typically has fever, chills, tachycardia, tachypnea, and dyspnea along with crackles, rhonchi, and chest pain that worsens during deep breathing. He may also be fatigued and anorexic and have a productive cough with green or yellow mucus or rust-colored sputum.

● *Pneumothorax.* Entrapment of air in the pleural space can cause chest lag at end-inspiration. Pneumothorax is a life-threatening condition that also causes sudden, stabbing chest pain that may radiate to the arms, face, back, or abdomen and dyspnea unrelated to the chest pain's severity. Other findings include tachypnea, decreased tactile fremitus, tympany on percussion, decreased or absent breath sounds over the trapped air, tachycardia, restlessness, and anxiety.

With tension pneumothorax, the same signs and symptoms occur as in pneumothorax, but they're much more severe. A tension pneumothorax rapidly compresses the heart and great vessels, causing cyanosis, hypotension, tachycardia, restlessness, and anxiety. The patient may also develop subcutaneous crepitation of the upper trunk, neck, and face and mediastinal and tracheal deviation away from the affected side. You may auscultate a crunching sound over the precordium with each heartbeat; this indicates pneumomediastinum.

● *Poliomyelitis.* With poliomyelitis — a rare disorder — paralysis of the chest wall muscles and diaphragm produces chest-abdomen asynchrony ("abdominal paradox"), fever, muscle pain, and weakness. Other findings include decreased reflex response in the affected muscles and impaired swallowing and speaking.

● *Pulmonary embolism.* Pulmonary embolism is an acute, life-threatening disorder that causes chest lag; sudden, stabbing chest pain; and tachycardia. The patient usually has severe dyspnea, blood-tinged sputum, pleural friction rub, and acute anxiety.

OTHER CAUSES

● *Medical treatments.* Asymmetrical chest expansion can result from pneumonectomy and surgical removal of several ribs. Chest lag or the absence of chest movement may also result from intubation of a mainstem bronchus, a serious complication typically due to incorrect insertion of an endotracheal tube or tube movement while it's in the trachea.

NURSING CONSIDERATIONS

Because asymmetrical chest expansion increases the work of breathing, supplemental oxygen is usually given during acute events. Assess the patient's respiratory status frequently.

If the patient is intubated, regularly auscultate breath sounds in the lung peripheries to ensure equal ventilation. Maintain the ventilator settings and alarms, as ordered.

PATIENT TEACHING

Explain all procedures and tests, especially if the patient is intubated. Teach the patient and his family early signs of infection.

Chest pain

Disorders that affect thoracic or abdominal organs—the heart, pleurae, lungs, esophagus, rib cage, gallbladder, pancreas, or stomach—are typical causes of chest pain. It can also result from a musculoskeletal or hematologic disorder, anxiety, and drug therapy. Chest pain is an important indicator of several acute and life-threatening cardiopulmonary and GI disorders.

The onset of chest pain can be sudden or gradual, and its cause may initially be difficult to ascertain. Chest pain can radiate to the arms, neck, jaw, or back. It can be steady or intermittent, mild or acute. And it can range in character from a sharp shooting sensation to a feeling of heaviness, fullness, or even indigestion. Chest pain can be provoked or aggravated by stress, anxiety, exertion, deep breathing, or eating certain foods.

Act now *Sudden, severe chest pain requires prompt evaluation and treatment because it may herald a life-threatening disorder. (See* Managing severe chest pain, *pages 76 and 77.) Standardized algorithms are used to address the*

treatment regimen of the patient with chest pain. Determine the time of onset and whether it was sudden or gradual. Ask the patient about precipitating, alleviating, or aggravating factors, if the pain radiates, and associated signs and symptoms. Ask him to rate the pain using a standardized pain rating scale. Obtain a 12-lead electrocardiogram (ECG) and a blood sample for serum testing. Administer oxygen through a nasal cannula. Place the patient on a cardiac monitor and establish I.V. access. If test results indicate an acute myocardial infarction (MI), the patient will require emergency percutaneous coronary intervention or fibrinolytic therapy. Be prepared to administer emergency care if the patient experiences cardiopulmonary arrest.

ASSESSMENT
History

Ask the patient to rate the pain using a standardized pain rating scale. Is the pain a dull, aching, pressurelike sensation, or sharp, stabbing, and knifelike? Is it constant or intermittent? If it's intermittent, ask how long an episode lasts. Ask him about precipitating, aggravating, or alleviating factors. Review the patient's history for cardiac or pulmonary disease, chest trauma, intestinal disease, or sickle cell anemia. Ask about medications he's taking, if any, including recent dosage or schedule changes.

Alert *Chest pain in perimenopausal women may be difficult to diagnose because it may present atypically. Fatigue, nausea, dyspnea, and shoulder or neck pain are symptoms more likely to signal an MI in women than in men.*

Physical examination

Take the patient's vital signs, noting tachypnea, fever, tachycardia, oxygen saturation, paradoxical pulse, and hypertension or hypotension. Check for jugular vein distention and peripheral edema. Observe the patient's breathing pattern, and inspect his chest for asymmetrical expansion. Auscultate his lungs for pleural friction rub, crackles, rhonchi, wheezing, or diminished or absent breath sounds. Next, auscultate for murmurs, clicks, gallops, or pericardial friction rub. Palpate for lifts, heaves, thrills, gallops, tactile fremitus, and abdominal masses or tenderness.

Pediatric pointers

Even a child old enough to talk may have difficulty describing chest pain, so stay alert for nonverbal clues, such as restlessness, facial grimaces, or holding the painful area. Ask the child to point to the painful area and then to where the pain goes (to find out if it's radiating). Assess the severity of the pain by asking the parents whether the pain interferes with the child's normal activities and behavior. Remember, a child may complain of chest pain in an attempt to get attention or to avoid attending school.

Geriatric pointers

Remember to carefully evaluate chest pain in elderly patients, who have a higher risk of developing life-threatening conditions, such as an MI, angina, and aortic dissection.

MEDICAL CAUSES

See *Chest pain: Causes and associated findings,* pages 78 to 81.

● *Angina pectoris.* With angina pectoris, the patient may experience a feeling of tightness or pressure in the chest that he describes as pain or a sensation of indigestion or expansion. The pain usually occurs in the retrosternal region over a palm-sized or larger area. It may radiate to the neck, jaw, and arms — classically, to the inner aspect of the left arm. Angina tends to begin gradually, build to its maximum, and then slowly subside. Provoked by exertion, emotional stress, or a heavy meal, the pain typically lasts 2 to 10 minutes, usually no longer than 20 minutes. Associated findings include dyspnea, nausea, vomiting, tachycardia, dizziness, diaphoresis, belching, and palpitations. You may hear an atrial gallop (a fourth heart sound) or murmur during an anginal episode.

With Prinzmetal's angina, caused by vasospasm of coronary vessels, chest pain typically occurs when the patient is at rest — or it may awaken him. It may be accompanied by shortness of breath, nausea, vomiting, dizziness, and palpitations. During an attack, you may hear an atrial gallop.

● *Anthrax (inhalation).* Anthrax is an acute infectious disease that's caused by the gram-positive, spore-forming bacterium *Bacillus anthracis.* Although the disease most commonly occurs in wild and domestic grazing animals, such as cattle, sheep, and goats, the spores can live in the soil for many years. The disease can occur in humans exposed to infected animals, tissue from infected animals, or biological warfare. Most natural cases occur in agricultural regions worldwide, and it may occur in cutaneous, inhalation, and GI forms.

Inhalation anthrax is caused by inhalation of aerosolized spores. Initial signs and symptoms are flulike and include fever, chills, weakness, cough, and chest pain. The disease generally occurs in two stages with a period of recovery after the initial signs and symptoms. The second stage develops abruptly with rapid deterioration marked by fever, dyspnea, stridor, and hypotension, generally leading to death within 24 hours. Radiologic findings include mediastinitis and symmetric mediastinal widening.

● *Anxiety.* Acute anxiety — or, more commonly, *panic attacks* — can produce intermittent, sharp, stabbing pain, commonly located behind the left breast. This pain isn't related to exertion and lasts only a few seconds, but the patient may experience a precordial ache or a sensation of heaviness that lasts for hours or days. Associated signs and symptoms include precordial tenderness, palpitations, fatigue, headache, insomnia, breathlessness, nausea, vomiting, diarrhea, and tremors. Panic attacks may be associated with agoraphobia — fear of leaving home or being in open places with other people.

● *Aortic aneurysm (dissecting).* The chest pain associated with aortic aneurysm — a life-threatening disorder — usually begins suddenly and is most severe at its onset. The patient describes an excruciating tearing, ripping, stabbing pain in his chest and neck that radiates to his upper back, abdomen, and lower back. He may exhibit abdominal tenderness, a palpable abdominal mass, tachycardia, murmurs, syncope, blindness, loss of consciousness, weakness or transient paralysis of the arms or legs, a systolic bruit, systemic hypotension, asymmetrical brachial pulses, lower blood pressure in the legs than in the arms, and weak or absent femoral or pedal pulses. His skin is pale, cool, diaphoretic, and mottled below the waist. Capillary refill time is increased in the toes, and palpation reveals decreased pulsation in one or both carotid arteries.

● *Asthma.* In a life-threatening asthma attack, diffuse and painful chest tightness arises suddenly along with a dry cough and mild wheezing, which progress to a productive cough, audible wheezing, and severe dyspnea. Related respiratory findings include rhonchi, crackles, prolonged expirations, intercostal and supraclavicular retractions on inspiration, accessory muscle use, flaring nostrils, and tachypnea. The patient may

Managing severe chest pain

Sudden, severe chest pain may result from any one of several life-threatening disorders. Your evaluation and interventions will vary, depending on the pain's location and character. The flowchart below will help you establish priorities for managing this emergency successfully.

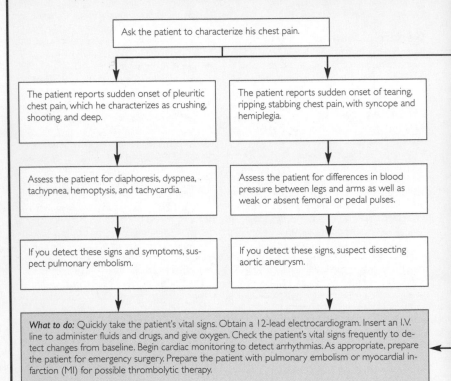

Ask the patient to characterize his chest pain.

The patient reports sudden onset of pleuritic chest pain, which he characterizes as crushing, shooting, and deep.

The patient reports sudden onset of tearing, ripping, stabbing chest pain, with syncope and hemiplegia.

Assess the patient for diaphoresis, dyspnea, tachypnea, hemoptysis, and tachycardia.

Assess the patient for differences in blood pressure between legs and arms as well as weak or absent femoral or pedal pulses.

If you detect these signs and symptoms, suspect pulmonary embolism.

If you detect these signs, suspect dissecting aortic aneurysm.

What to do: Quickly take the patient's vital signs. Obtain a 12-lead electrocardiogram. Insert an I.V. line to administer fluids and drugs, and give oxygen. Check the patient's vital signs frequently to detect changes from baseline. Begin cardiac monitoring to detect arrhythmias. As appropriate, prepare the patient for emergency surgery. Prepare the patient with pulmonary embolism or myocardial infarction (MI) for possible thrombolytic therapy.

also experience anxiety, tachycardia, diaphoresis, flushing, and cyanosis.

• *Blastomycosis.* Besides pleuritic chest pain, blastomycosis initially produces signs and symptoms that mimic those of viral upper respiratory tract infection: a dry, hacking, or productive cough (and sometimes hemoptysis), fever, chills, anorexia, weight loss, fatigue, night sweats, and malaise.

• *Bronchitis.* In its acute form, bronchitis produces burning chest pain or a sensation of substernal tightness. It also produces a cough, initially dry but later productive, that worsens the chest pain. Other findings include low-grade fever, chills, sore throat, tachycardia, muscle and back pain, rhonchi,

crackles, and wheezing. Severe bronchitis causes a fever of 101° to 102° F (38.3° to 38.9° C) and possible bronchospasm with worsening wheezing and increased coughing.

• *Cardiomyopathy.* With hypertrophic cardiomyopathy, angina-like chest pain may occur with dyspnea, cough, dizziness, syncope, gallops, murmurs, and bradycardia associated with tachycardia.

• *Cholecystitis.* Cholecystitis typically produces abrupt epigastric or right upper quadrant pain, which may be sharp or intensely aching. Steady or intermittent pain may radiate to the back or right shoulder. Commonly associated findings include nausea, vomiting,

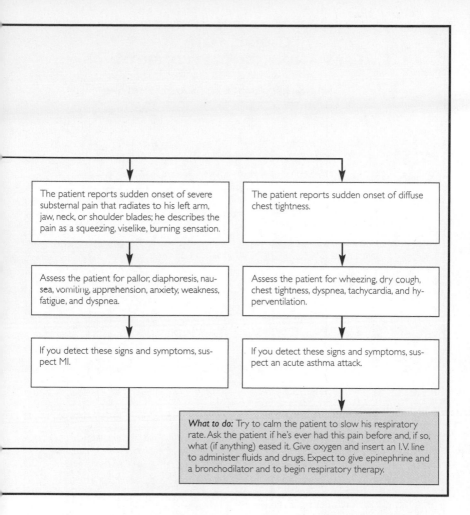

The patient reports sudden onset of severe substernal pain that radiates to his left arm, jaw, neck, or shoulder blades; he describes the pain as a squeezing, viselike, burning sensation.

↓

Assess the patient for pallor, diaphoresis, nausea, vomiting, apprehension, anxiety, weakness, fatigue, and dyspnea.

↓

If you detect these signs and symptoms, suspect MI.

The patient reports sudden onset of diffuse chest tightness.

↓

Assess the patient for wheezing, dry cough, chest tightness, dyspnea, tachycardia, and hyperventilation.

↓

If you detect these signs and symptoms, suspect an acute asthma attack.

↓

What to do: Try to calm the patient to slow his respiratory rate. Ask the patient if he's ever had this pain before and, if so, what (if anything) eased it. Give oxygen and insert an I.V. line to administer fluids and drugs. Expect to give epinephrine and a bronchodilator and to begin respiratory therapy.

fever, diaphoresis, and chills. Palpation of the right upper quadrant may reveal an abdominal mass, rigidity, distention, or tenderness. Murphy's sign — inspiratory arrest elicited when the examiner palpates the right upper quadrant as the patient takes a deep breath — may also occur.

● *Coccidioidomycosis.* With coccidioidomycosis, pleuritic chest pain occurs with a dry or slightly productive cough. Other effects include fever, rhonchi, wheezing, occasional chills, sore throat, backache, headache, malaise, marked weakness, anorexia, and macular rash.

● *Costochondritis.* Pain and tenderness occur at the costochondral junctions, especially at the second costicartilage. The pain usually can be elicited by palpating the inflamed joint.

● *Distention of colon's splenic flexure.* Central chest pain may radiate to the left arm in patients with distention of colon's splenic flexure. The pain may be relieved by defecation or passage of flatus.

● *Esophageal spasm.* With esophageal spasm, substernal chest pain may last up to an hour and can radiate to the neck, jaw, arms, or back. It commonly mimics angina — a squeezing or dull sensation. Associated signs and symptoms include dysphagia for solid foods, bradycardia, and nodal rhythm.

CHEST PAIN:
CAUSES AND ASSOCIATED FINDINGS

MAJOR ASSOCIATED SIGNS AND SYMPTOMS

COMMON CAUSES	Abdominal mass	Abdominal tenderness	Atrial gallop	Breath sounds, decreased	Cough	Crackles	Cyanosis	Diaphoresis	Dizziness	Dyspnea	Fever	Hemoptysis	Murmur
Angina pectoris			●					●	●	●			●
Anthrax (inhalation)					●					●	●		
Anxiety									●	●			
Aortic aneurysm (dissecting)	●	●						●					●
Asthma					●	●	●	●		●			
Blastomycosis					●			●			●		
Bronchitis					●	●					●		
Cardiomyopathy			●		●				●	●			●
Cholecystitis	●	●						●			●		
Coccidioidomycosis					●						●		
Costochondritis										●			
Distention of colon's splenic flexure		●						●					
Esophageal spasm										●			
Herpes zoster (shingles)											●		
Hiatal hernia													
Interstitial lung disease					●	●	●			●			
Legionnaires' disease						●		●		●	●	●	
Lung abscess				●	●	●		●		●	●	●	
Lung cancer						●				●	●	●	
Mediastinitis											●		
Mitral valve prolapse									●	●			●

	Nausea and vomiting	Pericardial friction rub	Pleural friction rub	Skin mottling	Syncope	Tachycardia	Tachypnea	Wheezing
	•					•		
	•					•	•	
				•	•	•		
						•	•	•
						•		•
					•			
	•							
								•
	•							
	•							
	•					•	•	
				•				
								•
						•		

(continued)

- *Herpes zoster (shingles).* The pain of pre-eruptive herpes zoster may mimic that of an MI. Initially, the pain is characteristically sharp, shooting, and unilateral. About 4 to 5 days after its onset, small, red, nodular lesions erupt on the painful areas—usually the thorax, arms, and legs—and chest pain becomes burning. Associated findings include fever, malaise, pruritus, and paresthesia or hyperesthesia of the affected areas.

- *Hiatal hernia.* Typically, hiatal hernia produces an angina-like sternal burning (heartburn), ache, or pressure that may radiate to the left shoulder and arm. The discomfort commonly occurs after a meal when the patient bends over or lies down. Other findings include a bitter taste and pain while eating or drinking, especially hot drinks and spicy foods.

- *Interstitial lung disease.* As interstitial lung disease advances, the patient may experience pleuritic chest pain along with progressive dyspnea, cellophane-type crackles, nonproductive cough, fatigue, weight loss, decreased exercise tolerance, clubbing, and cyanosis.

- *Legionnaires' disease.* Legionnaires' disease produces pleuritic chest pain, in addition to malaise, headache and, possibly, diarrhea, anorexia, diffuse myalgia, and general weakness. Within 12 to 24 hours, the patient develops a sudden high fever, chills, and a nonproductive cough that progresses to mucoid and then to mucopurulent sputum, possibly with hemoptysis. Patients may also experience flushed skin, mild diaphoresis, prostration, nausea and vomiting, mild temporary amnesia, confusion, dyspnea, crackles, tachypnea, and tachycardia.

- *Lung abscess.* Pleuritic chest pain develops insidiously in lung abscess along with a pleural friction rub and cough that raises copious amounts of purulent, foul-smelling, blood-tinged sputum. The affected side is dull on percussion, and decreased breath sounds and crackles may be heard. The patient also displays diaphoresis, anorexia, weight loss, fever, chills, fatigue, weakness, dyspnea, and clubbing.

- *Lung cancer.* The chest pain associated with lung cancer is commonly described as an intermittent aching felt deep within the chest. If the tumor metastasizes to the ribs or vertebrae, the pain becomes localized, continuous, and gnawing. Associated findings include cough (sometimes bloody), wheez-

CHEST PAIN: CAUSES AND ASSOCIATED FINDINGS
(continued)

MAJOR ASSOCIATED SIGNS AND SYMPTOMS

COMMON CAUSES	Abdominal mass	Abdominal tenderness	Atrial gallop	Breath sounds, decreased	Cough	Crackles	Cyanosis	Diaphoresis	Dizziness	Dyspnea	Fever	Hemoptysis	Murmur
Muscle strain				●									
Myocardial infarction			●			●		●		●	●		●
Nocardiosis				●	●			●			●		
Pancreatitis		●				●					●		
Peptic ulcer		●											
Pericarditis										●	●		
Plague				●						●	●	●	●
Pleurisy				●		●	●			●	●		
Pneumonia				●	●	●	●	●		●	●		
Pneumothorax				●	●		●			●			
Psittacosis											●		
Pulmonary actinomycosis					●					●	●	●	
Pulmonary embolism (primary)					●	●	●	●		●	●	●	
Pulmonary hypertension (primary)					●					●			●
Q fever											●		
Rib fracture					●					●			
Sickle cell crisis		●								●	●		
Thoracic outlet syndrome										●			
Tuberculosis					●					●	●	●	
Tularemia				●						●	●		

ing, dyspnea, fatigue, anorexia, weight loss, and fever.

● *Mediastinitis.* Mediastinitis produces severe retrosternal chest pain that radiates to the epigastrium, back, or shoulder and may

Nausea and vomiting	Pericardial friction rub	Pleural friction rub	Skin mottling	Syncope	Tachycardia	Tachypnea	Wheezing
•							
•			•		•		
•							
	•				•		
						•	
		•				•	
					•	•	
						•	
		•			•	•	•
				•			
•							

- **Mitral valve prolapse.** Most patients with mitral valve prolapse are asymptomatic, but some may experience sharp, stabbing precordial chest pain or precordial ache. The pain can last for seconds or hours and occasionally mimics the pain of ischemic heart disease. The characteristic sign of mitral prolapse is a midsystolic click followed by a systolic murmur at the apex. The patient may experience cardiac awareness, migraine headache, dizziness, weakness, episodic severe fatigue, dyspnea, tachycardia, mood swings, and palpitations.
- **Muscle strain.** Strained chest, arm, or shoulder muscles may cause a superficial and continuous ache or "pulling" sensation in the chest. Lifting, pulling, or pushing heavy objects may aggravate this discomfort. With acute muscle strain, the patient may experience fatigue, weakness, and rapid swelling of the affected area.
- **Myocardial infarction (MI).** The chest pain during an MI lasts from 15 minutes to hours. Typically, crushing substernal pain, unrelieved by rest or nitroglycerin, may radiate to the patient's left arm, jaw, neck, or shoulder blades. Other findings include pallor, clammy skin, dyspnea, diaphoresis, nausea, vomiting, anxiety, restlessness, a feeling of impending doom, hypotension or hypertension, atrial gallop, murmurs, and crackles.
- **Nocardiosis.** Nocardiosis causes pleuritic chest pain with a cough that produces thick, tenacious, purulent or mucopurulent, and possibly blood-tinged sputum. Nocardiosis may also cause fever, night sweats, anorexia, malaise, weight loss, and diminished or absent breath sounds.
- **Pancreatitis.** In the acute form, pancreatitis usually causes intense pain in the epigastric area that radiates to the back and worsens when the patient is in a supine position. Nausea, vomiting, fever, abdominal tenderness and rigidity, diminished bowel sounds, and crackles at the lung bases may also occur. A patient with severe pancreatitis may be extremely restless and have mottled skin, tachycardia, and cold, sweaty extremities. Fulminant pancreatitis causes massive hemorrhage, resulting in shock and coma.
- **Peptic ulcer.** With peptic ulcer, sharp and burning pain usually arises in the epigastric region. This pain characteristically arises hours after food intake, commonly during the night. It lasts longer than angina-like pain and is relieved by food or an antacid. Other

worsen with breathing, coughing, or sneezing. Its accompanying signs and symptoms include chills, fever, and dysphagia.

findings include nausea, vomiting (sometimes with blood), melena, and epigastric tenderness.

- **Pericarditis.** Pericarditis produces precordial or retrosternal pain aggravated by deep breathing, coughing, position changes, and occasionally by swallowing. The pain is commonly sharp or cutting and radiates to the shoulder and neck. Associated signs and symptoms include pericardial friction rub, fever, tachycardia, and dyspnea. Pericarditis usually follows a viral illness, but several other causes should be considered.

- **Plague.** Plague is an acute bacterial infection caused by *Yersinia pestis*. It's one of the most virulent infections and, if untreated, one of the most potentially lethal diseases known. Most cases are sporadic, but the potential for epidemic spread still exists. Clinical forms include bubonic (the most common), septicemic, and pneumonic plagues. The bubonic form is transmitted to man when bitten by infected fleas. Signs and symptoms include fever, chills, and swollen, inflamed, and tender lymph nodes near the site of the fleabite. Septicemic plague develops as a fulminant illness generally with the bubonic form. The pneumonic form may be contracted from person-to-person through direct contact via the respiratory system or through biological warfare from aerosolization and inhalation of the organism. The onset is usually sudden with chills, fever, headache, and myalgia. Pulmonary signs and symptoms include productive cough, chest pain, tachypnea, dyspnea, hemoptysis, increasing respiratory distress, and cardiopulmonary insufficiency.

- **Pleurisy.** The chest pain of pleurisy arises abruptly and reaches maximum intensity within a few hours. The pain is sharp, even knifelike, usually unilateral, and located in the lower and lateral aspects of the chest. Deep breathing, coughing, or thoracic movement characteristically aggravates it. Auscultation over the painful area may reveal decreased breath sounds, inspiratory crackles, and a pleural friction rub. Dyspnea, rapid, shallow breathing, cyanosis, fever, and fatigue may also occur.

- **Pneumonia.** Pneumonia produces pleuritic chest pain that increases with deep inspiration and is accompanied by shaking chills and fever. The patient has a dry cough that later becomes productive. Other signs and symptoms include crackles, rhonchi, tachy-cardia, tachypnea, myalgia, fatigue, headache, dyspnea, abdominal pain, anorexia, cyanosis, decreased breath sounds, and diaphoresis.

- **Pneumothorax.** Spontaneous pneumothorax, a life-threatening disorder, causes sudden sharp chest pain that's severe, typically unilateral, and rarely localized; it increases with chest movement. When the pain is centrally located and radiates to the neck, it may mimic that of an MI. After the pain's onset, dyspnea and cyanosis progressively worsen. Breath sounds are decreased or absent on the affected side with hyperresonance or tympany, subcutaneous crepitation, and decreased vocal fremitus. Asymmetrical chest expansion, accessory muscle use, nonproductive cough, tachypnea, tachycardia, anxiety, and restlessness also occur.

- **Psittacosis.** Psittacosis may produce pleuritic chest pain on rare occasions. It typically begins abruptly with chills, fever, headache, myalgia, epistaxis, and prostration.

- **Pulmonary actinomycosis.** Pulmonary actinomycosis causes pleuritic chest pain with a cough that's initially dry but later produces purulent sputum. The patient may also display hemoptysis, fever, weight loss, fatigue, weakness, dyspnea, and night sweats. Multiple sinuses may extend through the chest wall and drain externally.

- **Pulmonary embolism.** Pulmonary embolism produces chest pain or a choking sensation. Typically, the patient first experiences sudden dyspnea with intense angina-like or pleuritic pain aggravated by deep breathing and thoracic movement. Other findings include tachycardia, tachypnea, cough (nonproductive or producing blood-tinged sputum), low-grade fever, restlessness, diaphoresis, crackles, pleural friction rub, diffuse wheezing, dullness on percussion, signs of circulatory collapse (weak, rapid pulse; hypotension), paradoxical pulse, signs of cerebral ischemia (transient unconsciousness, coma, seizures), signs of hypoxia (restlessness) and, particularly in the elderly, hemiplegia and other focal neurologic deficits. Less common signs include massive hemoptysis, chest splinting, and leg edema. A patient with a large embolus may have cyanosis and jugular vein distention.

- **Pulmonary hypertension (primary).** Angina-like pain develops late in patients with pulmonary hypertension, usually on exertion. The precordial pain may radiate to the neck but doesn't characteristically radiate to the arms. Typical accompanying signs and symptoms include exertional dyspnea, fatigue, syncope, weakness, cough, and hemoptysis.

● *Q fever.* Q fever is a Rickettsial disease caused by *Coxiella burnetii.* The primary source of human infection results from exposure to infected animals. Cattle, sheep, and goats are most likely to carry the organism. Human infection results from exposure to contaminated milk, urine, feces, or other fluids from infected animals. Infection may also result from inhalation of contaminated barnyard dust. *C. burnetii* is highly infectious and is considered a possible airborne agent for biological warfare. Signs and symptoms include fever, chills, severe headache, malaise, chest pain, nausea, vomiting, and diarrhea. The fever may last for up to 2 weeks. In severe cases, the patient may develop hepatitis or pneumonia.

● *Rib fracture.* The chest pain due to fractured ribs is usually sharp, severe, and aggravated by inspiration, coughing, or pressure on the affected area. Besides shallow, splinted respirations, dyspnea, and cough, the patient experiences tenderness and slight edema at the fracture site.

● *Sickle cell crisis.* Chest pain associated with sickle cell crisis typically has a bizarre distribution. It may start as a vague pain, commonly located in the back, hands, or feet. As the pain worsens, it becomes generalized or localized to the abdomen or chest, causing severe pleuritic pain. The presence of chest pain and difficulty breathing requires prompt intervention. The patient may also have abdominal distention and rigidity, dyspnea, fever, and jaundice.

● *Thoracic outlet syndrome.* Commonly causing paresthesia along the ulnar distribution of the arm, thoracic outlet syndrome can be confused with angina, especially when it affects the left arm. The patient usually experiences angina-like pain after lifting his arms above his head, working with his hands above his shoulders, or lifting a weight. The pain disappears as soon as he lowers his arms. Other signs and symptoms include pale skin and a difference in blood pressure between both arms.

● *Tuberculosis.* In a patient with tuberculosis, pleuritic chest pain and fine crackles occur after coughing. Associated signs and symptoms include night sweats, anorexia, weight loss, fever, malaise, dyspnea, easy fatigability, mild to severe productive cough, occasional hemoptysis, dullness on percussion, increased tactile fremitus, and amphoric breath sounds.

● *Tularemia.* Also known as *rabbit fever,* tularemia is caused by the gram-negative, nonspore forming bacterium *Francisella tularensis.* It's typically a rural disease found in wild animals, water, and moist soil. It's transmitted to humans through the bite of an infected insect or tick, handling infected animal carcasses, drinking contaminated water, or inhaling the bacteria. It's considered a possible airborne agent for biological warfare. Signs and symptoms following inhalation of the organism include the abrupt onset of fever, chills, headache, generalized myalgia, nonproductive cough, dyspnea, pleuritic chest pain, and empyema.

OTHER CAUSES

● *Chinese restaurant syndrome.* Chinese restaurant syndrome, which stems from a reaction to excessive ingestion of monosodium glutamate (a common additive in Chinese foods), is a benign condition that mimics the signs of an acute MI. The patient may complain of retrosternal burning, ache, or pressure; a burning sensation over his arms, legs, and face; a sensation of facial pressure; headache, shortness of breath; and tachycardia.

● *Drugs.* Abrupt withdrawal of a beta-adrenergic blocker can cause rebound angina if the patient has coronary heart disease—especially if he has received high doses for a prolonged period.

NURSING CONSIDERATIONS

As needed, prepare the patient for cardiopulmonary studies, such as an ECG and a lung scan. Perform a venipuncture to collect a serum sample for cardiac enzyme and other studies. Assess the cardiovascular system frequently. Interpret changes in cardiac rhythm. Be prepared for emergency procedures.

Keep in mind that a patient with chest pain may deny his discomfort, so stress the importance of reporting symptoms to allow adjustment of his treatment.

PATIENT TEACHING

Explain the purpose and procedure of each diagnostic test to the patient to help alleviate his anxiety. Prepare him if cardiac catheterization or fibrinolytic therapy is indicated. Explain the purpose of any prescribed drugs and make sure that he understands the dosage, schedule, and possible adverse effects. Teach the patient with coronary artery disease to recognize the typical features of cardiac ischemia as well as symptoms that require prompt medical attention. Teach him how to administer sublingual nitroglycerin and advise him to seek medical attention if the pain lasts more than 20 minutes, fails to respond to nitroglycerin, or has a different pattern than the usual angina.

Cheyne-Stokes respirations

Cheyne-Stokes respirations are characterized by a waxing and waning period of hyperpnea that alternates with a shorter period of apnea. It's the most common pattern of periodic breathing. This pattern can occur normally in patients with heart or lung disease. It usually indicates increased intracranial pressure (ICP) from a deep cerebral or brain stem lesion or a metabolic disturbance in the brain.

Cheyne-Stokes respirations may indicate a major change in the patient's condition — usually for the worse. For example, in a patient who has had head trauma or brain surgery, Cheyne-Stokes respirations may signal increasing ICP. Cheyne-Stokes respirations can occur normally in patients who live at high altitudes.

Act now *If Cheyne-Stokes respirations occur in a patient with a history of head trauma, recent brain surgery, or another brain insult, quickly take his vital signs. Keep his head elevated 30 degrees, and perform a rapid neurologic examination to obtain baseline data. Reevaluate the patient's neurologic status frequently. If ICP continues to rise, you'll detect changes in the patient's level of consciousness (LOC), pupillary reactions, and ability to move his extremities. ICP monitoring is indicated.*

Time the periods of hyperpnea and apnea for 3 to 4 minutes to evaluate respirations and to obtain baseline data. Stay alert for prolonged periods of apnea. Frequently check blood pressure; also check skin color to detect signs of hypoxemia. Maintain air-way patency and administer oxygen as needed. If the patient's condition worsens, endotracheal intubation is necessary.

ASSESSMENT
History
Determine the onset of abnormal respirations as well as associated changes in the patient's LOC or mentation. Ask about a history of head trauma. Also, ask the patient about drug use, including prescription, over-the-counter, and illicit drugs. Obtain a complete medication history.

Physical examination
Obtain the patient's vital signs. Perform complete neurologic and respiratory assessments. Stay alert for signs of hypoxemia — peripheral or central cyanosis, dyspnea, or changes in mentation.

Pediatric pointers
Cheyne-Stokes respirations rarely occur in children, except during late heart failure.

Geriatric pointers
Cheyne-Stokes respirations can occur normally in elderly patients during sleep.

MEDICAL CAUSES
● *Adams-Stokes attacks.* Cheyne-Stokes respirations may follow an Adams-Stokes attack — a syncopal episode associated with atrioventricular block. The patient is hypotensive, with a heart rate of 20 to 50 beats/minute. He may also appear pale, shaking, and confused.
● *Heart failure.* With left-sided heart failure, Cheyne-Stokes respirations may occur with exertional dyspnea and orthopnea. Related findings include fatigue, weakness, tachycardia, tachypnea, and crackles. The patient may also have a cough, generally nonproductive but occasionally producing clear or blood-tinged sputum.
● *Hypertensive encephalopathy.* With hypertensive encephalopathy — a life-threatening disorder — severe hypertension precedes Cheyne-Stokes respirations. The patient's LOC is decreased, and he may experience vomiting, seizures, severe headaches, vision disturbances (including transient blindness), or transient paralysis.
● *Increased ICP.* As ICP rises, Cheyne-Stokes is the first irregular respiratory pattern to occur. It's preceded by a decreased LOC

and accompanied by hypertension, headache, vomiting, impaired or unequal motor movement, and vision disturbances (blurring, diplopia, photophobia, and pupillary changes). In late stages of increased ICP, bradycardia and widened pulse pressure occur.

● *Renal failure.* With end-stage chronic renal failure, Cheyne-Stokes respirations may occur in addition to bleeding gums, oral lesions, ammonia breath odor, and marked changes in every body system.

OTHER CAUSES
● *Drugs.* Large doses of an opioid, hypnotic, or barbiturate can precipitate Cheyne-Stokes respirations.

NURSING CONSIDERATIONS
Obtain the patient's vital signs, noting respiratory rate and pattern. When evaluating Cheyne-Stokes respirations, be careful not to mistake periods of hypoventilation or decreased tidal volume for complete apnea.

PATIENT TEACHING
Advise the patient and his family that sleep apnea differs from Cheyne-Stokes respirations in both causes and methods of treatment.

Cough, barking

Resonant, brassy, and harsh, a barking cough is part of a complex of signs and symptoms that characterize croup syndrome, a group of pediatric disorders marked by varying degrees of respiratory distress. Croup syndrome is most common in boys. It's most prevalent in the fall and may recur.

A barking cough indicates edema of the larynx and surrounding tissue. Because children's airways are smaller in diameter than those of adults, edema can rapidly lead to airway occlusion — a life-threatening emergency.

Act now When a child presents with barking cough, quickly evaluate his respiratory status. Then take his vital signs. Stay particularly alert for tachycardia and signs of hypoxemia. Also, check for a decreased level of consciousness. Try to determine if the child has been playing with a small object that he may have aspirated.

Check for cyanosis in the lips and nail beds. Observe the patient for sternal or intercostal retractions or nasal flaring. Next, note the depth and rate of respirations, which become increasingly shallow as respiratory distress increases. Observe the child's body position. Is he sitting up, leaning forward, and struggling to breathe? Observe his activity level and facial expression. As respiratory distress increases from airway edema, the child will become restless and have a frightened, wide-eyed expression. As air hunger continues, the child will become lethargic and difficult to arouse.

If the child shows signs of severe respiratory distress, try to calm him, maintain airway patency, and provide oxygen. Endotracheal intubation or a tracheotomy may be necessary.

ASSESSMENT
History
Determine when the barking cough began and other associated signs and symptoms. Determine when the child first appeared to be ill and ask if there have been previous episodes of croup syndrome.

Spasmodic croup and epiglottiditis typically occur in the middle of the night. The child with spasmodic croup has no fever, but the child with epiglottiditis has a high fever of sudden onset. An upper respiratory tract infection typically is followed by laryngotracheobronchitis.

Physical examination
Assess the respiratory system, noting rate and pattern of respirations. Assess the patient for signs of hypoxia. Stay alert for signs of airway obstruction (nasal flaring, sternal retraction, stridor).

Pediatric pointers
In children, respiratory status and airway maintenance can disintegrate rapidly. In children who are too young to speak, close observation is of utmost importance.

Geriatric pointers
A barking cough is generally not seen in elderly patients.

MEDICAL CAUSES
● *Aspiration of foreign body.* Partial obstruction of the upper airway first produces sudden hoarseness, and then a barking cough and inspiratory stridor. Other effects of this life-threatening condition include gagging,

tachycardia, dyspnea, decreased breath sounds, wheezing and, possibly, cyanosis.

● *Epiglottiditis.* Epiglottiditis is a life-threatening disorder that has become less common since the use of influenza vaccines. It occurs nocturnally, heralded by a barking cough and high fever. The child is hoarse, dysphagic, dyspneic, and restless and appears extremely ill and panicky. The cough may progress to severe respiratory distress with sternal and intercostal retractions, nasal flaring, cyanosis, and tachycardia. The child will struggle to get sufficient air as epiglottic edema increases. Epiglottiditis is a true medical emergency.

● *Laryngotracheobronchitis (acute).* Also known as *viral croup,* laryngotracheobronchitis is most common in children between ages 9 and 18 months and usually occurs in the fall and early winter. It initially produces low to moderate fever, runny nose, poor appetite, and infrequent cough. When the infection descends into the laryngotracheal area, barking cough, hoarseness, and inspiratory stridor occur.

As respiratory distress progresses, substernal and intercostal retractions occur along with tachycardia and shallow, rapid respirations. Sleeping in a dry room worsens these signs. The patient becomes restless, irritable, pale, and cyanotic.

● *Spasmodic croup.* Acute spasmodic croup usually occurs during sleep with the abrupt onset of a barking cough that awakens the child. Typically, he doesn't have fever but may be hoarse, restless, and dyspneic. As his respiratory distress worsens, the child may exhibit sternal and intercostal retractions, nasal flaring, tachycardia, cyanosis, and an anxious, frantic appearance. The signs usually subside within a few hours, but attacks tend to recur.

NURSING CONSIDERATIONS

Don't attempt to inspect the throat of a child with a barking cough unless intubation equipment is available. If the child isn't in severe respiratory distress, a lateral neck X-ray may be done to visualize epiglottal edema; a negative X-ray doesn't completely rule out epiglottal edema. A chest X-ray may also be done to rule out lower respiratory tract infection. Depending on the child's age and degree of respiratory distress, oxygen may be administered. Rapid-acting epinephrine (racemic epinephrine) and a steroid should be considered.

Be sure to observe the child frequently, and monitor the oxygen level if used. Provide the child with periods of rest with minimal interruptions. Maintain a calm, quiet environment and offer reassurance. Encourage the parents to stay with the child to help alleviate stress.

PATIENT TEACHING

Teach the parents how to evaluate and treat recurrent episodes of croup syndrome. For example, creating steam by running hot water in a sink or shower and sitting with the child in the closed bathroom may help relieve subsequent attacks. The child may also benefit from being brought outdoors (properly dressed) to breathe cold night air.

Cough, productive

Productive coughing is the body's mechanism for clearing airway passages of accumulated secretions that normal mucociliary action doesn't remove. It's a sudden, forceful, noisy expulsion of air (from the lungs) that contains sputum, blood, or both. The sputum's color, consistency, and odor provide important clues about the patient's condition. A productive cough can occur as a single cough or as paroxysmal coughing, and it can be voluntarily induced, although it's usually a reflexive response to stimulation of the airway mucosa.

Usually due to a cardiovascular or respiratory disorder, productive coughing commonly results from an acute or chronic infection that causes inflammation, edema, and increased mucus production in the airways. However, this sign can also result from acquired immunodeficiency syndrome. Inhalation of antigenic or irritating substances or foreign bodies also can cause a productive cough. In fact, the most common cause of chronic productive coughing is cigarette smoking, which produces mucoid sputum ranging in color from clear to yellow to brown. (See *Productive cough: Causes and associated findings.*)

Many patients minimize or overlook a chronic productive cough or accept it as normal. Such patients may not seek medical attention until an associated problem — such as dyspnea, hemoptysis, chest pain,

PRODUCTIVE COUGH:
CAUSES AND ASSOCIATED FINDINGS

MAJOR ASSOCIATED SIGNS AND SYMPTOMS

COMMON CAUSES	Chest pain	Crackles	Cyanosis	Decreased breath sounds	Dyspnea	Fatigue	Fever	Rhonchi	Sore throat	Tachycardia	Tachypnea	Weight loss	Wheezing
Actinomycosis	●				●	●	●					●	
Aspiration pneumonitis		●	●		●	●	●	●		●	●		●
Asthma (acute)	●	●	●		●			●		●	●		●
Bronchiectasis		●			●	●	●	●				●	●
Bronchitis (chronic)		●	●		●			●			●		●
Chemical pneumonitis		●			●		●	●			●		●
Common cold						●	●		●				
Legionnaires' disease	●	●			●	●	●			●	●		
Lung abscess (ruptured)	●	●			●	●	●					●	
Lung cancer	●				●	●	●					●	●
Nocardiosis	●			●	●		●					●	
North American blastomycosis	●					●	●					●	
Plague	●				●		●				●		
Pneumonia (bacterial)	●	●	●		●	●	●	●		●	●		
Pneumonia (mycoplasma)	●	●				●	●		●				
Psittacosis	●	●					●				●		
Pulmonary coccidioidomycosis	●						●	●	●				●
Pulmonary edema		●	●		●	●	●			●	●		
Pulmonary embolism	●	●	●		●					●	●		●
Pulmonary emphysema				●	●			●			●	●	
Pulmonary tuberculosis	●	●			●	●	●	●				●	
Silicosis		●			●	●				●	●		
Tracheobronchitis	●	●					●	●	●				●

weight loss, or recurrent respiratory tract infections — develops. The delay can have serious consequences because productive coughing is associated with several life-threatening disorders and can also herald airway occlusion from excessive secretions.

Act now   *A patient with a productive cough can develop acute respiratory distress from thick or excessive secretions, bronchospasm, or fatigue, so examine him before you take his history. Take his vital signs and check the rate, depth, and rhythm of respirations. Keep his airway patent, and be prepared to provide supplemental oxygen if he becomes restless or confused or if his respirations become shallow, irregular, rapid, or slow. Look for stridor, wheezing, choking, or gurgling. Stay alert for nasal flaring and cyanosis.*

ASSESSMENT
History
Determine the onset of the cough and amount of daily sputum production. (The normal tracheobronchial tree can produce up to 3 oz [89 ml] of sputum per day.) Determine the time of day that the most sputum is produced and relationship of food to sputum production. Also ask about the color, odor, and consistency of the sputum. Blood-tinged or rust-colored sputum may result from trauma due to coughing or from an underlying condition, such as a pulmonary infection or tumor. Foul-smelling sputum may result from an anaerobic infection, such as bronchitis or lung abscess.

Determine cough characteristics. A hacking cough results from laryngeal involvement, whereas a "brassy" cough indicates major airway involvement. Ask the patient about cigarette, drug, and alcohol use and if there has been weight or appetite changes. Find out if he has a history of asthma, allergies, or respiratory disorders, and ask about recent illnesses, surgery, or trauma. Determine a medication history, including over-the-counter medications. Ask the patient if his work involves chemicals or respiratory irritants.

Physical examination
Examine the patient's mouth and nose for congestion, drainage, or inflammation. Note breath odor: Halitosis can be a sign of pulmonary infection. Inspect his neck for jugular vein distention, and palpate for tenderness and masses or enlarged lymph nodes. Observe his chest for accessory muscle use, re-

tractions, and uneven chest expansion, and percuss for dullness, tympany, or flatness. Finally, auscultate for pleural friction rub and abnormal breath sounds — rhonchi, crackles, or wheezes.

Pediatric pointers
Because his airway is narrow, a child with a productive cough can quickly develop airway occlusion and respiratory distress from thick or excessive secretions. Causes of a productive cough in children include asthma, bronchiectasis, bronchitis, acute bronchiolitis, cystic fibrosis, and pertussis.

When caring for a child with a productive cough, administer expectorants, but don't expect to give a cough suppressant. To soothe inflamed mucous membranes and prevent drying of secretions, provide humidified air or oxygen. Remember, high humidity can induce bronchospasm in a hyperactive child or produce overhydration in an infant.

Geriatric pointers
Always ask elderly patients about a productive cough, which may indicate a serious acute or chronic illness.

MEDICAL CAUSES
● *Actinomycosis.* Actinomycosis begins with a cough that produces purulent sputum. Fever, weight loss, fatigue, weakness, dyspnea, night sweats, pleuritic chest pain, and hemoptysis may also occur.
● *Aspiration pneumonitis.* Aspiration pneumonitis causes coughing that produces pink, frothy, and possibly purulent sputum. The patient also has marked dyspnea, fever, tachypnea, tachycardia, wheezing, and cyanosis.
● *Asthma (acute).* A severe asthma attack, which can be life-threatening, may produce mucoid, tenacious sputum and mucus plugs. Such an attack typically starts with a dry cough and mild wheezing, and then progresses to severe dyspnea, audible wheezing, chest tightness, and a productive cough. Other findings include apprehension, prolonged expirations, intercostal and supraclavicular retraction on inspiration, accessory muscle use, rhonchi, crackles, flaring nostrils, tachypnea, tachycardia, diaphoresis, and flushing or cyanosis. Attacks commonly occur at night or during sleep.
● *Bronchiectasis.* The chronic cough of bronchiectasis produces copious, mucopuru-

lent sputum that has characteristic layering (top, frothy; middle, clear; bottom, dense with purulent particles). The patient has halitosis; his sputum may smell foul or sickeningly sweet. Other characteristic findings include hemoptysis, persistent coarse crackles over the affected lung area, occasional wheezing, rhonchi, exertional dyspnea, weight loss, fatigue, malaise, weakness, recurrent fever, and late-stage finger clubbing.

● *Bronchitis (chronic).* Bronchitis causes a cough that may be nonproductive initially. Eventually, however, it produces mucoid sputum that becomes purulent. Secondary infection can also cause mucopurulent sputum, which may be blood-tinged and foul-smelling. The coughing, which may be paroxysmal during exercise, usually occurs when the patient is recumbent or rises from sleep.

The patient also exhibits prolonged expirations, increased use of accessory muscles for breathing, barrel chest, tachypnea, cyanosis, wheezing, exertional dyspnea, scattered rhonchi, coarse crackles (which can be precipitated by coughing), and late-stage clubbing.

● *Chemical pneumonitis.* Chemical pneumonitis causes a cough with purulent sputum. It can also cause dyspnea, wheezing, orthopnea, fever, malaise, and crackles; mucous membrane irritation of the conjunctivae, throat, and nose; laryngitis; or rhinitis. Signs and symptoms may increase for 24 to 48 hours after exposure, and then resolve; if severe, however, they may recur 2 to 5 weeks later.

● *Common cold.* When the common cold causes productive coughing, the sputum is mucoid or mucopurulent. Early indications of the common cold include a dry, hacking cough, sneezing, headache, malaise, fatigue, rhinorrhea (watery to tenacious mucopurulent secretions), nasal congestion, sore throat, myalgia, and arthralgia.

● *Legionnaires' disease.* Legionnaires' disease causes a cough that produces scant mucoid, nonpurulent, and possibly blood-streaked sputum. Prodromal signs and symptoms typically include malaise, fatigue, weakness, anorexia, diffuse myalgia and, possibly, diarrhea. Then, within 48 hours, the patient develops a dry cough and sudden high fever with chills. Many patients also have pleuritic chest pain, headache, tachypnea, tachycardia, nausea, vomiting, dyspnea,

crackles, mild temporary amnesia, disorientation, confusion, flushing, mild diaphoresis, and prostration.

● *Lung abscess (ruptured).* The cardinal sign of ruptured lung abscess is coughing that produces copious amounts of purulent, foul-smelling, and possibly blood-tinged sputum. A ruptured abscess can also cause diaphoresis, anorexia, clubbing, weight loss, weakness, fatigue, fever with chills, dyspnea, headache, malaise, pleuritic chest pain, halitosis, inspiratory crackles, and tubular or amphoric breath sounds. The patient's chest is dull on percussion on the affected side.

● *Lung cancer.* One of the earliest signs of bronchogenic carcinoma is a chronic cough that produces small amounts of purulent (or mucopurulent), blood-streaked sputum. In a patient with bronchoalveolar cancer, however, coughing produces large amounts of frothy sputum. Other signs and symptoms include dyspnea, anorexia, fatigue, weight loss, chest pain, fever, diaphoresis, wheezing, and clubbing.

● *Nocardiosis.* Nocardiosis causes a productive cough with purulent, thick, tenacious, and possibly blood-tinged sputum and fever that may last several months. Other findings include night sweats, pleuritic pain, anorexia, malaise, fatigue, weight loss, and diminished or absent breath sounds. The patient's chest is dull on percussion.

● *North American blastomycosis.* With North American blastomycosis—a chronic disorder—coughing is dry and hacking, or produces bloody or purulent sputum. Other findings include pleuritic chest pain, fever, chills, anorexia, weight loss, malaise, fatigue, night sweats, cutaneous lesions (small, painless, nonpruritic macules or papules), and prostration.

● *Plague.* Plague is an acute bacterial infection caused by *Yersinia pestis.* It's one of the most virulent infections and, if untreated, one of the most potentially lethal diseases known. Most cases are sporadic, but the potential for epidemic spread still exists. Clinical forms include bubonic (the most common), septicemic, and pneumonic plagues. The bubonic form is transmitted to man when bitten by infected fleas. Signs and symptoms include fever, chills, and swollen, inflamed, and tender lymph nodes near the site of the fleabite. Septicemic plague develops as a fulminant illness generally with the bubonic form. The pneumonic form may be contracted from person-to-person through direct contact via the respiratory system or through biological warfare from aerosolization and inhalation of the organism. The onset is usually sudden with chills, fever, headache, and myalgia. Pulmonary signs and symptoms include productive cough, chest pain, tachypnea, dyspnea, hemoptysis, increasing respiratory distress, and cardiopulmonary insufficiency.

● *Pneumonia.* Bacterial pneumonia initially produces a dry cough that becomes productive. Associated signs and symptoms develop suddenly and include shaking chills, high fever, myalgia, headache, pleuritic chest pain that increases with chest movement, tachypnea, tachycardia, dyspnea, cyanosis, diaphoresis, decreased breath sounds, fine crackles, and rhonchi.

Mycoplasma pneumonia may cause a cough that produces scant blood-flecked sputum. Most common, however, is a nonproductive cough that starts 2 to 3 days after the onset of malaise, headache, fever, and sore throat. Paroxysmal coughing causes substernal chest pain. Patients may develop crackles but generally don't appear seriously ill.

● *Psittacosis.* As psittacosis progresses, the characteristic hacking cough, nonproductive at first, may later produce a small amount of mucoid, blood-streaked sputum. The infection may begin abruptly, with chills, fever, headache, myalgia, and prostration. Other signs and symptoms include tachypnea, fine crackles, chest pain (rare), epistaxis, photophobia, abdominal distention and tenderness, nausea, vomiting, and a faint macular rash. Severe infection may produce stupor, delirium, and coma.

● *Pulmonary coccidioidomycosis.* Pulmonary coccidioidomycosis causes a nonproductive or slightly productive cough with fever, occasional chills, pleuritic chest pain, sore throat, headache, backache, malaise, marked weakness, anorexia, hemoptysis, and an itchy macular rash. Rhonchi and wheezing may be heard. The disease may spread to other areas, causing arthralgia, swelling of the knees and ankles, and erythema nodosum or erythema multiforme.

● *Pulmonary edema.* When severe, pulmonary edema — a life-threatening disorder — causes a cough that produces frothy, bloody sputum. Early signs and symptoms include exertional dyspnea as well as paroxysmal nocturnal dyspnea, followed by orthopnea. Coughing may be nonproductive initially. Other signs and symptoms include fever, fatigue, tachycardia, tachypnea, dependent crackles, and ventricular gallop. As the patient's respirations become increasingly rapid and labored, he develops more diffuse crackles and productive cough, worsening tachycardia and, possibly, arrhythmias. The patient's skin becomes cold, clammy, and cyanotic, his blood pressure falls, and his pulse becomes thready.

● *Pulmonary embolism.* Pulmonary embolism is a life-threatening disorder that causes a cough that may be nonproductive or may produce blood-tinged sputum. Usually, the first symptom of pulmonary embolism is severe dyspnea, which may be accompanied by angina or pleuritic chest pain. The patient experiences marked anxiety, low-grade fever, tachycardia, tachypnea, and diaphoresis. Less-common signs include massive hemoptysis, chest splinting, leg edema and, with a large embolus, cyanosis, syncope, and jugular vein distention. The patient may also have pleural friction rub, diffuse wheezing, crackles, chest dullness on percussion, decreased breath sounds, and signs of circulatory collapse.

● *Pulmonary emphysema.* Pulmonary emphysema causes a chronic productive cough with scant, mucoid, translucent, grayish white sputum that can become mucopurulent. The patient is thin and has the characteristic "pink puffer" appearance with weight loss, increased accessory muscle use, tachypnea, grunting expirations through pursed lips, diminished breath sounds, exertional dyspnea, rhonchi, barrel chest, and anorexia. Clubbing is a late sign.

● *Pulmonary tuberculosis.* Pulmonary tuberculosis causes a mild to severe productive cough along with some combination of hemoptysis, malaise, dyspnea, and pleuritic chest pain. Sputum may be scant and mucoid or copious and purulent. Typically, the patient experiences night sweats, easy fatigability, and weight loss. His breath sounds are amphoric. He may have chest dullness on percussion and, after coughing, increased tactile fremitus with crackles.

● *Silicosis.* A productive cough with mucopurulent sputum is the earliest sign of silicosis. The patient also has exertional dyspnea, tachypnea, weight loss, fatigue, general weakness, and recurrent respiratory infections. Auscultation reveals end-inspiratory, fine crackles at the lung bases.

● *Tracheobronchitis.* Inflammation initially causes a nonproductive cough that later — following the onset of chills, sore throat, slight fever, muscle and back pain, and sub-sternal tightness — becomes productive as secretions increase. Sputum is mucoid, mu-copurulent, or purulent. The patient typically has rhonchi and wheezes; he may also develop crackles. Severe tracheobronchitis may cause a fever of 101° to 102° F (38.3° to 38.9° C) and bronchospasm.

OTHER CAUSES

● *Diagnostic tests.* Bronchoscopy and pulmonary function tests may increase productive coughing.

● *Drugs.* Expectorants, of course, increase productive coughing. These include ammonium chloride, calcium iodide, guaifenesin, iodinated glycerol, potassium iodide, and terpin hydrate.

● *Respiratory therapy.* Intermittent positive-pressure breathing, nebulizer therapy, and incentive spirometry can help loosen secretions and cause or increase productive coughing.

NURSING CONSIDERATIONS

Obtain the patient's vital signs and note signs of infection. Assess the respiratory system frequently, noting signs of respiratory distress. Avoid taking measures to suppress a productive cough because retention of sputum may interfere with alveolar aeration or impair pulmonary resistance to infection. Expect to give a mucolytic and an expectorant, and increase the patient's intake of oral fluids to thin his secretions and increase their flow. In addition, you may give a bronchodilator to relieve bronchospasms and open airways. An antibiotic may be ordered to treat underlying infection.

Humidify the air around the patient; this will relieve mucous membrane inflammation and also help loosen dried secretions. Provide pulmonary physiotherapy, such as postural drainage with vibration and percussion, to loosen secretions. Aerosol therapy may be necessary.

Provide the patient with uninterrupted rest periods. If bed rest is ordered, change the position often to promote the drainage of secretions.

Prepare the patient for diagnostic tests, such as chest X-ray, bronchoscopy, lung scan, and pulmonary function tests. Collect sputum samples for culture and sensitivity testing.

PATIENT TEACHING

Encourage the patient not to smoke because doing so can aggravate his condition. Explain that quitting even after decades of use is helpful. Teach the patient how to breathe deeply, to cough effectively and, if appropriate, to splint his incision when he coughs. Teach the patient and his family how to use chest percussion to loosen secretions.

Tell the patient to cover his mouth and nose with a tissue when he coughs and to dispose of contaminated tissues properly, to protect himself and others from the cough and secretions. Be sure to provide a container for tissues and sputum.

Crackles

A common finding in patients with certain cardiovascular and pulmonary disorders, crackles are nonmusical clicking or rattling noises heard during auscultation of breath sounds. Crackles, sometimes called *rales* or *crepitus*, usually occur during inspiration and recur constantly from one respiratory cycle to the next. They're classified as unilateral or bilateral, moist or dry. Crackles are characterized by pitch, loudness, location, persistence, and occurrence during the respiratory cycle.

Crackles indicate abnormal movement of air through fluid-filled airways. They can be irregularly dispersed, as in pneumonia, or localized, as in bronchiectasis. (A few basilar crackles can be heard in normal lungs after prolonged shallow breathing. These normal crackles clear with a few deep breaths.) Usually, crackles indicate the degree of an underlying illness. When crackles result from a generalized disorder, they usually occur in the less distended and more dependent areas of the lungs such as the lung bases when the patient is standing. Crackles due to air passing through inflammatory exudate may not be audible if the involved portion of the lung isn't being ventilated because of shallow respirations. (See *How crackles occur*, page 92.)

HOW CRACKLES OCCUR

Crackles occur when air passes through fluid-filled airways, causing collapsed alveoli to pop open as the airway pressure equalizes. They can also occur when membranes lining the chest cavity and lungs become inflamed. The illustrations below show a normal alveolus and two pathologic alveolar changes that cause crackles.

Normal alveolus

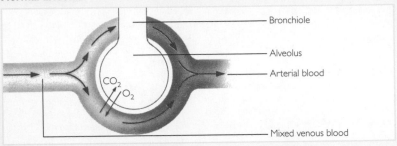

- Bronchiole
- Alveolus
- Arterial blood
- Mixed venous blood

Alveolus in pulmonary edema

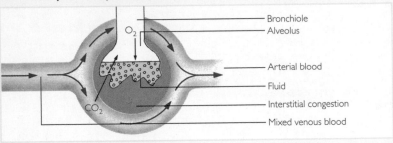

- Bronchiole
- Alveolus
- Arterial blood
- Fluid
- Interstitial congestion
- Mixed venous blood

Alveolus in inflammation

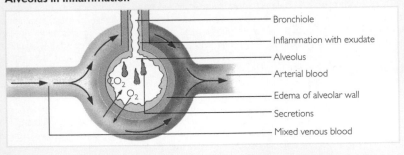

- Bronchiole
- Inflammation with exudate
- Alveolus
- Arterial blood
- Edema of alveolar wall
- Secretions
- Mixed venous blood

Act now *If you detect crackles after auscultating the patient's lungs and visible shortness of breath without significant exertion, quickly take the patient's vital signs and examine him for signs of respiratory distress or airway obstruction. Check for increased accessory muscle use and chest wall motion, retractions, stridor, or nasal flaring. Provide supplemental oxygen. Endotracheal intubation may be necessary.*

ASSESSMENT
History

Determine the onset of cough and if it's constant or intermittent. Determine what the cough sounds like and whether there are associated signs and symptoms. If the cough is productive, determine the sputum's consistency, amount, odor, and color.

If there's pain, determine its onset, radiation, location, and precipitating, alleviating, and aggravating factors. Determine any underlying cancer or known respiratory or cardiovascular problem. Ask about recent surgery, trauma, or illness. Ask about a smoking or alcohol history. Obtain a medication history, including over-the-counter medications. Check about associated symptoms, such as recent weight loss, anorexia, nausea, vomiting, fatigue, weakness, vertigo, and syncope.

Physical examination

Examine the patient's nose and mouth for signs of infection, such as inflammation or increased secretions. Note his breath odor: Halitosis could indicate pulmonary infection. Check his neck for masses, tenderness, swelling, lymphadenopathy, or venous distention.

Inspect the patient's chest for abnormal configuration or uneven expansion. Percuss for dullness, tympany, or flatness. Auscultate his lungs for other abnormal, diminished, or absent breath sounds. Listen to his heart for abnormal sounds, and check his hands and feet for edema or clubbing.

Pediatric pointers

Crackles in an infant or a child may indicate a serious cardiovascular or respiratory disorder. Pneumonias produce diffuse, sudden crackles in children. Esophageal atresia and tracheoesophageal fistula can cause bubbling, moist crackles due to aspiration of food or secretions into the lungs—especially in a neonate. Pulmonary edema causes fine crackles at the bases of the lungs, and bronchiectasis produces moist crackles. Cystic fibrosis produces widespread, fine to coarse inspiratory crackles and wheezing in an infant. Sickle cell anemia may produce crackles when it causes pulmonary infarction or infection.

Geriatric pointers

Crackles that clear after deep breathing may indicate mild basilar atelectasis. In older patients, auscultate lung bases before and after auscultating apices.

MEDICAL CAUSES

See *Crackles: Causes and associated findings,* page 94.

- *Acute respiratory distress syndrome (ARDS).* ARDS—a life-threatening disorder—causes diffuse, fine to coarse crackles usually heard in the dependent portions of the lungs. It also produces cyanosis, nasal flaring, tachypnea, tachycardia, grunting respirations, rhonchi, dyspnea, anxiety, and decreased level of consciousness.
- *Asthma (acute).* A severe asthma attack usually occurs at night or during sleep, causing dry, whistling crackles. An attack typically starts with a dry cough and mild wheezing and progresses to severe dyspnea, audible wheezing, chest tightness, and productive cough. Other findings include apprehension, prolonged expirations, rhonchi, intercostal and supraclavicular retraction on inspiration, accessory muscle use, flaring nostrils, tachypnea, tachycardia, diaphoresis, and flushing or cyanosis.
- *Bronchiectasis.* With bronchiectasis, persistent, coarse crackles are heard over the affected area of the lung. They're accompanied by a chronic cough that produces copious amounts of mucopurulent sputum. Other characteristics include halitosis, occasional wheezes, exertional dyspnea, rhonchi, weight loss, fatigue, malaise, weakness, recurrent fever, and late-stage clubbing.
- *Bronchitis (chronic).* Bronchitis causes coarse crackles that are usually heard at the lung bases. Prolonged expirations, wheezing, rhonchi, exertional dyspnea, tachypnea, and persistent, productive cough occur because of increased bronchial secretions. Clubbing and cyanosis may occur.
- *Chemical pneumonitis.* With acute chemical pneumonitis, diffuse, fine to coarse, moist crackles accompany a productive cough with purulent sputum, dyspnea, wheezing, orthopnea, fever, malaise, and mucous membrane irritation. Signs and symptoms may worsen for 24 to 48 hours after exposure, and then resolve; if severe, however, they may recur 2 to 5 weeks later.
- *Interstitial fibrosis of the lungs.* With interstitial fibrosis of the lungs, cellophane-like crackles can be heard over all lobes. As the disease progresses, a nonproductive cough,

CRACKLES:
CAUSES AND ASSOCIATED FINDINGS

MAJOR ASSOCIATED SIGNS AND SYMPTOMS

COMMON CAUSES	Chest pain	Cough	Cyanosis	Dyspnea	Fatigue	Fever	Hemoptysis	Rhonchi	Tachycardia	Tachypnea	Vomiting	Weakness	Weight loss
Acute respiratory distress syndrome			●	●				●	●	●			
Asthma	●	●	●	●				●	●	●			
Bronchiectasis		●		●	●	●		●				●	●
Bronchitis (chronic)		●	●	●			●	●		●			
Chemical pneumonitis		●				●		●					
Interstitial fibrosis of the lungs	●	●	●	●						●			●
Legionnaires' disease	●	●		●	●	●	●		●	●	●	●	
Lung abscess	●	●		●	●	●	●					●	●
Pneumonia (bacterial)	●	●	●	●	●	●		●	●	●			
Pneumonia (mycoplasma)		●				●	●			●			
Pneumonia (viral)		●				●				●			
Psittacosis	●					●				●	●		
Pulmonary edema		●	●	●				●	●	●			
Pulmonary embolism	●	●	●	●			●		●	●			
Pulmonary tuberculosis	●	●		●	●	●	●					●	●
Sarcoidosis		●		●	●					●		●	●
Silicosis		●		●	●					●		●	●
Tracheobronchitis	●					●		●					

dyspnea, fatigue, weight loss, cyanosis, and pleuritic chest pain develop.

● *Legionnaires' disease.* Legionnaires' disease produces diffuse moist crackles and cough that produces scant mucoid, nonpurulent, and possibly blood-streaked sputum.

Usually, prodromal signs and symptoms occur, including malaise, fatigue, weakness, anorexia, diffuse myalgia and, possibly, diarrhea. Within 12 to 48 hours, the patient develops a dry cough and sudden high fever with chills. He may also have pleuritic chest pain, headache, tachypnea, tachycardia, nausea, vomiting, dyspnea, mild temporary amnesia, confusion, flushing, mild diaphoresis, and prostration.

● *Lung abscess.* Lung abscess produces fine to medium and moist inspiratory crackles. The onset is insidious; signs and symptoms include sweating, anorexia, weight loss, fever, fatigue, weakness, dyspnea, clubbing, pleuritic chest pain, pleural friction rub, and a cough producing copious amounts of foul-smelling, purulent sputum that may be blood-tinged. The patient's breath sounds are hollow and tubular or amphoric; the affected side of his chest is dull on percussion.

● *Pneumonia.* Bacterial pneumonia produces diffuse fine crackles, sudden onset of shaking chills, high fever, tachypnea, pleuritic chest pain, cyanosis, grunting respirations, nasal flaring, decreased breath sounds, myalgia, headache, tachycardia, dyspnea, cyanosis, diaphoresis, and rhonchi. The patient also has a dry cough that later becomes productive.

Mycoplasma pneumonia produces medium to fine crackles together with a nonproductive cough, malaise, sore throat, headache, and fever. The patient may have blood-flecked sputum. Viral pneumonia causes gradually developing, diffuse crackles. The patient may also have a nonproductive cough, malaise, headache, anorexia, low-grade fever, and decreased breath sounds.

● *Psittacosis.* As psittacosis progresses, diffuse fine crackles may be heard. Accompanying findings include a characteristic hacking, productive cough, chills, fever, headache, myalgia, and prostration. Other features include tachypnea, chest pain (rare), epistaxis, photophobia, abdominal distention and tenderness, nausea, vomiting, and a faint macular rash.

● *Pulmonary edema.* Moist, bubbling crackles on inspiration are one of the first signs of pulmonary edema—a life-threatening disorder. Other early findings include exertional dyspnea; paroxysmal nocturnal dyspnea, then orthopnea; and coughing, which may be initially nonproductive but later produces frothy, bloody sputum. Related clinical effects include tachycardia, tachypnea, and a third heart sound (S_3 gallop). As the patient's respirations become increasingly rapid and labored, he develops more diffuse crackles, worsening tachycardia, hypotension, rapid

and thready pulse, cyanosis, and cold, clammy skin.

● *Pulmonary embolism.* Pulmonary embolism is a life-threatening disorder that can cause fine to coarse crackles and a cough that may be dry or produce blood-tinged sputum. Usually, the first sign of pulmonary embolism is severe dyspnea, which may be accompanied by angina or pleuritic chest pain. The patient has marked anxiety, low-grade fever, tachycardia, tachypnea, and diaphoresis. Less common signs include massive hemoptysis, chest splinting, leg edema and, with a large embolus, cyanosis, syncope, and jugular vein distention. The patient may also have a pleural friction rub, diffuse wheezing, chest dullness on percussion, decreased breath sounds, and signs of circulatory collapse.

● *Pulmonary tuberculosis.* With pulmonary tuberculosis, fine crackles occur after coughing. The patient has some combination of hemoptysis, malaise, dyspnea, and pleuritic chest pain. Sputum may be scant and mucoid or copious and purulent. Typically, the patient is easily fatigued and experiences night sweats, weakness, and weight loss. His breath sounds are amphoric.

● *Sarcoidosis.* Sarcoidosis produces fine, bibasilar, end-inspiratory crackles and, rarely, wheezing. The patient doesn't have a fever but does have malaise, fatigue, weakness, weight loss, cough, dyspnea, and tachypnea.

● *Silicosis.* Silicosis produces end-inspiratory, fine crackles heard at the lung bases. It also causes a productive cough with mucopurulent sputum—the earliest sign of this disorder. The patient also exhibits exertional dyspnea, tachypnea, weight loss, fatigue, general weakness, and recurrent respiratory tract infections.

● *Tracheobronchitis.* In its acute form, tracheobronchitis produces moist or coarse crackles along with a productive cough, chills, sore throat, slight fever, muscle and back pain, and substernal tightness. The patient typically has rhonchi and wheezes. Severe tracheobronchitis may cause moderate fever and bronchospasm.

NURSING CONSIDERATIONS

To keep the patient's airway patent and facilitate his breathing, elevate the head of his bed. To liquefy thick secretions and relieve mucous membrane inflammation, administer fluids, humidified air, or oxygen. Diuretics may be needed if crackles result from cardiogenic pulmonary edema. Turn the patient every 1 to 2 hours, and encourage him to breathe deeply.

Plan daily uninterrupted rest periods to help the patient relax and sleep. Prepare the patient for diagnostic tests, such as chest X-rays, a lung scan, and sputum analysis.

PATIENT TEACHING
Teach the patient how to cough effectively and splint incision areas if appropriate. Encourage him to avoid smoking and using aerosols, powders, or other products that might irritate his airways.

Crepitation, subcutaneous

When bubbles of air or other gases, such as carbon dioxide, are trapped in subcutaneous tissue, palpation or stroking of the skin produces a crackling sound called subcutaneous crepitation or subcutaneous emphysema. The bubbles feel like small, unstable nodules and aren't painful, even though subcutaneous crepitation is commonly associated with painful disorders. Usually, the affected tissue is visibly edematous; this can lead to life-threatening airway occlusion if the edema affects the neck or upper chest.

The air or gas bubbles enter the tissues through open wounds from the action of anaerobic microorganisms or from traumatic or spontaneous rupture or perforation of pulmonary or GI organs.

Act now Subcutaneous crepitation can impede structures lying underneath. If subcutaneous crepitation is located in the chest area, note respiratory or cardiac distress. Be prepared for emergency intervention, if necessary.

ASSESSMENT
History
Because subcutaneous crepitation can indicate a life-threatening disorder, you'll need to perform a rapid initial evaluation and intervene if necessary. (See *Managing subcutaneous crepitation.*) Ask the patient if he's experiencing pain or having difficulty breathing. If he's in pain, find out where the pain is located, how severe it is, and when it began. Ask

about recent thoracic surgery, diagnostic tests, and respiratory therapy or a history of trauma or chronic pulmonary disease.

Physical examination
Obtain the patient's vital signs. Perform a respiratory and cardiac assessment. Note location of crepitus, recording the location, extent, and associated symptoms.

When the patient's condition permits, palpate the affected skin to evaluate the location and extent of subcutaneous crepitation and to obtain baseline information. Repalpate frequently to determine if the subcutaneous crepitation is increasing.

Pediatric pointers
Children may develop subcutaneous crepitation in the neck from ingestion of corrosive substances that perforate the esophagus.

Geriatric pointers
Elderly patients with pre-existing disease may experience the sudden onset of subcutaneous crepitation following blunt or tissue trauma.

MEDICAL CAUSES
● *Gas gangrene.* Subcutaneous crepitation is the hallmark of gas gangrene — a rare, but commonly fatal, infection that's caused by anaerobic microorganisms. It's accompanied by local pain, swelling, and discoloration, with the formation of bullae and necrosis. The skin over the wound may rupture, revealing dark red or black necrotic muscle and producing foul-smelling, watery or frothy discharge. Related findings include tachycardia, tachypnea, moderate fever, cyanosis, and lassitude.
● *Orbital fracture.* An orbital fracture allows air from the nasal sinuses to escape into subcutaneous tissue, causing subcutaneous crepitation of the eyelid and orbit. The most common sign of orbital fracture is periorbital ecchymosis. Visual acuity is usually normal, although a swollen lid may prevent accurate testing. The patient has facial edema, diplopia, a hyphema and, occasionally, a dilated or unreactive pupil on the affected side. Extraocular movements may also be affected.
● *Pneumothorax.* Severe pneumothorax produces subcutaneous crepitation in the upper chest and neck. In many cases, the patient has chest pain that's unilateral, rarely localized initially, and increased on inspiration.

Act now

MANAGING SUBCUTANEOUS CREPITATION

Subcutaneous crepitation occurs when air or gas bubbles escape into tissues. It may signal life-threatening rupture of an air-filled or gas-producing organ or a fulminating anaerobic infection.

ORGAN RUPTURE

If the patient shows signs of respiratory distress — such as severe dyspnea, tachypnea, accessory muscle use, nasal flaring, air hunger, or tachycardia — quickly test for Hamman's sign to detect trapped air bubbles in the mediastinum.

To test for Hamman's sign, help the patient assume a left-lateral recumbent position. Then place your stethoscope over the precordium. If you hear a loud crunching sound that synchronizes with his heartbeat, the patient has a positive Hamman's sign.

Depending on which organ is ruptured, be prepared for endotracheal intubation, an emergency tracheotomy, or chest tube insertion. Start administering supplemental oxygen immediately. Start an I.V. line to administer fluids and medication, and connect the patient to a cardiac monitor.

ANAEROBIC INFECTION

If the patient has an open wound with a foul odor and local swelling and discoloration, you must act quickly. Take the patient's vital signs, checking especially for fever, tachycardia, hypotension, and tachypnea. Next, start an I.V. line to administer fluids and medication, and provide supplemental oxygen.

In addition, be prepared for emergency surgery to drain and debride the wound. If the patient's condition is life-threatening, you may need to prepare him for transfer to a facility with a hyperbaric chamber.

Dyspnea, anxiety, restlessness, tachypnea, cyanosis, tachycardia, accessory muscle use, asymmetrical chest expansion, and a nonproductive cough can also occur. On the affected side, breath sounds are absent or decreased, hyperresonance or tympany may be heard, and decreased vocal fremitus may be present.

● *Rupture of the esophagus.* A ruptured esophagus usually produces subcutaneous crepitation in the neck, chest wall, or supraclavicular fossa, although this sign doesn't always occur. With rupture of the cervical esophagus, the patient has excruciating pain in the neck or supraclavicular area, his neck is resistant to passive motion, and he has local tenderness, soft-tissue swelling, dysphagia, odynophagia, and orthostatic vertigo.

Life-threatening rupture of the intrathoracic esophagus can produce mediastinal emphysema confirmed by a positive Hamman's sign. The patient has severe retrosternal, epigastric, neck, or scapular pain and edema of the chest wall and neck. He may also display dyspnea, tachypnea, asymmetrical chest expansion, nasal flaring, cyanosis, diaphoresis, tachycardia, hypotension, dysphagia, and fever.

● *Rupture of the trachea or major bronchus.* Rupture of the trachea or major bronchus is a life-threatening injury that produces abrupt subcutaneous crepitation of the neck and anterior chest wall. The patient has severe dyspnea with nasal flaring, tachycardia, accessory muscle use, hypotension, cyanosis, extreme anxiety and, possibly, hemoptysis and mediastinal emphysema, with a positive Hamman's sign.

OTHER CAUSES

● *Diagnostic tests.* Endoscopic tests, such as bronchoscopy and upper GI tract endoscopy, can cause rupture or perforation of respiratory or GI organs, producing subcutaneous crepitation.

● *Respiratory treatments.* Mechanical ventilation and intermittent positive-pressure breathing can rupture alveoli, producing subcutaneous crepitation.

● *Thoracic surgery.* If air escapes into the tissue in the area of the incision, subcutaneous crepitation can occur.

NURSING CONSIDERATIONS

Monitor the patient's vital signs frequently, especially respirations. Because excessive edema from subcutaneous crepitation in the neck and upper chest can cause airway obstruction, stay alert for signs of respiratory distress such as dyspnea.

PATIENT TEACHING

Warn the patient with asthma or chronic bronchitis to stay alert for subcutaneous crepitation, which can signal pneumothorax, a dangerous complication. Explain to the patient that the affected tissues will eventually absorb the air or gas bubbles, so the subcutaneous crepitation will decrease.

Cullen's sign

Cullen's sign is ecchymosis around the umbilicus associated with severe intraperitoneal bleeding. It develops gradually and may not be seen until a few days after the injury.

Blood travels from a retroperitoneal organ or structure to the periumbilical area, where it diffuses through subcutaneous tissues. It's seen with ruptured ectopic pregnancy, duodenal ulcer perforation, rupture or obstruction of the common bile duct or gallbladder, hepatoma, ruptured aortic aneurysm, and rectus sheath hematoma.

The extent of discoloration depends on the extent of bleeding. In time, the bluish discoloration fades to greenish yellow and then yellow before disappearing. It may be difficult to detect in dark-skinned individuals.

Act now The patient with Cullen's sign — which indicates bleeding with possible rupture or obstruction of an organ — should be evaluated for shock immediately. Obtain his vital signs; he may require immediate emergency care if he exhibits tachycardia, hypotension, cool and clammy skin, or changes in his level of consciousness. Start an I.V. line with fluids infusing at a rapid rate. Administer oxygen and monitor the patient's respiratory status. Monitor laboratory tests for signs of bleeding, and be prepared to administer blood and blood products.

ASSESSMENT
History

Determine whether the patient had surgery recently or has experienced abdominal pain or discomfort. Has he noted any bleeding? Ask about a history of gallbladder or ulcer disease. Ask about medication history, including over-the-counter medications. Ask the female patient about the possibility of pregnancy and the first day of her last menses.

Physical examination

Complete a full GI assessment, inspecting the skin in the periumbilical and flank areas. Palpate peripheral pulses, noting strength and symmetry of pulses in the lower extremities. Note color and temperature of lower extremities.

Pediatric pointers

While some of the precipitating effects are not commonly seen in children, Cullen's sign can occur in children with internal hemorrhage or acute pancreatitis.

Geriatric pointers

Elderly patients experiencing gradual and continuous bleeding may exhibit signs of shock earlier than other patients. Treatment of shock may exacerbate pre-existing conditions such as heart failure.

MEDICAL CAUSES

● *Duodenal ulcer perforation.* Duodenal ulcers are characterized by abdominal pain, which is described as steady, gnawing, burning, or hungerlike. It occurs in the high to midepigastrium. The pain typically begins 2 to 4 hours after a meal and can cause nocturnal awakening. Ingestion of food or antacids bring relief until the cycle starts again. The main cause of ulcer disease is *Helicobacter pylori,* which weakens the protective mucus coating the stomach. Perforation can lead to acute bleeding, with or without signs of shock.

● *Pancreatitis.* Pancreatitis is an acute inflammation of the pancreas that occurs suddenly, lasts for a short time, and resolves quickly. Signs and symptoms include abdominal and back pain, hypotension, dehydration, fever, nausea and vomiting, and flank mass. Abnormally elevated amylase and lipase levels are seen. Gallstones need to be ruled out. Treatment includes hydration and pain relief.

● *Ruptured aortic aneurysm.* Progressive weakening of the aortic wall will result in an outpouching or "ballooning" of the wall. As it dilates further and grows, life-threatening rupture may occur. Massive blood loss occurs with typical signs of refractory shock. For patients with known aneurysms, elective surgery is safe and effective. Endovascular grafting has made the treatment regimen much less invasive.

- **Ruptured ectopic pregnancy.** Ectopic pregnancy occurs when a developing embryo implants itself at a site other than the inside wall of the uterus; the fallopian tube is the most common site of an ectopic pregnancy. Generally, the embryo won't survive. Ectopic pregnancies can result in a rupture of the organ of implantation, which can precipitate severe internal bleeding, shock, and possible death of the mother.

Associated signs and symptoms include amenorrhea, abdominal mass, nausea and vomiting, tachycardia, and urinary frequency.

NURSING CONSIDERATIONS

Monitor the patient and assess his vital signs frequently. Prepare him for laboratory tests and radiologic procedures. Maintain I.V. access and administer fluids and blood products, as necessary. Administer pain medications, as ordered.

PATIENT TEACHING

Explain all tests and procedures. Instruct the patient to report signs of bleeding. For female patients with ruptured ectopic pregnancy, offer emotional support and guidance. Refer the patient and her spouse to a grief support group.

Cyanosis

Cyanosis — a bluish or bluish black discoloration of the skin and mucous membranes — results from excessive concentration of unoxygenated hemoglobin in the blood. This common sign may develop abruptly or gradually. It can be classified as central or peripheral, although the two types may coexist.

Central cyanosis reflects inadequate oxygenation of systemic arterial blood caused by right-to-left cardiac shunting, pulmonary disease, or hematologic disorders. It may occur anywhere on the skin and also on the mucous membranes of the mouth, lips, and conjunctiva.

Peripheral cyanosis reflects sluggish peripheral circulation caused by vasoconstriction, reduced cardiac output, or vascular occlusion. It may be widespread or may occur locally in one extremity; however, it doesn't affect mucous membranes. Typically, peripheral cyanosis appears on exposed areas, such as the fingers, nail beds, feet, nose, and ears.

Although cyanosis is an important sign of cardiovascular and pulmonary disorders, it isn't always an accurate gauge of oxygenation. Several factors contribute to its development: hemoglobin concentration and oxygen saturation (SaO_2), cardiac output, and partial pressure of arterial oxygen (PaO_2). Cyanosis is usually undetectable until the SaO_2 of hemoglobin falls below 80%. Severe cyanosis is quite obvious, whereas mild cyanosis is more difficult to detect, even in natural, bright light. In dark-skinned patients, cyanosis is most apparent in the mucous membranes and nail beds.

Transient, nonpathologic cyanosis may result from environmental factors. For example, peripheral cyanosis may result from cutaneous vasoconstriction following a brief exposure to cold air or water. Central cyanosis may result from reduced PaO_2 at high altitudes.

Act now *If the patient displays sudden, localized cyanosis and other signs of arterial occlusion, protect the affected limb from injury; however, don't massage the limb. If you see central cyanosis stemming from a pulmonary disorder or shock, perform a rapid evaluation. Take immediate steps to maintain a patent airway, assist breathing, and monitor circulation.*

ASSESSMENT
History

Ask the patient about cardiac, pulmonary, and hematologic disorders or previous surgeries. Ask whether he's experiencing chest pain; if so, ask him to rate its severity using a standardized pain rating scale. Note precipitating, aggravating, or alleviating factors and whether the pain radiates. Determine when the patient first noticed the cyanosis and precipitating, aggravating, or alleviating factors; ask whether it's intermittent or constant. Does the patient have a history of headaches, dizziness, blurred vision, or pain or abnormal sensations in the extremities? Does he have a cough and if so, is it productive? Ask him to describe sputum. Inquire about a history of sleep apnea. Document the patient's medication history, including over-the-counter medications.

Physical examination

Obtain the patient's vital signs. Inspect the skin and mucous membranes to determine the extent of cyanosis. Assess the skin for coolness, pallor, redness, pain, and ulceration. Note the presence of clubbing.

Evaluate the patient's level of consciousness and test motor strength. Palpate peripheral pulses and test capillary refill time. Auscultate heart rate and rhythm, especially noting gallops and murmurs. Auscultate the abdominal aorta and femoral arteries to detect bruits.

Evaluate respiratory rate and rhythm. Check for nasal flaring and accessory muscle use. Inspect the patient for asymmetrical chest expansion or barrel chest. Percuss the lungs for dullness or hyperresonance, and auscultate for decreased or adventitious breath sounds.

Inspect the abdomen for ascites, and test for shifting dullness or fluid wave. Percuss and palpate for liver enlargement and tenderness.

Pediatric pointers

Many pulmonary disorders responsible for cyanosis in adults also cause cyanosis in children. In addition, central cyanosis may result from cystic fibrosis, asthma, airway obstruction by a foreign body, acute laryngotracheobronchitis, or epiglottiditis. It may also result from a congenital heart defect, such as transposition of the great vessels, that causes right-to-left intracardiac shunting.

In children, circumoral cyanosis may precede generalized cyanosis. Acrocyanosis (also called "glove and bootee" cyanosis) may occur in infants because of excessive crying or exposure to cold. Exercise and agitation enhance cyanosis, so provide comfort and regular rest periods. Also, administer supplemental oxygen during cyanotic episodes.

Geriatric pointers

Because elderly patients have reduced tissue perfusion, peripheral cyanosis can present even with a slight decrease in cardiac output or systemic blood pressure.

MEDICAL CAUSES

● *Arteriosclerotic occlusive disease (chronic).* With arteriosclerotic occlusive disease, peripheral cyanosis occurs in the legs whenever they're in a dependent position. Associated signs and symptoms include intermittent claudication and burning pain at rest, paresthesia, pallor, muscle atrophy, weak leg pulses, and impotence. Late signs are leg ulcers and gangrene.

● *Bronchiectasis.* Bronchiectasis produces chronic central cyanosis. Its classic sign, however, is chronic productive cough with copious, foul-smelling, mucopurulent sputum or hemoptysis. Auscultation reveals rhonchi and coarse crackles during inspiration. Other signs and symptoms include dyspnea, recurrent fever and chills, weight loss, malaise, clubbing, and signs of anemia.

● *Buerger's disease.* With Buerger's disease, exposure to cold initially causes the feet to become cold, cyanotic, and numb; later, they redden, become hot, and tingle. Intermittent claudication of the instep is characteristic; it's aggravated by exercise and smoking and relieved by rest. Associated signs and symptoms include weak peripheral pulses and, in later stages, ulceration, muscle atrophy, and gangrene.

● *Chronic obstructive pulmonary disease (COPD).* Chronic central cyanosis occurs in advanced stages of COPD and may be aggravated by exertion. Associated signs and symptoms include exertional dyspnea, productive cough with thick sputum, anorexia, weight loss, pursed-lip breathing, tachypnea, and accessory muscle use. Examination reveals wheezing and hyperresonant lung fields. Barrel chest and clubbing are late signs. Tachycardia, diaphoresis, and flushing may also accompany COPD.

● *Deep vein thrombosis.* With deep vein thrombosis, acute peripheral cyanosis occurs in the affected extremity associated with tenderness, painful movement, edema, warmth, and prominent superficial veins. Homans' sign can also be elicited.

● *Heart failure.* Acute or chronic cyanosis may occur in patients with heart failure. Typically, it's a late sign and may be central, peripheral, or both. With left-sided heart failure, central cyanosis occurs with tachycardia, fatigue, dyspnea, cold intolerance, orthopnea, cough, ventricular or atrial gallop, bibasilar crackles, and diffuse apical impulse. With right-sided heart failure, peripheral cyanosis occurs with fatigue, peripheral edema, ascites, jugular vein distention, and hepatomegaly.

● *Lung cancer.* Lung cancer causes chronic central cyanosis accompanied by fever, weakness, weight loss, anorexia, dyspnea, chest pain, hemoptysis, and wheezing. Atelectasis causes mediastinal shift, decreased diaphragmatic excursion, asymmetrical chest expansion, a dull percussion note, and diminished breath sounds.

● *Peripheral arterial occlusion (acute).* Peripheral arterial occlusion produces acute cyanosis of one arm or leg or, occasionally, of both legs. The cyanosis is accompanied by sharp or aching pain that worsens when the patient moves. The affected extremity also exhibits paresthesia, weakness, and pale, cool skin. Examination reveals decreased or absent pulse and increased capillary refill time.

● *Pneumonia.* With pneumonia, acute central cyanosis is usually preceded by fever, shaking chills, cough with purulent sputum, crackles, rhonchi, and pleuritic chest pain that's exacerbated by deep inspiration. Associated signs and symptoms include tachycardia, dyspnea, tachypnea, diminished breath sounds, diaphoresis, myalgia, fatigue, headache, and anorexia.

● *Pneumothorax.* A cardinal sign of pneumothorax, acute central cyanosis is accompanied by sharp chest pain that's exacerbated by movement, deep breathing, and coughing. The patient exhibits asymmetrical chest wall expansion, shortness of breath, and pallor. He may also experience jugular vein distention, anxiety, absence of breath sounds over the affected lobe, and rapid, shallow respirations. His pulse may be weak and rapid.

● *Polycythemia vera.* A ruddy complexion that can appear cyanotic is characteristic in polycythemia vera — a chronic myeloproliferative disorder. Other findings include hepatosplenomegaly, headache, dizziness, fatigue, aquagenic pruritus, blurred vision, chest pain, intermittent claudication, and coagulation defects.

● *Pulmonary edema.* With pulmonary edema, acute central cyanosis occurs with dyspnea, orthopnea, tachycardia, tachypnea, dependent crackles, ventricular gallop, hypotension, confusion, and frothy, blood-tinged sputum. The patient may exhibit cold, clammy skin and a weak, thready pulse.

● *Pulmonary embolism.* Acute central cyanosis occurs when a large embolus causes significant obstruction of the pulmonary circulation. Syncope and jugular vein distention may also occur. Other common signs and symptoms include dyspnea, chest pain, tachycardia, paradoxical pulse, dry or productive cough with blood-tinged sputum, low-grade fever, restlessness, and diaphoresis.

● *Raynaud's disease.* With Raynaud's disease, exposure to cold or stress causes the fingers or hands to blanch and turn cold, become cyanotic, and finally redden with return of normal temperature. Numbness and tingling may also occur. Raynaud's phenomenon describes the same presentation when associated with other disorders, such as rheumatoid arthritis, scleroderma, or lupus erythematosus.

● *Shock.* With shock, acute peripheral cyanosis develops in the hands and feet, which may also be cold, clammy, and pale. Other characteristic signs and symptoms include lethargy, confusion, increased capillary refill time, and a rapid, weak pulse. Tachypnea, hyperpnea, and hypotension may also be present.

● *Sleep apnea.* When chronic and severe, sleep apnea causes pulmonary hypertension and cor pulmonale (right-sided heart failure), which can produce chronic cyanosis.

NURSING CONSIDERATIONS

Provide supplemental oxygen to relieve shortness of breath, improve oxygenation, and decrease cyanosis. However, deliver small doses (2 L/minute) in the patient with COPD, who may retain carbon dioxide. Use a low-flow oxygen rate for mild COPD exacerbations. However, for acute situations, a high-flow oxygen rate may be needed initially. Simply remember to be attentive to the patient's respiratory drive and adjust the amount of oxygen accordingly. Position the patient comfortably to ease breathing. Administer a diuretic, bronchodilator, antibiotic, or cardiac drug as needed. Make sure that the patient gets sufficient rest between activities to prevent dyspnea.

Prepare the patient for such tests as arterial blood gas analysis and complete blood count to determine the cause of cyanosis.

PATIENT TEACHING

Teach patients with chronic cardiopulmonary diseases, such as heart failure, asthma, or COPD, to recognize cyanosis as a sign of severe disease requiring immediate medical attention.

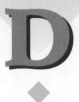

Decerebrate posture

[Decerebrate rigidity, abnormal extensor reflex]

Decerebrate posture is characterized by adduction (internal rotation) and extension of the arms, with the wrists pronated and the fingers flexed. The legs are stiffly extended, with forced plantar flexion of the feet. In severe cases, the back is acutely arched (opisthotonos). Decerebrate posture indicates upper brain stem damage, which may result from primary lesions, such as infarction, hemorrhage, or tumor. Other causes include metabolic encephalopathy, head injury, and brain stem compression associated with increased intracranial pressure (ICP).

Decerebrate posture may be elicited by noxious stimuli or may occur spontaneously. It may be unilateral or bilateral. With concurrent brain stem and cerebral damage, decerebrate posture may affect only the arms, with the legs remaining flaccid. Decerebrate posture may also affect one side of the body and decorticate posture the other. The two postures may also alternate as the patient's neurologic status fluctuates. Generally, the duration of each posturing episode correlates with the severity of brain stem damage. (See *Comparing decerebrate and decorticate postures.*)

Act now Upon initial assessment of the decerebrate posture, your first priority is to ensure a patent airway. Insert an artificial airway and institute measures to prevent aspiration. (Don't disrupt spinal alignment if you suspect spinal cord injury.) Suction the patient as necessary.

Next, examine spontaneous respirations. Give supplemental oxygen, and ventilate the patient with a handheld resuscitation bag, if necessary. Intubation and mechanical ventilation may be indicated. Keep emergency resuscitation equipment handy. Be sure to check the patient's chart for a do-not-resuscitate order.

ASSESSMENT
History

After the patient's airway has been stabilized, assess the history of the patient's coma. If a family member is available, ask about any accident or trauma responsible for the coma, and find out when the patient's level of consciousness (LOC) began deteriorating. Did it occur abruptly? Did the patient express presence of any symptoms, such as headache, nausea, or visual or behavioral changes, before he lost consciousness? Does he have a history of diabetes, liver disease, cancer, blood clots, or aneurysm? If you're unable to obtain this information, look for clues to the causative disorder, such as hepatomegaly, cyanosis, diabetic skin changes, needle tracks, or obvious trauma.

Physical examination

After taking the patient's vital signs, determine his LOC. Use the Glasgow Coma Scale as a reference. Evaluate the pupils for size, equality, and response to light. Test deep tendon reflexes and cranial nerve reflexes, and check for doll's eye sign. (See *Testing for absent doll's eye sign,* page 104.)

Pediatric pointers

Children younger than age 2 may not display decerebrate posture because the nervous sys-

COMPARING DECEREBRATE AND DECORTICATE POSTURES

Decerebrate posture results from damage to the upper brain stem. In this posture, the arms are adducted and extended, with the wrists pronated and the fingers flexed. The legs are stiffly extended, with plantar flexion of the feet.

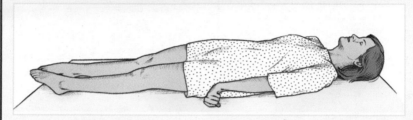

Decorticate posture results from damage to one or both corticospinal tracts. In this posture, the arms are adducted and flexed, with the wrists and fingers flexed on the chest. The legs are stiffly extended and internally rotated, with plantar flexion of the feet.

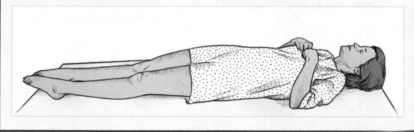

tem is still immature. However, if the posture occurs, it's usually the more severe opisthotonos. In fact, opisthotonos is more common in infants and young children than in adults and is usually a terminal sign. In children, the most common cause of decerebrate posture is head injury. It also occurs with Reye's syndrome — the result of increased ICP causing brain stem compression.

MEDICAL CAUSES

● *Brain stem infarction.* When brain stem infarction — a primary lesion — produces a coma, decerebrate posture may be elicited. Associated signs and symptoms vary with the severity of the infarct and may include cranial nerve palsies, bilateral cerebellar ataxia, and sensory loss. With deep coma, all normal reflexes are usually lost, resulting in absence of doll's eye sign, a positive Babinski's reflex, and flaccidity.
● *Brain stem tumor.* With brain stem tumor, decerebrate posture is a late sign that accom-

panies coma. Commonly, the posture is preceded by hemiparesis or quadriparesis, cranial nerve palsies, vertigo, dizziness, ataxia, and vomiting.
● *Cerebral lesion.* Whether the cause is trauma, tumor, abscess, or infarction, any cerebral lesion that increases ICP may also produce decerebrate posture. Typically, this posture is a late sign. Associated findings vary with the lesion's site and extent but commonly include coma, abnormal pupil size and response to light, and the classic triad of increased ICP — bradycardia, increasing systolic blood pressure, and widening pulse pressure.
● *Hepatic encephalopathy.* A late sign in hepatic encephalopathy, decerebrate posture occurs with coma resulting from increased ICP and ammonia toxicity. Associated signs include fetor hepaticus (foul-smelling breath), a positive Babinski's reflex, and hyperactive deep tendon reflexes.

TESTING FOR ABSENT DOLL'S EYE SIGN

To evaluate the patient's oculocephalic reflex, hold her upper eyelids open and quickly (but gently) turn her head from side to side, noting eye movements with each head turn.

With absent doll's eye sign, the eyes remain fixed in midposition.

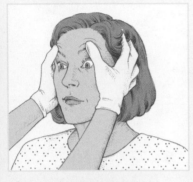

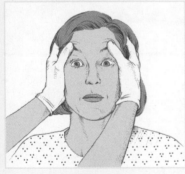

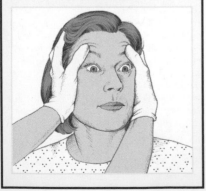

• *Hypoglycemic encephalopathy.* Characterized by extremely low blood glucose levels, hypoglycemic encephalopathy may produce decerebrate posture and coma. It also causes dilated pupils, slow respirations, and bradycardia. Muscle spasms, twitching, and seizures eventually progress to flaccidity.

• *Hypoxic encephalopathy.* Severe hypoxia may produce decerebrate posture — the result of brain stem compression associated with anaerobic metabolism and increased ICP. Other findings include coma, a positive Babinski's reflex, absence of doll's eye sign, hypoactive deep tendon reflexes and, possibly, fixed pupils and respiratory arrest.

• *Pontine hemorrhage.* Typically, pontine hemorrhage — a life-threatening disorder — rapidly leads to decerebrate posture with coma. Accompanying signs include total paralysis, absence of doll's eye sign, a positive Babinski's reflex, and small, reactive pupils.

• *Posterior fossa hemorrhage.* Posterior fossa hemorrhage is a subtentorial lesion that causes decerebrate posture. Early signs and symptoms include vomiting, headache, vertigo, ataxia, stiff neck, drowsiness, papilledema, and cranial nerve palsies. The patient eventually slips into coma and may experience respiratory arrest.

OTHER CAUSES

• *Diagnostic tests.* Relief of high ICP by removal of spinal fluid during a lumbar puncture may precipitate cerebral compression of the brain stem and cause decerebrate posture and coma.

NURSING CONSIDERATIONS

Help prepare the patient for diagnostic tests that will determine the cause of his decerebrate posture; these can include skull X-rays, computed tomography scan, magnetic resonance imaging, cerebral angiography, digital subtraction angiography, electroencephalogram, brain scan, and ICP monitoring.

Monitor the patient's neurologic status and vital signs every 30 minutes or as indicated. Also, be alert for signs of increased ICP (bradycardia, increasing systolic blood pressure, and widening pulse pressure) and neurologic deterioration (altered respiratory pattern and abnormal temperature).

PATIENT TEACHING

Inform the patient and his family that decerebrate posture is a reflex response, not a voluntary response to pain or a sign of recovery. Offer emotional support. Refer the patient and his family to a mental health worker or spiritual counselor, if indicated.

Decorticate posture

[Decorticate rigidity, abnormal flexor response]

A sign of corticospinal damage, decorticate posture is characterized by adduction of the arms and flexion of the elbows, with wrists and fingers flexed on the chest. The legs are extended and internally rotated, with plantar flexion of the feet. This posture may occur unilaterally or bilaterally. It usually results from stroke or head injury. It may be elicited by noxious stimuli or may occur spontaneously. The intensity of the required stimulus, the duration of the posture, and the frequency of spontaneous episodes vary with the severity and location of cerebral injury.

Although a serious sign, decorticate posture carries a more favorable prognosis than decerebrate posture. However, if the causative disorder extends lower in the brain stem, decorticate posture may progress to decerebrate posture. (See *Comparing decerebrate and decorticate postures,* page 103.)

Act now Obtain vital signs and evaluate the patient's level of consciousness (LOC). If his consciousness is impaired, insert an oropharyngeal airway, and take measures to prevent aspiration (unless spinal cord injury is suspected). Evaluate the patient's respiratory rate, rhythm, and depth. Prepare to assist respirations with a handheld resuscitation bag or with intubation and mechanical ventilation, if necessary. Also, institute seizure precautions.

ASSESSMENT
History

Obtain a history from the patient (if possible) or his family. Did the patient complain about headache, dizziness, nausea, changes in vision, and numbness or tingling? When did he first notice these symptoms? Did the family observe any behavioral changes?

Ask about a history of cerebrovascular disease, cancer, meningitis, encephalitis, up-

per respiratory tract infection, bleeding or clotting disorders, or recent trauma.

Physical examination

Test the patient's motor and sensory functions. Evaluate pupil size, equality, and response to light. Test cranial nerve function and deep tendon reflexes. Perform a complete neurologic examination and continue to perform frequent neurologic checks. Assess the patient's respiratory function.

Alert Abnormal respirations may indicate a breakdown in the brain's respiratory center and an impending tentorial herniation — a neurologic emergency.

Pediatric pointers

Decorticate posture is an unreliable sign before age 2 because of nervous system immaturity. Head injury and Reye's syndrome can, however, cause decorticate posture in children.

MEDICAL CAUSES

● **Brain abscess.** Decorticate posture may occur with brain abscess. Accompanying findings vary on the size and location of the abscess but may include aphasia, hemiparesis, headache, dizziness, seizures, nausea, and vomiting. The patient may also experience behavioral changes, altered vital signs, and decreased LOC.

● **Brain tumor.** Brain tumor may produce decorticate posture that's usually bilateral — the result of increased intracranial pressure (ICP) associated with tumor growth. Related signs and symptoms include headache, behavioral changes, memory loss, diplopia, blurred vision or vision loss, seizures, ataxia, dizziness, apraxia, aphasia, paresis, sensory loss, paresthesia, vomiting, papilledema, and signs of hormonal imbalance.

● **Head injury.** Decorticate posture may be among the variable features of a head injury, depending on the site and severity of head injury. Associated signs and symptoms include headache, nausea and vomiting, dizziness, irritability, decreased LOC, aphasia, hemiparesis, unilateral numbness, seizures, and pupillary dilation.

● **Stroke.** Typically, a stroke involving the cerebral cortex produces unilateral decorticate posture, also called *spastic hemiplegia.* Other signs and symptoms include hemiplegia (contralateral to the lesion), dysarthria, dysphagia, unilateral sensory loss, apraxia, agnosia, aphasia, memory loss, decreased LOC, urine retention, urinary incontinence, and constipation. Ocular effects include homonymous hemianopsia, diplopia, and blurred vision.

NURSING CONSIDERATIONS

Monitor neurologic status and vital signs every 30 minutes to 2 hours. Be alert for signs of increased ICP, including bradycardia, increasing systolic blood pressure, and widening pulse pressure.

PATIENT TEACHING

Instruct the patient and his family about the signs and symptoms of decreased LOC and seizures. Explain to the family or caregiver how to keep the patient safe, especially during a seizure. Discuss quality of life concerns, if appropriate. Provide referrals to other health care services and professionals, as indicated.

Diarrhea

Usually a chief sign of an intestinal disorder, diarrhea is an increase in the volume of stools compared with the patient's normal bowel habits. It varies in severity and may be acute or chronic. Acute diarrhea may result from acute infection, stress, fecal impaction, or the effect of a drug. Chronic diarrhea may result from chronic infection, obstructive and inflammatory bowel disease, malabsorption syndrome, an endocrine disorder, or GI surgery. Periodic diarrhea may result from food intolerance or from ingestion of spicy or high-fiber foods or caffeine.

One or more pathophysiologic mechanisms may contribute to diarrhea. (See *What causes diarrhea.*) The fluid and electrolyte imbalances it produces may precipitate life-threatening arrhythmias or hypovolemic shock.

Act now *If the patient's diarrhea is profuse, check for signs of shock—tachycardia, hypotension, and cool, pale, clammy skin. If you detect these signs, place the patient in the supine position and elevate his legs 20 degrees. Insert an I.V. line for fluid replacement. Monitor him for electrolyte imbalances, and look for an irregular pulse, muscle weakness, anorexia, and nausea and vom-*

iting. Keep emergency resuscitation equipment handy.

ASSESSMENT
History

Obtain the patient's history. Does he have abdominal pain and cramps? Difficulty breathing? Is he weak or fatigued? Ask about his drug history. Has he had GI surgery or radiation therapy recently? Ask the patient to briefly describe his diet. Does he have any known food allergies? Lastly, find out if he's under unusual stress.

Physical examination

If the patient isn't in shock, proceed with a brief physical examination. Evaluate hydration, check skin turgor and mucous membranes, and take blood pressure with the patient lying, sitting, and standing. Inspect the abdomen for distention, and palpate for tenderness. Auscultate bowel sounds. Check for tympany over the abdomen. Take the patient's temperature, and note any chills. Also, look for a rash. Conduct a rectal examination and a pelvic examination if indicated.

Pediatric pointers

Diarrhea in children commonly results from infection, although chronic diarrhea may result from malabsorption syndrome, an anatomic defect, or allergies. Because dehydration and electrolyte imbalance occur rapidly in children, diarrhea can be life-threatening. Diligently monitor all episodes of diarrhea, and immediately replace lost fluids.

Geriatric pointers

In elderly patients with new-onset segmental colitis, rule out ischemia before considering a diagnosis of Crohn's disease.

MEDICAL CAUSES
- *Anthrax, GI.* GI anthrax manifests after the patient has eaten contaminated meat from an animal infected with *Bacillus anthracis*. Early signs and symptoms include decreased appetite, nausea, vomiting, and fever. Later signs and symptoms include severe bloody diarrhea, abdominal pain, and hematemesis.
- *Carcinoid syndrome.* With carcinoid syndrome, severe diarrhea occurs with flushing — usually of the head and neck — that's commonly caused by emotional stimuli or the ingestion of food, hot water, or alcohol.

WHAT CAUSES DIARRHEA

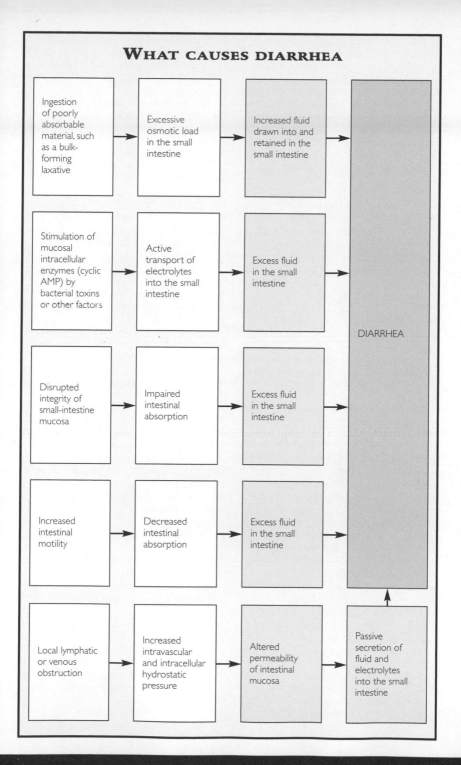

Ingestion of poorly absorbable material, such as a bulk-forming laxative	Excessive osmotic load in the small intestine	Increased fluid drawn into and retained in the small intestine	
Stimulation of mucosal intracellular enzymes (cyclic AMP) by bacterial toxins or other factors	Active transport of electrolytes into the small intestine	Excess fluid in the small intestine	
Disrupted integrity of small-intestine mucosa	Impaired intestinal absorption	Excess fluid in the small intestine	DIARRHEA
Increased intestinal motility	Decreased intestinal absorption	Excess fluid in the small intestine	
Local lymphatic or venous obstruction	Increased intravascular and intracellular hydrostatic pressure	Altered permeability of intestinal mucosa	Passive secretion of fluid and electrolytes into the small intestine

Associated signs and symptoms include abdominal cramps, dyspnea, weight loss, anorexia, weakness, palpitations, valvular heart disease, and depression.

● *Cholera.* After ingesting water or food contaminated by the bacterium *Vibrio cholerae,* the patient experiences abrupt watery diarrhea and vomiting. Other signs and symptoms include thirst (due to severe water and electrolyte loss), weakness, muscle cramps, decreased skin turgor, oliguria, tachycardia, and hypotension. Without treatment, death can occur within hours.

● *Clostridium difficile infection.* The patient may be asymptomatic or may have soft, unformed stools or watery diarrhea that may be foul-smelling or grossly bloody; abdominal pain, cramping, and tenderness; fever; and a white blood cell count as high as 20,000/µl. In severe cases, the patient may develop toxic megacolon, colonic perforation, or peritonitis.

● *Crohn's disease.* Crohn's disease is a recurring inflammatory disorder that produces diarrhea accompanied by abdominal pain with guarding and tenderness, and nausea. The patient may also display fever, chills, weakness, anorexia, and weight loss.

● **Escherichia coli O157:H7.** Watery or bloody diarrhea, nausea, vomiting, fever, and abdominal cramps occur after the patient eats undercooked beef or other foods contaminated with *E. coli* O157:H7. Hemolytic uremic syndrome, which causes red blood cell destruction and eventually acute renal failure, is a complication of *E. coli* O157:H7 in children age 5 and younger and elderly people.

● *Infections.* Acute viral, bacterial, and protozoal infections (such as cryptosporidiosis) cause the sudden onset of watery diarrhea as well as abdominal pain, cramps, nausea, vomiting, and fever. Significant fluid and electrolyte loss may cause signs of dehydration and shock. Chronic tuberculosis and fungal and parasitic infections may produce a less severe but more persistent diarrhea, accompanied by epigastric distress, vomiting, weight loss and, possibly, passage of blood and mucus.

● *Intestinal obstruction.* Partial intestinal obstruction increases intestinal motility, resulting in diarrhea, abdominal pain with tenderness and guarding, nausea and, possibly, distention.

● *Irritable bowel syndrome.* Diarrhea alternates with constipation or normal bowel function. Related findings include abdominal pain, tenderness, and distention; dyspepsia; and nausea.

● *Ischemic bowel disease.* Ischemic bowel disease is a life-threatening disorder that causes bloody diarrhea with abdominal pain. If severe, shock may occur, requiring surgery.

● *Lactose intolerance.* Diarrhea occurs within several hours of ingesting milk or milk products. It's accompanied by cramps, abdominal pain, borborygmi, bloating, nausea, and flatus.

● *Large-bowel cancer.* With large-bowel cancer, bloody diarrhea is seen with a partial obstruction. Other signs and symptoms include abdominal pain, anorexia, weight loss, weakness, fatigue, exertional dyspnea, and depression.

● *Lead poisoning.* Alternating diarrhea and constipation occur with lead poisoning. Other GI effects include abdominal pain, anorexia, nausea, and vomiting. The patient complains of a metallic taste, headache, and dizziness and displays a bluish gingival lead line.

● *Listeriosis.* With listeriosis — an infectious disease — diarrhea occurs in conjunction with fever, myalgias, abdominal pain, nausea, and vomiting. Fever, headache, nuchal rigidity, and altered level of consciousness may occur if the infection spreads to the nervous system and causes meningitis. This infection, caused by the ingestion of food contaminated with the bacterium *Listeria monocytogenes* primarily affects pregnant females, neonates, and those with weakened immune systems.

● *Malabsorption syndrome.* Occurring after meals, diarrhea is accompanied by steatorrhea, abdominal distention, and muscle cramps. The patient also displays anorexia, weight loss, bone pain, anemia, weakness, and fatigue. He may bruise easily and have night blindness.

● *Pseudomembranous enterocolitis.* Pseudomembranous enterocolitis is a potentially life-threatening disorder that commonly follows antibiotic administration. It produces copious watery, green, foul-smelling, bloody diarrhea that rapidly precipitates signs of shock. Other signs and symptoms include colicky abdominal pain, distention, fever, and dehydration.

- *Q fever.* Q fever is caused by the bacterium *Coxiella burnetii* and causes diarrhea along with fever, chills, severe headache, malaise, chest pain, and vomiting. In severe cases, hepatitis or pneumonia may occur.
- *Rotavirus gastroenteritis.* Rotavirus gastroenteritis commonly starts with a fever, nausea, and vomiting, followed by diarrhea. The illness can range from mild to severe and last from 3 to 9 days. Diarrhea and vomiting may result in dehydration.
- *Thyrotoxicosis.* With thyrotoxicosis, diarrhea is accompanied by nervousness, tremors, diaphoresis, weight loss despite increased appetite, dyspnea, palpitations, tachycardia, enlarged thyroid, heat intolerance and, possibly, exophthalmos.
- *Ulcerative colitis.* The hallmark of ulcerative colitis is recurrent bloody diarrhea with pus or mucus. Other signs and symptoms include tenesmus, hyperactive bowel sounds, cramping lower abdominal pain, low-grade fever, anorexia and, at times, nausea and vomiting. Weight loss, anemia, and weakness are late findings.

OTHER CAUSES

- *Drugs.* Many antibiotics — such as ampicillin, cephalosporins, tetracyclines, and clindamycin — cause diarrhea. Other drugs that may cause diarrhea include magnesium-containing antacids, colchicine, guanethidine, lactulose, dantrolene, ethacrynic acid, mefenamic acid, methotrexate, metyrosine and, in high doses, cardiac glycosides and quinidine. Laxative abuse can cause acute or chronic diarrhea.
- *Foods.* Foods that contain certain oils may inhibit absorption of food causing acute uncontrollable diarrhea and rectal leakage.
- *Herbal remedies.* Certain herbal remedies, such as ginkgo biloba, ginseng, and licorice, may cause diarrhea.
- *Medical treatments.* Gastrectomy, gastroenterostomy, and pyloroplasty may produce diarrhea. High-dose radiation therapy may produce enteritis associated with diarrhea.

NURSING CONSIDERATIONS

Administer an analgesic for pain and an opioid to decrease intestinal motility, unless the patient has a possible or confirmed stool infection. Ensure the patient's privacy during defecation, and empty bedpans promptly.

Clean the perineum thoroughly, and apply ointment to prevent skin breakdown.

Alert *Excessive diarrhea may cause skin breakdown and excoriation. To decrease excoriation and facilitate drainage measurement, insert a rectal tube or large indwelling catheter.*

Help the patient maintain adequate hydration, administering I.V. fluid replacements. Measure liquid stools, and weigh the patient daily. Monitor electrolyte levels and hematocrit.

Quantify the amount of liquid stool and carefully observe intake and output.

PATIENT TEACHING

Explain the purpose of diagnostic tests to the patient. These tests may include blood studies, stool cultures, X-rays, and endoscopy.

Advise the patient to avoid spicy or high-fiber foods (such as fruits), caffeine, high-fat foods, and milk. Suggest smaller, more frequent meals if he has had GI surgery or disease. If appropriate, teach the patient stress-reducing exercises, such as guided imagery and deep-breathing techniques, or recommend counseling.

Stress the need for medical follow-up to patients with inflammatory bowel disease (particularly ulcerative colitis), who have an increased risk of developing colon cancer.

Dizziness

A common symptom, dizziness is a sensation of imbalance or faintness, sometimes associated with giddiness, weakness, confusion, and blurred or double vision. Episodes of dizziness are usually brief; they may be mild or severe with abrupt or gradual onset. Dizziness may be aggravated by standing up quickly and alleviated by lying down and by rest.

Dizziness typically results from inadequate blood flow and oxygen supply to the cerebrum and spinal cord. It may occur with anxiety, respiratory and cardiovascular disorders, and postconcussion syndrome. It's a key symptom in certain serious disorders, such as hypertension and vertebrobasilar artery insufficiency.

Dizziness is commonly confused with vertigo — a sensation of revolving in space or of surroundings revolving about oneself.

However, unlike dizziness, vertigo is commonly accompanied by nausea, vomiting, nystagmus, staggering gait, and tinnitus or hearing loss. Dizziness and vertigo may occur together, as in postconcussion syndrome. (See *Understanding concussion*.)

Act now If the patient complains of dizziness, first ensure his safety by providing a safe environment to prevent falls. Then determine the severity and onset of the dizziness. Ask the patient to describe it. Is the dizziness associated with headache or blurred vision? Next, take the patient's blood pressure while he's lying, sitting, and standing to check for orthostatic hypotension. Ask about a history of high blood pressure. Determine if the patient is at risk for hypoglycemia. Tell the patient to lie down, and recheck his vital signs every 15 minutes. Start an I.V. line, and prepare to administer medications as ordered.

ASSESSMENT
History

Ask about a history of diabetes and cardiovascular disease. Is the patient taking drugs prescribed for high blood pressure? If so, when did he take his last dose?

If the patient's blood pressure is normal, obtain a more complete history. Ask about myocardial infarction, heart failure, kidney disease, or atherosclerosis, which may predispose the patient to cardiac arrhythmias, hypertension, and a transient ischemic attack. Does he have a history of anemia, chronic obstructive pulmonary disease (COPD), anxiety disorders, or head injury? Obtain a complete drug history.

Explore the patient's dizziness. How often does it occur? How long does each episode last? Does the dizziness abate spontaneously? Does it lead to loss of consciousness? Find out if dizziness is triggered by sitting or standing up suddenly or stooping over. Does being in a crowd make the patient feel dizzy? Ask about emotional stress. Has the patient been irritable or anxious lately? Does he have insomnia or difficulty concentrating? Look for fidgeting and eyelid twitching. Does the patient startle easily? Also, ask about palpitations, chest pain, diaphoresis, shortness of breath, and chronic cough.

Physical examination

Perform a physical examination. Begin with a quick neurocheck, assessing the patient's level of consciousness (LOC), motor and sensory functions, and reflexes. Then inspect for poor skin turgor and dry mucous membranes, signs of dehydration. Auscultate heart rate and rhythm. Inspect for barrel chest, clubbing, cyanosis, and use of accessory muscles. Also auscultate breath sounds. Take the patient's blood pressure while he's lying, sitting, and standing to check for orthostatic hypotension. Test capillary refill time in the extremities, and palpate for edema.

Pediatric pointers

Dizziness is less common in children than in adults. Many children have difficulty describing this symptom and instead complain of tiredness, stomachache, or feeling sick. If you suspect dizziness, assess the patient for vertigo as well. A more common symptom in children, vertigo may result from a vision disorder, an ear infection, or antibiotic therapy.

MEDICAL CAUSES

● *Anemia.* Typically, anemia causes dizziness that's aggravated by postural changes or exertion. Other signs and symptoms include pallor, dyspnea, fatigue, tachycardia, and bounding pulse. Capillary refill time is increased.

● *Cardiac arrhythmias.* Dizziness lasts for several seconds or longer and may precede fainting in arrhythmias. The patient may experience palpitations; irregular, rapid, or thready pulse; and possibly hypotension. He may also experience weakness, blurred vision, paresthesia, and confusion.

● *Carotid sinus hypersensitivity.* Carotid sinus hypersensitivity is characterized by brief episodes of dizziness that usually terminate in fainting. These episodes are precipitated by stimulation of one or both carotid arteries by seemingly minor sensations or actions, such as wearing a tight collar or moving the head. Associated signs and symptoms include sweating, nausea, and pallor.

● *Emphysema.* Dizziness may follow exertion or the chronic productive cough in patients with emphysema. Associated signs and symptoms include dyspnea, anorexia, weight loss, malaise, use of accessory muscles, pursed-lip breathing, tachypnea, peripheral cyanosis, and diminished breath sounds. Barrel chest and clubbing may be seen.

● *Generalized anxiety disorder.* Generalized anxiety disorder produces continuous dizziness that may intensify as the disorder worsens. Associated signs and symptoms are persistent anxiety (for at least 1 month), insomnia, difficulty concentrating, and irritability. The patient may show signs of motor tension — for example, twitching or fidgeting, muscle aches, furrowed brow, and a tendency to be startled. He may also display signs of autonomic hyperactivity, such as diaphoresis, palpitations, cold and clammy hands, dry mouth, paresthesia, indigestion, hot or cold flashes, frequent urination, diarrhea, a lump in the throat, pallor, and increased pulse and respiratory rates.

● *Hypertension.* With hypertension, dizziness may precede fainting, but it may also be relieved by rest. Other common signs and symptoms include headache and blurred vision. Retinal changes include hemorrhage, sclerosis of retinal blood vessels, exudate, and papilledema.

● *Hyperventilation syndrome.* Episodes of hyperventilation cause dizziness that usually lasts a few minutes; however, if these episodes occur frequently, dizziness may persist between them. Other effects include apprehension, diaphoresis, pallor, dyspnea, chest tightness, palpitations, trembling, fatigue, and peripheral and circumoral paresthesia.

● *Hypoglycemia.* Dizziness is a central nervous system (CNS) disturbance that can occur due to fasting hypoglycemia. It's generally accompanied by headache, clouding of vision, restlessness, and mental status changes.

● *Hypovolemia.* Dizziness is caused by a lack of circulating volume and may be accompanied by other signs of fluid volume deficit (dry mucous membranes, decreased blood pressure, increased heart rate).

● *Orthostatic hypotension.* Orthostatic hypotension produces dizziness that may terminate in fainting or disappear with rest. Related findings include dim vision, spots before the eyes, pallor, diaphoresis, hypotension, tachycardia and, possibly, signs of dehydration.

● *Panic disorder.* Dizziness may accompany acute attacks of panic in patients with panic disorder. Other findings include anxiety, dyspnea, palpitations, chest pain, a choking or smothering sensation, vertigo, paresthesia, hot and cold flashes, diaphoresis, and trembling or shaking. The patient may have the sensation of dying or losing his mind.

● *Postconcussion syndrome.* Occurring from the time of injury to 3 weeks after a head injury, postconcussion syndrome is marked by dizziness, headache (throbbing, aching, bandlike, or stabbing), emotional lability, alcohol intolerance, fatigue, anxiety and, possibly, vertigo. Dizziness and other symptoms are intensified by mental or physical stress. The syndrome may persist for years, but symptoms eventually abate.

● *Rift Valley fever.* Typical signs and symptoms of Rift Valley fever include dizziness, fever, myalgia, weakness, and back pain. A small percentage of patients may develop encephalitis or may progress to hemorrhagic fever that can lead to shock and hemorrhage. Inflammation of the retina may result in some permanent vision loss.

- *Transient ischemic attack (TIA).* Lasting from a few seconds to 24 hours, a TIA commonly signals impending stroke. Besides dizziness of varying severity, TIAs are accompanied by unilateral or bilateral diplopia, blindness or visual field deficits, ptosis, tinnitus, hearing loss, paresis, and numbness. Other findings include dysarthria, dysphagia, vomiting, hiccups, confusion, decreased LOC, and pallor.

OTHER CAUSES

- *Drugs.* Anxiolytics, CNS depressants, opioids, decongestants, antihistamines, antihypertensives, and vasodilators commonly cause dizziness.
- *Herbal remedies.* St. John's wort can produce dizziness.

NURSING CONSIDERATIONS

Prepare the patient for diagnostic tests, such as blood studies, arteriography, computed tomography scan, electroencephalograph, magnetic resonance imaging, and tilt-table studies.

PATIENT TEACHING

Teach the patient ways to control dizziness. If he's hyperventilating, have him breathe and rebreathe into his cupped hands or a paper bag. If he experiences dizziness in an upright position, tell him to lie down and rest and then to rise slowly. Advise the patient with carotid sinus hypersensitivity to avoid wearing garments that fit tightly at the neck. Instruct the patient who risks a TIA from vertebrobasilar insufficiency to turn his body instead of sharply turning his head to one side.

Dysarthria

Dysarthria, poorly articulated speech, is characterized by slurring and labored, irregular rhythm. It may be accompanied by nasal voice tone caused by palate weakness. Whether it occurs abruptly or gradually, dysarthria is usually evident in ordinary conversation. It's confirmed by asking the pa-

tient to produce a few simple sounds and words, such as "ba," "sh," and "cat." However, dysarthria is occasionally confused with aphasia, loss of the ability to produce or comprehend speech.

Dysarthria results from damage to the brain stem that affects cranial nerves IX, X, or XII. Degenerative neurologic disorders and cerebellar disorders commonly cause dysarthria. In fact, dysarthria is a chief sign of olivopontocerebellar degeneration. It may also result from ill-fitting dentures.

Act now If the patient displays dysarthria, ask him about associated difficulty swallowing. Then determine respiratory rate and depth. Measure vital capacity with a Wright respirometer, if available. Assess blood pressure and heart rate. Usually, tachycardia, slightly increased blood pressure, and shortness of breath are early signs of respiratory muscle weakness.

Ensure a patent airway. Place the patient in Fowler's position and suction him if necessary. Administer oxygen, and keep emergency resuscitation equipment nearby. Anticipate intubation and mechanical ventilation in progressive respiratory muscle weakness. Withhold oral fluids in the patient with associated dysphagia.

If dysarthria isn't accompanied by respiratory muscle weakness and dysphagia, continue to assess for other neurologic deficits. Compare muscle strength and tone in the limbs. Then evaluate tactile sensation. Ask the patient about numbness or tingling. Test deep tendon reflexes (DTRs), and note gait ataxia. (See *Documenting deep tendon reflexes.*) Assess cerebellar function by observing rapid alternating movement, which should be smooth and coordinated. Next, test visual fields and ask about double vision. Check for signs of facial weakness, such as ptosis. Finally, determine level of consciousness (LOC) and mental status.

ASSESSMENT
History

Obtain a history of the condition. When did it begin? Has it gotten better? Ask if dysarthria worsens during the day. Then obtain a drug and alcohol history. Also, ask about a history of seizures.

Physical examination

Explore dysarthria completely. Speech improves with resolution of a transient ischemic attack, but not in a completed stroke.

DOCUMENTING DEEP TENDON REFLEXES

Record the patient's deep tendon reflex scores by drawing a stick figure and entering the grades on this scale at the proper location. The figure shown here indicates hypoactive deep tendon reflexes in the legs; other reflexes are normal.

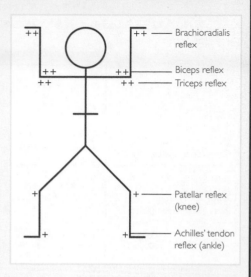

- Brachioradialis reflex
- Biceps reflex
- Triceps reflex
- Patellar reflex (knee)
- Achilles' tendon reflex (ankle)

Key:
0	= absent
+	= hypoactive (diminished)
++	= normal
+++	= brisk (increased)
++++	= hyperactive (clonus may be present)

Observe dentures for a proper fit. Ask the patient to produce a few simple sounds and words. Compare muscle strength and tone in the limbs on one side of the body with the other. Assess the patient's tactile sense, DTRs, and note gait ataxia. Assess cerebellar function, test visual fields, and ask about the presence of double vision. Check for signs of facial weakness. Evaluate LOC and mental status.

Pediatric pointers

Dysarthria in children usually results from brain stem glioma, a slow-growing tumor that primarily affects children. It may also result from cerebral palsy.

Dysarthria may be difficult to detect, especially in an infant or a young child who hasn't perfected speech. Be sure to look for other neurologic deficits, too. Encourage speech in a child with dysarthria; a child's potential for rehabilitation is typically greater than an adult's.

MEDICAL CAUSES

See *Dysarthria: Causes and associated findings,* pages 114 and 115.
- *Alcoholic cerebellar degeneration.* Alcoholic cerebellar degeneration commonly causes chronic, progressive dysarthria along

with ataxia, diplopia, ophthalmoplegia, hypotension, and altered mental status.
- *Amyotrophic lateral sclerosis (ALS).* Dysarthria occurs when ALS affects the bulbar nuclei; it may worsen as the disease progresses. Other signs and symptoms include dysphagia; difficulty breathing; muscle atrophy and weakness, especially of the hands and feet; fasciculations; spasticity; hyperactive DTRs in the legs; and occasionally excessive drooling. Progressive bulbar palsy may cause crying spells or inappropriate laughter.
- *Basilar artery insufficiency.* Basilar artery insufficiency causes random, brief episodes of bilateral brain stem dysfunction, resulting in dysarthria. Accompanying it are diplopia, vertigo, facial numbness, ataxia, paresis, and visual field loss, all of which last for minutes to hours.
- *Botulism.* The hallmark of botulism is acute cranial nerve dysfunction causing dysarthria, dysphagia, diplopia, and ptosis. Early findings include dry mouth, sore throat, weakness, vomiting, and diarrhea. Later, descending weakness or paralysis of muscles in the extremities and trunk causes hyporeflexia and dyspnea.
- *Manganese poisoning.* Chronic manganese poisoning causes progressive dys-

DYSARTHRIA:
CAUSES AND ASSOCIATED FINDINGS

MAJOR ASSOCIATED SIGNS AND SYMPTOMS

COMMON CAUSES	Aphasia	Ataxia	Bradykinesia	Diplopia	Drooling	Dysphagia	Dyspnea	Fasciculations	Gait, propulsive	Hyperreflexia	Hypotension	Level of consciousness, decreased
Alcoholic cerebellar degeneration		●		●							●	●
Amyotrophic lateral sclerosis					●	●	●	●		●		
Basilar artery insufficiency		●		●								
Botulism				●		●	●					
Manganese poisoning					●				●			●
Mercury poisoning		●										●
Multiple sclerosis		●		●		●				●		
Myasthenia gravis				●	●	●	●					
Olivopontocerebellar degeneration		●										
Parkinson's disease			●		●	●			●			
Shy-Drager syndrome		●	●								●	
Stroke (brain stem)				●	●	●	●					●
Stroke (cerebral)	●				●	●				●		

arthria accompanied by weakness, fatigue, confusion, hallucinations, drooling, hand tremors, limb stiffness, spasticity, gross rhythmic movements of the trunk and head, and propulsive gait.

● *Mercury poisoning.* Chronic mercury poisoning also causes progressive dysarthria accompanied by weakness, fatigue, depression, lethargy, irritability, confusion, ataxia, and tremors.

● *Multiple sclerosis.* When demyelination affects the brain stem and cerebellum, the patient displays dysarthria accompanied by nystagmus, blurred or double vision, dysphagia, ataxia, and intention tremor. Exacerbations and remissions of these signs and symptoms are common. Other findings include paresthesia, spasticity, intention tremor, hyperreflexia, muscle weakness or paralysis, constipation, emotional lability, and urinary frequency, urgency, and incontinence.

● *Myasthenia gravis.* Myasthenia gravis is a neuromuscular disorder that causes dysarthria associated with a nasal voice tone. Typically, the dysarthria worsens during the day

	Masklike facies	Muscle atrophy	Muscle weakness	Ptosis	Spasticity	Tremor	Vertigo	Visual field deficits
		●	●		●			
			●				●	●
			●	●				
			●		●	●		
			●			●		
			●		●	●		
			●	●				
						●		
	●		●			●		
	●							
					●	●		
					●	●		

and may temporarily improve with short rest periods. Other findings include dysphagia, drooling, facial weakness, diplopia, ptosis, dyspnea, and muscle weakness.

- *Olivopontocerebellar degeneration.* Dysarthria, a major sign, accompanies cerebellar ataxia and spasticity.
- *Parkinson's disease.* Parkinson's disease produces dysarthria and a monotone voice. It also produces muscle rigidity, bradykinesia, involuntary tremor usually beginning in the fingers, difficulty in walking, muscle weakness, and stooped posture. Other find-

ings include masklike facies, dysphagia, and occasionally drooling.

- *Shy-Drager syndrome.* Marked by chronic orthostatic hypotension, Shy-Drager syndrome eventually causes dysarthria as well as cerebellar ataxia, bradykinesia, masklike facies, dementia, impotence and, possibly, stooped posture and incontinence.
- *Stroke (brain stem).* Brain stem stroke is characterized by bulbar palsy, resulting in the triad of dysarthria, dysphonia, and dysphagia. The dysarthria is most severe at onset; it may lessen or disappear with rehabilitation and training. Other findings include facial weakness, diplopia, hemiparesis, spasticity, drooling, dyspnea, and decreased LOC.
- *Stroke (cerebral).* A massive bilateral stroke causes pseudobulbar palsy. Bilateral weakness produces dysarthria that's most severe at onset. This sign is accompanied by dysphagia, drooling, dysphonia, bilateral hemianopsia, and aphasia. Sensory loss, spasticity, and hyperreflexia may also occur.

OTHER CAUSES

- *Drugs.* Dysarthria can occur when anticonvulsant dosage is too high. Ingestion of large doses of barbiturates may also cause dysarthria.

NURSING CONSIDERATIONS

Encourage the patient with dysarthria to speak slowly so that he can be understood. Give him time to express himself, and encourage him to use gestures. Dysarthria usually requires consultation with a speech pathologist.

PATIENT TEACHING

Instruct the patient and his family about communication techniques. Encourage the patient to express his feelings. Provide guidelines on foods or liquids that should be avoided due to risk for aspiration. Refer the patient to a speech therapist.

Dysphagia

Dysphagia — difficulty swallowing — is a common symptom that's usually easy to localize. It may be constant or intermittent and is classified by the phase of swallowing it affects. (See *Classifying dysphagia,* page 116.)

Classifying dysphagia

Because swallowing occurs in three distinct phases, dysphagia can be classified by the phase that it affects. Each phase suggests a specific pathology for dysphagia.

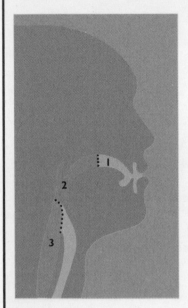

Phase 1
Swallowing begins in the *transfer phase* with chewing and moistening of food with saliva. The tongue presses against the hard palate to transfer the chewed food to the back of the throat; cranial nerve V then stimulates the swallowing reflex. Phase 1 dysphagia typically results from a neuromuscular disorder.

Phase 2
In the *transport phase*, the soft palate closes against the pharyngeal wall to prevent nasal regurgitation. At the same time, the larynx rises and the vocal cords close to keep food out of the lungs; breathing stops momentarily as the throat muscles constrict to move food into the esophagus. Phase 2 dysphagia usually indicates spasm or cancer.

Phase 3
Peristalsis and gravity work together in the *entrance phase* to move food through the esophageal sphincter and into the stomach. Phase 3 dysphagia results from lower esophageal narrowing by diverticula, esophagitis, and other disorders.

Among the factors that interfere with swallowing are severe pain, obstruction, abnormal peristalsis, impaired gag reflex, and excessive, scanty, or thick oral secretions.

Dysphagia is the most common—and sometimes the only—symptom of esophageal disorders. However, it may also result from oropharyngeal, respiratory, neurologic, and collagen disorders or from the effects of toxins and treatments. Dysphagia increases the risk of choking and aspiration and may lead to malnutrition and dehydration.

Act now *If the patient suddenly complains of dysphagia and displays signs of respiratory distress, such as dyspnea and stridor, suspect an airway obstruction and quickly perform abdominal thrusts. Prepare to administer oxygen by mask or nasal cannula, or to assist with endotracheal intubation.*

ASSESSMENT
History
If the patient's dysphagia doesn't suggest airway obstruction, begin a health history. Ask whether swallowing is painful and if so, is the pain constant or intermittent? Have the patient point to the location of the most intense dysphagia. Does eating alleviate or aggravate the symptom? Are solids or liquids more difficult to swallow? If the answer is liquids, ask if hot, cold, and lukewarm fluids affect him differently. Does the symptom disappear after he tries to swallow a few times? Is swallowing easier if he changes position? Ask if he has recently experienced vomiting, regurgitation, weight loss, anorexia, hoarseness, dyspnea, or a cough.

Physical examination
To evaluate the patient's swallowing reflex, place your finger along his thyroid notch and instruct him to swallow. If you feel his larynx rise, the reflex is intact. Next, have him cough to assess his cough reflex. Check his gag reflex if you're sure he has a good swallow or cough reflex. Listen closely to his speech for signs of muscle weakness. Does he have aphasia or dysarthria? Is his voice

nasal, hoarse, or breathy? Assess the patient's mouth carefully. Check for dry mucous membranes and thick, sticky secretions. Observe for tongue and facial weakness and obvious obstructions (for example, enlarged tonsils). Assess the patient for disorientation, which may make him neglect to swallow.

Pediatric pointers
In looking for dysphagia in an infant or a small child, be sure to pay close attention to his sucking and swallowing ability. Coughing, choking, or regurgitation during feeding suggests dysphagia.

Corrosive esophagitis and esophageal obstruction by a foreign body are more common causes of dysphagia in children than in adults. However, dysphagia may also result from congenital anomalies, such as annular stenosis, dysphagia lusoria, and esophageal atresia.

Geriatric pointers
In patients older than age 50, dysphagia is commonly the presenting complaint in cases of head or neck cancer. The incidence of such cancers increases markedly in this age-group.

MEDICAL CAUSES
● *Achalasia.* Most common in patients ages 20 to 40, achalasia produces phase 3 dysphagia for solids and liquids. The dysphagia develops gradually and may be precipitated or exacerbated by stress. Occasionally, it's preceded by esophageal colic. Regurgitation of undigested food, especially at night, may cause wheezing, coughing, or choking as well as halitosis. Weight loss, cachexia, hematemesis and, possibly, heartburn are late findings.

● *Airway obstruction.* Life-threatening upper airway obstruction is marked by signs of respiratory distress, such as crowing and stridor. Phase 2 dysphagia occurs with gagging and dysphonia. When hemorrhage obstructs the trachea, dysphagia is usually painless and rapid in onset. When inflammation causes the obstruction, dysphagia may be painful and develop slowly.

● *Amyotrophic lateral sclerosis (ALS).* Besides dysphagia, ALS causes muscle weakness and atrophy, fasciculations, dysarthria, dyspnea, shallow respirations, tachypnea, slurred speech, hyperactive deep tendon reflexes, and emotional lability.

● *Botulism.* Botulism causes phase 1 dysphagia and dysuria, usually within 36 hours of toxin ingestion. Other early findings include blurred or double vision, dry mouth, sore throat, nausea, vomiting, and diarrhea. Symmetrical descending weakness or paralysis occurs gradually.

● *Bulbar paralysis.* Phase 1 dysphagia occurs along with drooling, difficulty chewing, dysarthria, and nasal regurgitation. Dysphagia for both solids and liquids is painful and progressive. Accompanying features may include arm and leg spasticity, hyperreflexia, and emotional lability.

● *Dysphagia lusoria.* Dysphagia lusoria is caused by compression of the esophagus by a congenital vascular abnormality (usually an aberrant right subclavian artery arising from the left side of the aortic arch). Phase 3 dysphagia symptoms may occur in childhood or develop later from changes in the aberrant vessel such as arteriosclerosis.

● *Esophageal cancer.* Phases 2 and 3 dysphagia is the earliest and most common symptom of esophageal cancer. Typically, this painless, progressive symptom is accompanied by rapid weight loss. As the cancer advances, dysphagia becomes painful and constant. In addition, the patient complains of steady chest pain, cough with hemoptysis, hoarseness, and sore throat. He may also develop nausea and vomiting, fever, hiccups, hematemesis, melena, and halitosis.

● *Esophageal compression (external).* Usually caused by a dilated carotid or aortic aneurysm, external esophageal compression—a rare condition—causes phase 3 dysphagia as the primary symptom. Other features depend on the cause of the compression.

● *Esophageal diverticulum.* Esophageal diverticulum causes phase 3 dysphagia when the enlarged diverticulum obstructs the esophagus. Associated signs and symptoms include food regurgitation, chronic cough, hoarseness, chest pain, and halitosis.

● *Esophageal leiomyoma.* A relatively rare benign tumor, esophageal leiomyoma may cause phase 3 dysphagia along with retrosternal pain or discomfort. In addition, the patient experiences weight loss and a feeling of fullness.

● *Esophageal obstruction by foreign body.* Sudden onset of phase 2 or 3 dysphagia, gagging, coughing, and esophageal pain characterize esophageal obstruction by foreign body—a potentially life-threatening condition. Dyspnea may occur if the obstruction compresses the trachea.

● *Esophageal spasm.* The most striking symptoms of esophageal spasm are phase 2 dysphagia for solids and liquids and dull or squeezing substernal chest pain. The pain may last up to an hour and may radiate to the neck, arm, back, or jaw; however, it may be relieved by drinking a glass of water. Bradycardia may also occur.

● *Esophageal stricture.* Usually caused by a chemical ingestion or scar tissue, esophageal stricture causes phase 3 dysphagia. Drooling, tachypnea, and gagging may also be evident.

● *Esophagitis.* Corrosive esophagitis, resulting from ingestion of alkalies or acids, causes severe phase 3 dysphagia. Accompanying it are marked salivation, hematemesis, tachypnea, fever, and intense pain in the mouth and anterior chest that's aggravated by swallowing. Signs of shock, such as hypotension and tachycardia, may also occur.

Candidal esophagitis causes phase 2 dysphagia, sore throat and, possibly, retrosternal pain on swallowing. With reflux esophagitis, phase 3 dysphagia is a late symptom that usually accompanies stricture development. The patient complains of heartburn, which is aggravated by strenuous exercise, bending over, or lying down and is relieved by sitting up or taking an antacid.

Other features include regurgitation; frequent, effortless vomiting; a dry, nocturnal cough; and substernal chest pain that may mimic angina pectoris. If the esophagus ulcerates, signs of bleeding, such as melena and hematemesis, may occur along with weakness and fatigue.

● *Gastric carcinoma.* Infiltration of the cardia or esophagus by gastric carcinoma causes phase 3 dysphagia along with nausea, vomiting, and pain that may radiate to the neck, back, or retrosternum. In addition, perforation causes massive bleeding with coffee-ground vomitus or melena.

● *Hypocalcemia.* Although tetany is its primary sign, severe hypocalcemia may cause neuromuscular irritability, producing phase 1 dysphagia associated with numbness and tingling in the nose, ears, fingertips, and toes and around the mouth. Carpopedal spasms, muscle twitching, and laryngeal spasms may also occur.

● *Laryngeal cancer (extrinsic).* Phase 2 dysphagia and dyspnea develop late in extrinsic laryngeal cancer. Accompanying features include muffled voice, stridor, pain, halitosis, weight loss, ipsilateral otalgia, chronic cough, and cachexia. Palpation reveals enlarged cervical nodes.

● *Laryngeal nerve damage.* Commonly the result of radical neck surgery, superior laryngeal nerve damage may produce painless phase 2 dysphagia.

● *Lead poisoning.* Painless, progressive dysphagia may result from lead poisoning. Related findings include a lead line on the gums, metallic taste, papilledema, ocular palsy, footdrop or wristdrop, and signs of hemolytic anemia, such as abdominal pain and fever. The patient may be depressed and display severe mental impairment and seizures.

● *Lower esophageal ring.* Narrowing of the lower esophagus can cause an attack of phase 3 dysphagia that may recur several weeks or months later. During the attack, the patient complains of a foreign body in the lower esophagus, a sensation that may be relieved by drinking water or vomiting. Esophageal rupture produces severe lower chest pain followed by a feeling of something giving way.

● *Mediastinitis.* Varying with the extent of esophageal perforation, mediastinitis can cause insidious or rapid onset of phase 3 dysphagia. The patient displays chills, fever, and severe retrosternal chest pain that may radiate to the epigastrium, back, or shoulder. The pain may be aggravated by breathing, coughing, or sneezing. Other findings include tachycardia, subcutaneous crepitation in the suprasternal notch, and falling blood pressure.

● *Myasthenia gravis.* Fatigue and progressive muscle weakness characterize myasthenia gravis and account for painless phase 1 dysphagia and possibly choking. Typically, dysphagia follows ptosis and diplopia. Other features include masklike facies, nasal voice, frequent nasal regurgitation, and head bobbing. Shallow respirations and dyspnea may occur with respiratory muscle weakness. Signs and symptoms worsen during menses and with exposure to stress, cold, or infection.

● *Oral cavity tumor.* Painful phase 1 dysphagia develops along with hoarseness and ulcerating lesions.

● *Parkinson's disease.* Usually a late symptom, phase 1 dysphagia is painless but progressive and may cause choking. Other signs and symptoms include bradykinesia, tremors, muscle rigidity, dysarthria, masklike facies, muffled voice, increased salivation and lacrimation, constipation, stooped posture, propulsive gait, incontinence, and sexual dysfunction.

- **Pharyngitis (chronic).** Chronic pharyngitis causes painful phase 2 dysphagia for solids and liquids. Rarely serious, it's accompanied by a dry, sore throat; a cough; and thick mucus in the throat.
- **Plummer-Vinson syndrome.** Plummer-Vinson syndrome causes phase 3 dysphagia for solids in some females with severe iron deficiency anemia. Related features include upper esophageal pain; atrophy of the oral or pharyngeal mucous membranes; tooth loss; smooth, red, sore tongue; dry mouth; chills; inflamed lips; spoon-shaped nails; pallor; and splenomegaly.
- **Progressive systemic sclerosis.** Typically, dysphagia is preceded by Raynaud's phenomenon in patients with progressive systemic sclerosis. The dysphagia may be mild at first and described as a feeling of food sticking behind the breastbone. The patient also complains of heartburn after meals that's aggravated by lying down. As the disease progresses, dysphagia worsens until only liquids can be swallowed. It may be accompanied by other GI effects, including weight loss, abdominal distention, diarrhea, and malodorous, floating stools. Other characteristic late features include joint pain and stiffness and thickening of the skin that progresses to taut, shiny skin. The patient usually has masklike facies.
- **Rabies.** Severe phase 2 dysphagia for liquids results from painful pharyngeal muscle spasms occurring late in rabies — a rare, life-threatening disorder. In fact, the patient may become dehydrated and possibly apneic. Dysphagia also causes drooling, and in 50% of patients it's responsible for hydrophobia. Eventually, rabies causes progressive flaccid paralysis that leads to peripheral vascular collapse, coma, and death.
- **Syphilis.** Rarely, tertiary-stage syphilis causes ulceration and stricture of the upper esophagus, resulting in phase 3 dysphagia. The dysphagia may be accompanied by regurgitation after meals and heartburn that's aggravated by lying down or bending over.
- **Systemic lupus erythematosus (SLE).** SLE may cause progressive phase 2 dysphagia. However, its primary signs and symptoms include nondeforming arthritis, a characteristic butterfly rash, and photosensitivity.
- **Tetanus.** Phase 1 dysphagia usually develops about 1 week after the patient receives a puncture wound. Other characteristics include marked muscle hypertonicity, hyperactive deep tendon reflexes, tachycardia, diaphoresis, drooling, and low-grade fever. Painful, involuntary muscle spasms account for lockjaw (trismus), risus sardonicus, opisthotonos, boardlike abdominal rigidity, and intermittent tonic seizures.

OTHER CAUSES

- **Medical procedures.** Recent tracheostomy or repeated or prolonged intubation may cause temporary dysphagia.
- **Radiation therapy.** When directed against oral cancer, this therapy may cause scant salivation and temporary dysphagia.

NURSING CONSIDERATIONS

Stimulate salivation by talking with the patient about food, adding a lemon slice or dill pickle to his tray, and providing mouth care before and after meals. Moisten his food with a little liquid if salivation is decreased. Administer an anticholinergic or antiemetic to control excess salivation. If he has a weak or absent cough reflex, begin tube feedings or esophageal drips of special formulas.

Consult with the dietitian to select foods with distinct temperatures and textures. The patient should avoid sticky foods, such as bananas and peanut butter. If the patient has mucous production, avoid uncooked milk products. Consult a therapist to assess the patient for his aspiration risk and for swallowing exercises to possibly help decrease his risk. At mealtimes, take measures to minimize the patient's risk of choking and aspiration. Place the patient in an upright position, and have him flex his neck forward slightly and keep his chin at midline. Instruct the patient to swallow multiple times before taking the next bite or sip. Separate solids from liquids, which are harder to swallow.

Prepare the patient for diagnostic tests including endoscopy, esophageal manometry, esophagography, and esophageal acidity test to pinpoint the cause of dysphagia.

PATIENT TEACHING

Advise the patient to consume foods that are easy to swallow. Explain measures he can take to reduce the risk of choking and aspiration, such as positioning during eating and after the meal has been consumed. Encourage the patient's family or caregiver to take a first aid or cardiopulmonary course that provides techniques for managing choking.

Dyspnea

Typically a symptom of cardiopulmonary dysfunction, dyspnea is the sensation of difficult or uncomfortable breathing. It's usually reported as shortness of breath. Its severity varies greatly and is usually unrelated to the severity of the underlying cause. Dyspnea may arise suddenly or slowly and may subside rapidly or persist for years.

Most people normally experience dyspnea when they exert themselves, and its severity depends on their physical condition. In a healthy person, dyspnea is quickly relieved by rest. Pathologic causes of dyspnea include pulmonary, cardiac, neuromuscular, and allergic disorders. It may also be caused by anxiety.

Act now *If a patient complains of shortness of breath, quickly look for signs of respiratory distress, such as tachypnea, cyanosis, restlessness, and accessory muscle use. Prepare to administer oxygen by nasal cannula, mask, or endotracheal tube. Ensure patent I.V. access, and begin cardiac monitoring and oxygen saturation monitoring to detect arrhythmias and low oxygen saturation, respectively. Expect to insert a chest tube for severe pneumothorax and to administer continuous positive airway pressure or apply rotating tourniquets for pulmonary edema.*

ASSESSMENT
History
If the patient can answer questions without increasing his distress, take a complete history. Ask if the shortness of breath began suddenly or gradually. Is it constant or intermittent? Does it occur during activity or while at rest? If the patient has had dyspneic attacks before, ask if they're increasing in severity. Can he identify what aggravates or alleviates these attacks? Does he have a productive or nonproductive cough or chest pain? Ask about recent trauma, and note a history of upper respiratory tract infection, deep vein phlebitis, or other disorders. Ask the patient if he smokes or is exposed to toxic fumes or irritants on the job. Find out if he also has orthopnea, paroxysmal nocturnal dyspnea, or progressive fatigue.

Physical examination
During the physical examination, look for signs of chronic dyspnea such as accessory muscle hypertrophy (especially in the shoulders and neck). Also look for pursed-lip exhalation, clubbing, peripheral edema, barrel chest, diaphoresis, and jugular vein distention.

Check blood pressure and auscultate for crackles, abnormal heart sounds or rhythms, egophony, bronchophony, and whispered pectoriloquy. Finally, palpate the abdomen for hepatomegaly, and assess the patient for edema.

Pediatric pointers
Normally, an infant's respirations are abdominal, gradually changing to costal by age 7. Suspect dyspnea in an infant who breathes costally, in an older child who breathes abdominally, or in any child who uses his neck or shoulder muscles to help him breathe.

Both acute epiglottiditis and laryngotracheobronchitis (croup) can cause severe dyspnea in a child and may even lead to respiratory or cardiovascular collapse. Expect to administer oxygen, using a hood or cool mist tent.

Geriatric pointers
Older patients with dyspnea related to chronic illness may not be aware initially of a significant change in their breathing pattern.

MEDICAL CAUSES
See *Dyspnea: Causes and associated findings,* pages 122 to 125.
● *Acute respiratory distress syndrome (ARDS).* ARDS is a life-threatening form of noncardiogenic pulmonary edema that usually produces acute dyspnea as the first complaint. Progressive respiratory distress then develops with restlessness, anxiety, decreased mental acuity, tachycardia, and crackles and rhonchi in both lung fields. Other findings include cyanosis, tachypnea, motor dysfunction, and intercostal and suprasternal retractions. Severe ARDS can produce signs of shock, such as hypotension and cool, clammy skin.
● *Amyotrophic lateral sclerosis (ALS).* Also known as *Lou Gehrig disease,* ALS causes slow

onset of dyspnea that worsens with time. Other features include dysphagia, dysarthria, muscle weakness and atrophy, fasciculations, shallow respirations, tachypnea, and emotional lability.

● *Anemia.* Dyspnea usually develops gradually with anemia. Anemia commonly causes fatigue, weakness, and syncope; if severe, it may also cause tachycardia, tachypnea, restlessness, anxiety, and thirst.

● *Anthrax (inhalation).* Dyspnea is a symptom of the second stage of this inhalation anthrax, along with fever, stridor, and hypotension (the patient usually dies within 24 hours). Initial symptoms of this disorder, which are due to the inhalation of aerosolized spores (from infected animals or a result of bioterrorism) from the bacterium *Bacillus anthracis,* are flulike and include fever, chills, weakness, cough, and chest pain.

● *Aspiration of a foreign body.* Acute dyspnea marks aspiration of a foreign body — a life-threatening condition — along with paroxysmal intercostal, suprasternal, and substernal retractions. The patient may also display accessory muscle use, inspiratory stridor, tachypnea, decreased or absent breath sounds, possibly asymmetrical chest expansion, anxiety, cyanosis, diaphoresis, and hypotension.

● *Asthma.* Acute dyspneic attacks occur with this asthma — a chronic disorder — along with audible wheezing, dry cough, accessory muscle use, nasal flaring, intercostal and supraclavicular retractions, tachypnea, tachycardia, diaphoresis, prolonged expiration, flushing or cyanosis, and apprehension. Medications that block beta receptors can exacerbate asthma attacks.

● *Cardiac arrhythmia.* In a patient with arrhythmias, acute or gradual dyspnea can result from decreased cardiac output. The pulse rate may be rapid, slow, or irregular, with frequent premature or escape beats. Alternating pulse may be present. Other symptoms include palpitations, chest pain, diaphoresis, light-headedness, weakness, or vertigo.

● *Cor pulmonale.* Chronic dyspnea begins gradually with exertion and progressively worsens until it occurs even at rest. Underlying cardiac or pulmonary disease is usually present. The patient may have a chronic productive cough, wheezing, tachypnea, jugular vein distention, dependent edema, and he-patomegaly. He may also experience increasing fatigue, weakness, and light-headedness.

● *Emphysema.* Emphysema is a chronic disorder that gradually causes progressive exertional dyspnea. A history of smoking, an alpha$_1$-antitrypsin deficiency, or exposure to an occupational irritant usually accompanies barrel chest, accessory muscle hypertrophy, diminished breath sounds, anorexia, weight loss, malaise, peripheral cyanosis, tachypnea, pursed-lip breathing, prolonged expiration and, possibly, a chronic productive cough. Clubbing is a late sign.

● *Flail chest.* Sudden dyspnea results from multiple rib fractures and is accompanied by paradoxical chest movement, severe chest pain, hypotension, tachypnea, tachycardia, and cyanosis. Bruising and decreased or absent breath sounds occur over the affected side.

● *Guillain-Barré syndrome.* Usually following a fever and upper respiratory tract infection, Guillain-Barré syndrome causes slowly worsening dyspnea along with fatigue, ascending muscle weakness and, eventually, paralysis.

● *Heart failure.* Dyspnea usually develops gradually in patients with heart failure. Chronic paroxysmal nocturnal dyspnea, orthopnea, tachypnea, tachycardia, palpitations, ventricular gallop, fatigue, dependent peripheral edema, hepatomegaly, dry cough, weight gain, and loss of mental acuity may occur. With acute onset, heart failure may produce jugular vein distention, bibasilar rates, oliguria, and hypotension.

● *Inhalation injury.* Dyspnea may develop suddenly or gradually over several hours after inhalation of chemicals or hot gases. Increasing hoarseness, persistent cough, sooty or bloody sputum, and oropharyngeal edema may also be present. The patient may also exhibit thermal burns, singed nasal hairs, and orofacial burns as well as crackles, rhonchi, wheezing, and signs of respiratory distress.

● *Interstitial fibrosis.* Besides dyspnea, interstitial fibrosis causes chest pain, dry cough, crackles, weight loss and, possibly, cyanosis and pleural friction rub.

● *Lung cancer.* Dyspnea that develops slowly and progressively worsens occurs with late-stage lung cancer. Other findings include fever, hemoptysis, productive cough, wheezing, clubbing, chest pain, and pleural friction rub.

DYSPNEA:
CAUSES AND ASSOCIATED FINDINGS

MAJOR ASSOCIATED SIGNS AND SYMPTOMS

COMMON CAUSES	Accessory muscle use	Blood pressure decrease	Breath sounds, decreased	Chest pain	Cough, nonproductive	Cough, productive	Crackles	Cyanosis	Diaphoresis	Edema	Fasciculations	Fever	
Acute respiratory distress syndrome	●	●					●	●				●	
Amyotrophic lateral sclerosis											●		
Anemia													
Anthrax (inhalation)				●								●	
Aspiration of a foreign body	●	●	●		●			●	●				
Asthma	●				●			●	●				
Cardiac arrhythmia				●					●				
Cor pulmonale	●					●		●		●			
Emphysema	●		●		●								
Flail chest	●	●	●	●				●					
Guillain-Barré syndrome													
Heart failure	●	●			●					●			
Inhalation injury							●	●					
Interstitial fibrosis					●	●			●				
Lung cancer					●	●						●	
Myasthenia gravis													
Myocardial infarction		●		●					●				
Plague (*Yersinia pestis*)					●	●						●	
Pleural effusion			●	●								●	
Pneumonia			●	●		●	●	●	●			●	
Pneumothorax	●	●	●	●	●			●					

	Muscle weakness	Nausea	Jugular vein distention	Orthopnea	Stridor	Tachycardia	Tachypnea	Weight loss
						●	●	
	●						●	
	●					●	●	
					●			
						●	●	
						●	●	
						●		
				●			●	
						●	●	●
						●	●	
	●							
			●	●		●	●	
				●			●	
								●
								●
	●						●	
		●				●		
							●	
						●	●	
						●	●	
						●	●	

(continued)

● **Myasthenia gravis.** Myasthenia gravis is a neuromuscular disorder that causes bouts of dyspnea as the respiratory muscles weaken. With myasthenic crisis, acute respiratory distress may occur, with shallow respirations and tachypnea.

● **Myocardial infarction.** Sudden dyspnea occurs with crushing substernal chest pain that may radiate to the back, neck, jaw, and arms. Other signs and symptoms include nausea, vomiting, diaphoresis, vertigo, hypertension or hypotension, tachycardia, anxiety, and pale, cool, clammy skin.

● **Plague** (Yersinia pestis). Among the symptoms of the pneumonic form of plague are dyspnea, a productive cough, chest pain, tachypnea, hemoptysis, increasing respiratory distress, and cardiopulmonary insufficiency. The onset of this virulent infection is usually sudden and includes such signs and symptoms as chills, fever, headache, and myalgias. If untreated, plague is one of the most potentially lethal diseases known.

● **Pleural effusion.** Dyspnea develops slowly and becomes progressively worse with pleural effusion. Initial findings include a pleural friction rub accompanied by pleuritic pain that worsens with coughing or deep breathing. Other findings include dry cough; dullness on percussion; egophony, bronchophony, and whispered pectoriloquy; tachycardia; tachypnea; weight loss; and decreased chest motion, tactile fremitus, and decreased breath sounds. With infection, fever may occur.

● **Pneumonia.** Dyspnea occurs suddenly, usually accompanied by fever, shaking chills, pleuritic chest pain that worsens with deep inspiration, and a productive cough. Fatigue, headache, myalgia, anorexia, abdominal pain, crackles, rhonchi, tachycardia, tachypnea, cyanosis, decreased breath sounds, and diaphoresis may also occur.

● **Pneumothorax.** Pneumothorax is a life-threatening disorder that causes acute dyspnea unrelated to the severity of pain. Sudden, stabbing chest pain may radiate to the arms, face, back, or abdomen. Other signs and symptoms include anxiety, restlessness, dry cough, cyanosis, decreased vocal fremitus, tachypnea, tympany, decreased or absent breath sounds on the affected side, asymmetrical chest expansion, splinting, and accessory muscle use. In patients with tension pneumothorax, tracheal deviation occurs in addition to these typical findings. Decreased

MAJOR ASSOCIATED SIGNS AND SYMPTOMS

COMMON CAUSES	Accessory muscle use	Blood pressure decrease	Breath sounds, decreased	Chest pain	Cough, nonproductive	Cough, productive	Crackles	Cyanosis	Diaphoresis	Edema	Fasciculations	Fever
Poliomyelitis (bulbar)												●
Pulmonary edema	●	●			●	●	●	●	●			
Pulmonary embolism		●	●	●	●	●	●	●	●			●
Sepsis												●
Severe acute respiratory syndrome					●							●
Shock		●										
Tuberculosis						●	●		●			
Tularemia					●	●						●

blood pressure and tachycardia may also occur.

● *Poliomyelitis (bulbar).* Dyspnea develops gradually and progressively worsens. Additional signs and symptoms include fever, facial weakness, dysphasia, hypoactive deep tendon reflexes, decreased mental acuity, dysphagia, nasal regurgitation, and hypopnea.

● *Pulmonary edema.* Commonly preceded by signs of heart failure, such as jugular vein distention and orthopnea, pulmonary edema—a life-threatening disorder—causes acute dyspnea. Other features include tachycardia, tachypnea, crackles in both lung fields, a third heart sound (S_3 gallop), oliguria, thready pulse, hypotension, diaphoresis, cyanosis, and marked anxiety. The patient's cough may be dry or may produce copious amounts of pink, frothy sputum.

● *Pulmonary embolism.* Acute dyspnea that's usually accompanied by sudden pleuritic chest pain characterizes pulmonary embolism—a life-threatening disorder. Related findings include tachycardia, low-grade fever, tachypnea, nonproductive or productive cough with blood-tinged sputum, pleural friction rub, crackles, diffuse wheezing, dullness on percussion, decreased breath sounds, diaphoresis, restlessness, and acute anxiety. A massive embolism may cause signs of shock, such as hypotension and cool, clammy skin.

● *Sepsis.* Sepsis is a potentially fatal disorder that gradually causes dyspnea along with chills and sudden fever. As dyspnea worsens, it may be accompanied by tachycardia, tachypnea, restlessness, anxiety, decreased mental acuity, and warm, flushed, dry skin. Late findings include hypotension; oliguria; cool, clammy skin; and rapid, thready pulse.

● *Severe acute respiratory syndrome (SARS).* SARS is an acute infectious disease of unknown etiology; however, a novel coronavirus has been implicated as a possible cause. Although most cases have been re-

<table>

Muscle weakness	Nausea	Jugular vein distention	Orthopnea	Stridor	Tachycardia	Tachypnea	Weight loss
●							
		●	●		●	●	
					●	●	
					●	●	
					●	●	
							●

</table>

pepsia, palpitations on mild exertion, and dullness on percussion.

- *Tularemia.* Also known as *rabbit fever,* tularemia causes dyspnea along with fever, chills, headache, generalized myalgias, a nonproductive cough, pleuritic chest pain, and empyema.

NURSING CONSIDERATIONS

Monitor the dyspneic patient closely. Be as calm and reassuring as possible to reduce his anxiety, and help him into a comfortable position — usually high Fowler's or forward-leaning position. Support him with pillows, loosen his clothing, and administer oxygen if appropriate.

Prepare the patient for diagnostic studies, such as arterial blood gas analysis, chest X-rays, and pulmonary function tests. Administer a bronchodilator, an antiarrhythmic, a diuretic, and an analgesic, as needed, to dilate bronchioles, correct cardiac arrhythmias, promote fluid excretion, and relieve pain.

PATIENT TEACHING

Tell the patient that oxygen therapy isn't necessarily indicated for dyspnea. Encourage a patient with chronic dyspnea to pace his daily activities. Teach him about pursed-lip, diaphragmatic breathing and chest splinting. Instruct him to avoid chemical irritants, pollutants, and people with respiratory infections and discuss the importance of pneumococcal vaccination and influenza vaccination. Refer him to a respiratory therapist, as appropriate.

ported in Asia (China, Vietnam, Singapore, Thailand), cases have cropped up in Europe and North America. The incubation period is 2 to 7 days, and the illness generally begins with a fever (usually greater than 100.4° F [38° C]). Other symptoms include headache, malaise, a dry nonproductive cough, and dyspnea. The severity of the illness is highly variable, ranging from mild illness to pneumonia and, in some cases, progressing to respiratory failure and death.

- *Shock.* Dyspnea arises suddenly and worsens progressively in shock — a life-threatening disorder. Related findings include severe hypotension, tachypnea, tachycardia, decreased peripheral pulses, decreased mental acuity, restlessness, anxiety, and cool, clammy skin,

- *Tuberculosis.* Dyspnea commonly occurs with chest pain, crackles, and productive cough. Other findings are night sweats, fever, anorexia and weight loss, vague dys-

Edema, facial

Facial edema refers to either localized swelling—around the eyes, for example—or more generalized facial swelling that may extend to the neck and upper arms. Occasionally painful, this sign may develop gradually or abruptly. Sometimes it precedes onset of peripheral or generalized edema. Mild edema may be difficult to detect; the patient or someone who's familiar with his appearance may report it before it's noticed during assessment.

Facial edema results from disruption of the hydrostatic and osmotic pressures that govern fluid movement between the arteries, veins, and lymphatics. (See *Understanding fluid balance*.) It may result from venous, inflammatory, and certain systemic disorders; trauma; allergy; malnutrition; or the effects of certain drugs, tests, and treatments.

Act now *If the patient has facial edema associated with burns or if he reports recent exposure to an allergen, immediately evaluate his respiratory status: Edema may also affect his upper airway, causing life-threatening obstruction. If you detect audible wheezing, inspiratory stridor, or other signs of respiratory distress, administer epinephrine. For patients in severe distress—with absent breath sounds and cyanosis—tracheal intubation, cricothyroidotomy, or tracheotomy may be required. Always administer oxygen.*

ASSESSMENT
History
If the patient isn't in severe distress, take his health history. Ask if facial edema developed suddenly or gradually. Is it more prominent in early morning, or does it worsen throughout the day? Has the patient gained weight? If so, how much and over what length of time? Has he noticed a change in his urine color or output? In his appetite? Take a drug history and ask about recent facial trauma and dental procedures.

Physical examination
Begin the physical examination by characterizing the edema. Is it localized and distributed over one part of the face, or does it affect the entire face or other parts of the body? Determine if the edema is pitting or nonpitting, and grade its severity. (See *Edema: Pitting or nonpitting?* page 128.) Next, take vital signs, and assess neurologic status. Examine the oral cavity to evaluate dental hygiene and look for signs of infection. Visualize the oropharynx and look for any soft-tissue swelling.

Pediatric pointers
Normally, periorbital tissue pressure is lower in a child than in an adult. As a result, children are more likely to develop periorbital edema. In fact, periorbital edema is more common than peripheral edema in children with such disorders as heart failure and acute glomerulonephritis. Pertussis may also cause periorbital edema.

MEDICAL CAUSES
● *Abscess (periodontal).* Periodontal abscess is an infection that usually results from poor oral hygiene and is commonly caused by anaerobic organisms. It can cause edema of the side of the face, pain, warmth, erythema,

UNDERSTANDING FLUID BALANCE

Normally, fluid moves freely between the interstitial and intravascular spaces to maintain homeostasis. Four basic pressures control fluid shifts across the capillary membrane that separates these spaces:
◆ capillary hydrostatic pressure — the internal fluid pressure on the capillary membrane
◆ interstitial fluid pressure — the external fluid pressure on the capillary membrane
◆ osmotic pressure — the fluid-attracting pressure from protein concentration within the capillary
◆ interstitial osmotic pressure — the fluid-attracting pressure from protein concentration outside the capillary.

In homeostasis, capillary hydrostatic pressure is greater than plasma osmotic pressure at the capillary's arterial end, forcing fluid out of the capillary. The pressures are reversed at the capillary's venous end — plasma osmotic pressure is greater than capillary hydrostatic pressure — thereby drawing fluid into the capillary. The lymphatic system transports excess interstitial fluid back to the intravascular space.

Edema results when the balance is upset by increased capillary permeability, lymphatic obstruction, persistently increased capillary hydrostatic pressure, decreased plasma osmotic or interstitial fluid pressure, or dilation of precapillary sphincters.

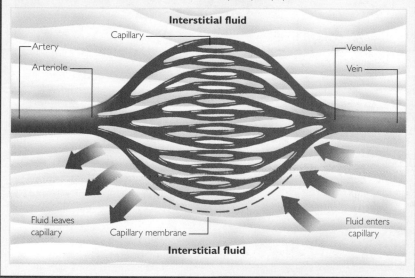

and purulent discharge around the affected tooth.
● *Abscess (peritonsillar).* Peritonsillar abscess is a complication of tonsillitis that may cause unilateral facial edema. Other key signs and symptoms include severe throat pain, neck swelling, drooling, cervical adenopathy, fever, chills, and malaise.
● *Allergic reaction.* Facial edema may characterize both local allergic reactions and anaphylaxis. With life-threatening anaphylaxis, angioneurotic facial edema may occur with urticaria and flushing. (See *Recognizing angioneurotic edema,* page 129.) Airway edema

causes hoarseness, stridor, and bronchospasm with dyspnea and tachypnea. Signs of shock, such as hypotension and cool, clammy skin, may also occur. A localized reaction produces facial edema, erythema, and urticaria.
● *Cavernous sinus thrombosis.* Cavernous sinus thrombosis is a rare but serious disorder that may begin with unilateral edema that quickly progresses to bilateral edema of the forehead, base of the nose, and eyelids. It may also produce chills, fever, headache, nausea, lethargy, exophthalmos, and eye pain.

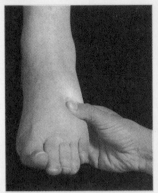
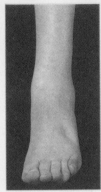
● *Chalazion.* A chalazion causes localized swelling and tenderness of the affected eyelid, accompanied by a small red lump on the conjunctival surface.

● *Conjunctivitis.* Conjunctivitis causes eyelid edema, excessive tearing, and itchy, burning eyes. Inspection reveals a thick purulent discharge, crusty eyelids, and conjunctival injection. Corneal involvement causes photophobia and pain.

● *Corneal ulcers (fungal).* Accompanying red, edematous eyelids in corneal ulcers are conjunctival injection, intense pain, photophobia, and severely impaired visual acuity. Copious, purulent eye discharge makes eyelids sticky and crusted. The characteristic dense, central ulcer grows slowly, is whitish gray, and is surrounded by progressively clearer rings.

● *Dacryoadenitis.* Severe periorbital swelling characterizes dacryoadenitis, which may also cause conjunctival injection, purulent discharge, and temporal pain.

● *Dacryocystitis.* Lacrimal sac inflammation causes prominent eyelid edema and constant tearing. With acute cases, pain and tenderness near the lacrimal sac accompany purulent discharge.

● *Dermatomyositis.* Periorbital edema and heliotropic rash develop gradually in dermatomyositis—a rare disease. An itchy, lilac-colored rash appears on the bridge of the nose, cheeks, and forehead. Localized or diffuse erythema, eye pain, and fever may also occur.

● *Facial burns.* Burns may cause extensive edema that impairs respiration. Additional findings include singed nasal hairs, red mucosa, sooty sputum, and signs of respiratory distress, such as inspiratory stridor.

● *Facial trauma.* The extent of edema varies with the type of injury. For example, a contusion may cause localized edema, whereas a nasal or maxillary fracture causes more generalized edema. Associated symptoms also depend on the type of injury.

● *Frontal sinus cancer.* Frontal sinus cancer is a rare form of cancer that causes cheek edema on the affected side, reddened skin over the sinus, unilateral nasal bleeding or discharge, and exophthalmos. Pain over the forehead and unilateral hypoesthesia or anesthesia may occur later.

● *Herpes zoster ophthalmicus (shingles).* With herpes zoster ophthalmicus, edematous and red eyelids are usually accompanied by excessive tearing and a serous discharge. Severe unilateral facial pain may occur several days before vesicles erupt.

● *Hordeolum (stye).* Typically, localized eyelid edema, erythema, and pain occur with a hordeolum.

● *Malnutrition.* Severe malnutrition causes facial edema followed by swelling of the feet and legs. Associated signs and symptoms include muscle atrophy and weakness; anorexia; diarrhea; lethargy; dry, wrinkled skin; sparse, brittle, easily plucked hair; and slowed pulse and respiratory rates.

- *Melkersson's syndrome.* Facial edema (especially of the lips), facial paralysis, and folds in the tongue are the three characteristic signs of Melkersson's syndrome.
- *Myxedema.* Myxedema eventually causes generalized facial edema, waxy dry skin, hair loss or coarsening, and other signs of hypothyroidism.
- *Nephrotic syndrome.* Commonly the first sign of nephrotic syndrome, periorbital edema precedes dependent and abdominal edema. Associated findings include weight gain, nausea, anorexia, lethargy, fatigue, and pallor.
- *Orbital cellulitis.* Sudden onset of periorbital edema marks orbital cellulitis. It may be accompanied by a unilateral purulent discharge, hyperemia, exophthalmos, conjunctival injection, impaired extraocular movements, fever, and extreme orbital pain.
- *Osteomyelitis.* When osteomyelitis affects the frontal bone, it may cause forehead edema as well as fever, chills, headache, and cool, pallid skin.
- *Preeclampsia.* Edema of the face, hands, and ankles is an early sign of preeclampsia — a disorder of pregnancy. Other characteristics include excessive weight gain, severe headache, blurred vision, hypertension, and midepigastric pain.
- *Rhinitis (allergic).* With rhinitis, red and edematous eyelids are accompanied by paroxysmal sneezing, itchy nose and eyes, and profuse, watery rhinorrhea. The patient may also develop nasal congestion, excessive tearing, headache, sinus pain, and sometimes malaise and fever.
- *Sinusitis.* Frontal sinusitis causes edema of the forehead and eyelids. Maxillary sinusitis produces edema in the maxillary area as well as malaise, gingival swelling, and trismus. Both types are also accompanied by facial pain, fever, nasal congestion, purulent nasal discharge, and red, swollen nasal mucosa.
- *Superior vena cava syndrome.* Superior vena cava syndrome gradually produces facial and neck edema accompanied by thoracic or jugular vein distention. It also causes central nervous system symptoms, such as headache, vision disturbances, and vertigo.

RECOGNIZING ANGIONEUROTIC EDEMA

Most dramatic in the lips, eyelids, and tongue, angioneurotic edema commonly results from an allergic reaction. It's characterized by rapid onset of painless, non-pitting, subcutaneous swelling that usually resolves in 1 to 2 days. This type of edema may also involve the hands, feet, genitalia, and viscera; laryngeal edema may cause life-threatening airway obstruction.

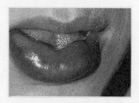

- *Trachoma.* With trachoma, edema affects the eyelid and conjunctiva and is accompanied by eye pain, excessive tearing, photophobia, and eye discharge. Examination reveals an inflamed preauricular node and visible conjunctival follicles.
- *Trichinosis.* Trichinosis is a relatively rare infectious disorder that causes sudden onset of eyelid edema with fever (102° to 104° F [38.9° to 40° C]), conjunctivitis, muscle pain, itching and burning skin, sweating, skin lesions, and delirium.

OTHER CAUSES
- *Diagnostic tests.* An allergic reaction to contrast media used in radiologic tests may produce facial edema.
- *Drugs.* Long-term use of glucocorticoids may produce facial edema. Any drug that causes an allergic reaction (aspirin, antipyretics, penicillin, and sulfa preparations, for example) may have the same effect.
- *Herbal remedies.* Ingestion of the fruit pulp of ginkgo biloba can cause severe erythema and edema and the rapid formation of vesicles. Feverfew and chrysanthemum parthenium can cause swelling of the lips, irritation of the tongue, and mouth ulcers. Licorice may cause facial edema and water retention or bloating, especially if used before menses.

- **Surgery and transfusion.** Cranial, nasal, or jaw surgery may cause facial edema, as may a blood transfusion that causes an allergic reaction.

NURSING CONSIDERATIONS
Administer an analgesic for pain, and apply an antipruritic cream to reduce itching. Unless contraindicated, apply cold compresses to the patient's eyes to decrease edema and promote comfort. Elevate the head of the bed to help drain the accumulated fluid. Urine and blood tests are commonly ordered to help diagnose the cause of facial edema. Cultures of eye exudate may be ordered.

PATIENT TEACHING
Explain the risks of delayed allergy symptoms, and the signs and symptoms the patient or his family should report. Discuss ways to avoid allergens and insect bites or stings. Emphasize the importance of having an anaphylaxis kit available at all times and of wearing a medical identification bracelet.

Edema, generalized

A common sign in severely ill patients, generalized edema is the excessive accumulation of interstitial fluid throughout the body. Its severity varies widely; slight edema may be difficult to detect, especially if the patient is obese, whereas massive edema is immediately apparent.

Generalized edema is typically chronic and progressive. It may result from cardiac, renal, endocrine, or hepatic disorders as well as from severe burns, malnutrition, or the effects of certain drugs and treatments.

Common factors responsible for edema are hypoalbuminemia and excess sodium ingestion or retention, both of which influence plasma osmotic pressure. (See *Understanding fluid balance,* page 127.) Cyclic edema associated with increased aldosterone secretion may occur in premenopausal females.

Act now Quickly determine the location and severity of edema, including the degree of pitting. (See Edema: Pitting or nonpitting? page 128.) If the patient has severe edema, promptly take his vital signs, and check for jugular vein distention and cyanotic lips. Auscultate the lungs and heart. Be alert for signs of cardiac failure or pulmonary congestion, such as crackles, muffled heart sounds, or ventricular gallop. Unless the patient is hypotensive, place him in Fowler's position to promote lung expansion. Prepare to administer oxygen and an I.V. diuretic. Have emergency resuscitation equipment nearby.

ASSESSMENT
History
When the patient's condition permits, obtain a complete medical history. First, note when and where the edema began. Does it move throughout the course of the day—for example, from the upper extremities to the lower, periorbitally, or within the sacral area? Is the edema worse in the morning or at the end of the day? Is it affected by position changes? Is it accompanied by shortness of breath or pain in the arms or legs? Find out how much weight the patient has gained. Has his urine output changed in quantity or quality?

Next, ask about previous burns or cardiac, renal, hepatic, endocrine, or GI disorders. Have the patient describe his diet so you can determine whether he suffers from protein malnutrition. Explore his drug history, and note recent I.V. therapy.

Physical examination
Begin the physical examination by comparing the patient's arms and legs for symmetrical edema. Also, note ecchymoses and cyanosis. Assess the back, sacrum, and hips of the bedridden patient for dependent edema. Palpate peripheral pulses, noting whether his hands and feet feel cold. Finally, perform a complete cardiac and respiratory assessment. Also, obtain a baseline weight for this patient.

Pediatric pointers
Renal failure in children commonly causes generalized edema. Monitor fluid balance closely. Remember that fever or diaphoresis can lead to fluid loss, so promote fluid intake.

Kwashiorkor—protein-deficiency malnutrition—is more common in children than in adults and causes anasarca.

Geriatric pointers
Elderly patients are more likely to develop edema for several reasons, including decreased cardiac and renal function and, in some cases, poor nutritional status. Use cau-

tion when giving older patients I.V. fluids or medications that can raise sodium levels and thereby increase fluid retention.

MEDICAL CAUSES

- *Angioneurotic edema or angioedema.* Recurrent attacks of acute, painless, nonpitting edema involving the skin and mucous membranes — especially those of the respiratory tract, face, neck, lips, larynx, hands, feet, genitalia, or viscera — may be the result of a food or drug allergy or emotional stress, or they may be hereditary. Abdominal pain, nausea, vomiting, and diarrhea accompany visceral edema; dyspnea and stridor accompany life-threatening laryngeal edema.
- *Burns.* Edema and associated tissue damage vary with the severity of the burn. Severe generalized edema (4+) may occur within 2 days of a major burn; localized edema may occur with a less severe burn.
- *Cirrhosis.* Edema that usually starts in the legs and thighs and may progress to the degree of anasarca. Edema is a late sign of cirrhosis — a chronic disease. Accompanying signs and symptoms include abdominal pain, anorexia, nausea and vomiting, hepatomegaly, ascites, jaundice, pruritus, bleeding tendencies, musty breath, lethargy, mental changes, and asterixis.
- *Heart failure.* Severe, generalized pitting edema — occasionally anasarca — may follow leg edema late in heart failure. Edema may improve with exercise or elevation of the limbs and is typically worse at the end of the day. Among other classic late findings are hemoptysis, cyanosis, marked hepatomegaly, clubbing, crackles, and a ventricular gallop. Typically, the patient has tachypnea, palpitations, hypotension, weight gain despite anorexia, nausea, slowed mental response, diaphoresis, and pallor. Dyspnea, orthopnea, tachycardia, and fatigue typify left-sided heart failure; jugular vein distention, enlarged liver, and peripheral edema typify right-sided heart failure.
- *Malnutrition.* Anasarca in malnutrition may mask dramatic muscle wasting. Malnutrition also typically causes muscle weakness; lethargy; anorexia; diarrhea; apathy; dry, wrinkled skin; and signs of anemia, such as dizziness and pallor.
- *Myxedema.* With myxedema — the severe form of hypothyroidism — generalized nonpitting edema is accompanied by dry, flaky, inelastic, waxy, pale skin, a puffy face,

and an upper eyelid droop. Assessment also reveals masklike facies, hair loss or coarsening, and psychomotor slowing. Associated findings include hoarseness, weight gain, fatigue, cold intolerance, bradycardia, hypoventilation, constipation, abdominal distention, menorrhagia, impotence, and infertility.
- *Nephrotic syndrome.* Although nephrotic syndrome is characterized by generalized pitting edema, the edema is initially localized around the eyes. With severe cases, anasarca develops, increasing body weight by up to 50%. Other common signs and symptoms are ascites, anorexia, fatigue, malaise, depression, and pallor.
- *Pericardial effusion.* With pericardial effusion, generalized pitting edema may be most prominent in the arms and legs. It may be accompanied by chest pain, dyspnea, orthopnea, nonproductive cough, pericardial friction rub, jugular vein distention, dysphagia, and fever.
- *Pericarditis (chronic constructive).* Resembling right-sided heart failure, pericarditis usually begins with pitting edema of the arms and legs that may progress to generalized edema. Other signs and symptoms include ascites, Kussmaul's sign, dyspnea, fatigue, weakness, abdominal distention, and hepatomegaly.
- *Protein-losing enteropathy.* Increased albumin levels lead to progressive generalized pitting edema in protein-losing enteropathy. The patient may also have mild fever and abdominal pain with bloody diarrhea and steatorrhea.
- *Renal failure.* With acute renal failure, generalized pitting edema occurs as a late sign. With chronic failure, edema is less likely to become generalized; its severity depends on the degree of fluid overload. Both forms of renal failure cause oliguria, anorexia, nausea and vomiting, drowsiness, confusion, hypertension, dyspnea, crackles, dizziness, and pallor.
- *Septic shock.* A late sign of septic shock — a life-threatening disorder — generalized edema typically develops rapidly. The edema is pitting and moderately severe. Accompanying it may be cool skin, hypotension, oliguria, tachycardia, cyanosis, thirst, anxiety, and signs of respiratory failure.

OTHER CAUSES

- *Drugs.* Any drug that causes sodium retention may aggravate or cause generalized edema. Examples include antihypertensives, corticosteroids, androgenic and anabolic steroids, estrogens, and nonsteroidal anti-inflammatories, such as celecoxib, ibuprofen, and naproxen.
- *Medical treatments.* I.V. saline solution infusions and internal feedings may cause sodium and fluid overload, resulting in generalized edema, especially in patients with cardiac or renal disease.

NURSING CONSIDERATIONS

Position the patient with his limbs above heart level to promote drainage unless positioning increases respiratory difficulty. Reposition him to avoid pressure ulcers at least every 2 hours. If the patient develops dyspnea, lower his limbs, elevate the head of the bed, and administer oxygen. Massage reddened areas, especially where dependent edema has formed (for example, the back, sacrum, hips, buttocks). Prevent skin breakdown in these areas by placing a pressure mattress, air mattress, or flotation ring on the patient's bed. Restrict fluids and sodium, and administer a diuretic or I.V. albumin.

Monitor intake and output and daily weight. Also monitor serum electrolyte levels — especially sodium and albumin. Prepare the patient for blood and urine tests, X-rays, echocardiography, or an electrocardiogram.

PATIENT TEACHING

Teach the patient with known heart failure or renal failure and the patient's caregivers to watch for edema; explain that it's an important sign of decompensation that indicates the need for immediate adjustment of therapy. Discuss foods and fluids he should avoid. Provide information related to medications prescribed and the importance of medication, diet, and activity compliance.

Epistaxis

[Nosebleed]

A common sign, epistaxis can be spontaneous or induced from the front or back of the nose. Most nosebleeds occur in the ante-rior-inferior nasal septum (Kiesselbach's plexus), but they may also occur at the point where the inferior turbinates meet the nasopharynx. Usually unilateral, they seem bilateral when blood runs from the bleeding side behind the nasal septum and out the opposite side. Epistaxis ranges from mild oozing to severe — possibly life-threatening — blood loss.

A rich supply of fragile blood vessels makes the nose particularly vulnerable to bleeding. Air moving through the nose can dry and irritate the mucous membranes, forming crusts that bleed when they're removed; dry mucous membranes are also more susceptible to infections, which can produce epistaxis as well. Trauma is another common cause of epistaxis. Additional causes include septal deviations; hematologic, coagulation, renal, and GI disorders; and certain drugs and treatments.

Act now   If your patient has severe epistaxis, quickly take his vital signs. Be alert for tachypnea, hypotension, and other signs of hypovolemic shock. Insert a large-gauge I.V. line for rapid fluid and blood replacement, and attempt to control bleeding by pinching the nares closed. (However, if you suspect a nasal fracture, don't pinch the nares. Instead, place gauze under the patient's nose to absorb the blood.)

Have a hypovolemic patient lie down and turn his head to the side to prevent blood from draining down the back of his throat, which could cause aspiration or vomiting of swallowed blood. If the patient isn't hypovolemic, have him sit upright and tilt his head forward. Constantly check airway patency. If the patient's condition is unstable, begin cardiac monitoring and give supplemental oxygen by mask.

ASSESSMENT
History

If your patient isn't in distress, take a history. Does he have a history of recent trauma? How often has he had nosebleeds in the past? Have the nosebleeds been long or unusually severe? Has the patient recently had surgery in the sinus area? Ask about a history of hypertension, bleeding, or liver disorders, and other recent illnesses. Ask if the patient bruises easily. Find out what drugs he uses, especially anti-inflammatories, such as aspirin, and anticoagulants such as warfarin.

Physical examination

Begin the physical examination by inspecting the patient's skin for other signs of bleeding, such as ecchymoses and petechiae, and noting any jaundice, pallor, or other abnormalities. When examining a trauma patient, look for associated injuries, such as eye trauma or facial fractures. Determine if the epistaxis is unilateral or bilateral. Inspect for blood seeping behind the nasal septum, in the middle ear, and in the corners of the eyes.

Pediatric pointers

Children are more likely to experience anterior nosebleeds, usually the result of nosepicking or allergic rhinitis. Biliary atresia, cystic fibrosis, hereditary afibrinogenemia, and nasal trauma due to a foreign body can also cause epistaxis. Rubeola may cause an oozing nosebleed along with the characteristic maculopapular rash. Two other childhood diseases — pertussis and diphtheria — can also cause oozing epistaxis.

Suspect a bleeding disorder if you see excess umbilical cord bleeding at birth or profuse bleeding during circumcision or other procedures. Epistaxis commonly begins at puberty in patients with hereditary hemorrhagic telangiectasia.

Geriatric pointers

Elderly patients are more likely to have posterior nosebleeds.

MEDICAL CAUSES

- *Angiofibroma (juvenile).* Angiofibroma is a rare disorder that usually occurs in males and is characterized by severe recurrent epistaxis and nasal obstruction.
- *Aplastic anemia.* Aplastic anemia develops insidiously, eventually producing nosebleeds as well as ecchymoses, retinal hemorrhages, menorrhagia, petechiae, bleeding from the mouth, and signs of GI bleeding. Fatigue, dyspnea, headache, tachycardia, and pallor may also occur.
- *Barotrauma.* Commonly seen in airline passengers and scuba divers, barotrauma may cause severe, painful epistaxis when the patient has an upper tract respiratory infection.
- *Biliary obstruction.* Biliary obstruction produces bleeding tendencies, including epistaxis. Typical features are colicky, right-upper-quadrant pain after eating fatty food,

nausea, vomiting, fever, flatulence and, possibly, jaundice.
- *Cirrhosis.* With cirrhosis, epistaxis is a late sign that occurs along with other bleeding tendencies (bleeding gums, easy bruising, hematemesis, melena). Other typical late findings include ascites, abdominal pain, shallow respirations, hepatomegaly or splenomegaly, and fever of 101° to 103° F (38.3° to 39.4° C). The patient may also exhibit muscle atrophy, enlarged superficial abdominal veins, severe pruritus, extremely dry skin, poor tissue turgor, abnormal pigmentation, spider angiomas, palmar erythema and, possibly, jaundice and central nervous system disturbances.
- *Coagulation disorders.* Such disorders as hemophilia and thrombocytopenic purpura can cause epistaxis along with ecchymoses, petechiae, and bleeding from the gums, mouth, and I.V. puncture sites. Menorrhagia and signs of GI bleeding, such as melena and hematemesis, can also occur.
- *Glomerulonephritis (chronic).* Glomerulonephritis produces nosebleeds as well as hypertension, proteinuria, hematuria, headache, edema, oliguria, hemoptysis, nausea, vomiting, pruritus, dyspnea, malaise, and fatigue.
- *Hepatitis.* When hepatitis interferes with the clotting mechanism, epistaxis and abnormal bleeding tendencies can result. Associated signs and symptoms typically include jaundice, clay-colored stools, pruritus, hepatomegaly, dry and flaky skin, abdominal pain, fever, fatigue, weakness, dark amber urine, anorexia, nausea, and vomiting.
- *Hereditary hemorrhagic telangiectasia (Rendu-Osler-Weber disease).* Rendu-Osler-Weber disease causes frequent, sometimes daily, epistaxis, as well as hemoptysis and GI bleeding. Telangiectases appear as pinpoint, purplish red spots or flat, spiderlike lesions on the mucous membranes of the lips, mouth, tongue, nose, and GI tract. They occasionally appear on the trunk and fingertips.
- *Hypertension.* Severe hypertension can produce extreme epistaxis, usually in the posterior nose, with pulsation above the middle turbinate. It may be accompanied by dizziness, a throbbing headache, anxiety, peripheral edema, nocturia, nausea, vomiting, drowsiness, and mental impairment.
- *Infectious mononucleosis.* In patients with infectious mononucleosis, blood may ooze from the nose. Characteristic features include

sore throat, cervical lymphadenopathy, and a fluctuating fever with an evening peak up to 101° to 102° F (38.3° to 38.9° C).

- *Influenza.* When influenza affects the capillaries, a slow, oozing nosebleed results. Other signs and symptoms of influenza include dry cough, chills, fever, malaise, myalgia, sore throat, hoarseness or loss of voice, conjunctivitis, facial flushing, headache, rhinitis, and rhinorrhea.
- *Leukemia.* With acute leukemia, sudden epistaxis is accompanied by a high fever and other types of abnormal bleeding, such as bleeding gums, ecchymoses, petechiae, easy bruising, and prolonged menses. These may follow less-noticeable signs and symptoms, such as weakness, lassitude, pallor, chills, recurrent infections, and low-grade fever. Acute leukemia may also cause dyspnea, fatigue, malaise, tachycardia, palpitations, a systolic ejection murmur, and abdominal or bone pain.

With chronic leukemia, epistaxis is a late sign that may be accompanied by other types of abnormal bleeding, extreme fatigue, weight loss, hepatosplenomegaly, bone tenderness, edema, macular or nodular skin lesions, pallor, weakness, dyspnea, tachycardia, palpitations, and headache.
- *Maxillofacial injury.* With a maxillofacial injury, a pumping arterial bleed usually causes severe epistaxis. Associated signs and symptoms include facial pain, numbness, swelling, asymmetry, open-bite malocclusion or inability to open the mouth, diplopia, conjunctival hemorrhage, lip edema, and buccal, mucosal, and soft-palatal ecchymoses.
- *Nasal fracture.* Unilateral or bilateral epistaxis occurs with nasal swelling, periorbital ecchymoses and edema, pain, nasal deformity, and crepitation of the nasal bones.
- *Nasal tumor.* Blood may ooze from the nose when a tumor disrupts the nasal vasculature. Benign tumors usually bleed when touched, but malignant tumors produce spontaneous unilateral epistaxis, along with a foul discharge, cheek swelling, and — in the late stage — pain.
- *Orbital floor fracture.* Orbital floor fracture is a type of trauma that may damage the maxillary sinus mucosa and, on rare occasions, cause epistaxis. More typical features include periorbital edema and ecchymoses, diplopia, infraorbital numbness, enophthal-

mos, limited eye movement, and facial asymmetry.
- *Polycythemia vera.* A common sign of polycythemia vera, spontaneous epistaxis may be accompanied by bleeding gums; ecchymoses; ruddy cyanosis of the face, nose, ears, and lips; and congestion of the conjunctiva, retina, and oral mucous membranes. Other signs and symptoms vary according to the affected body system but may include headache, dizziness, tinnitus, vision disturbances, hypertension, chest pain, intermittent claudication, early satiety and fullness, marked splenomegaly, epigastric pain, pruritus, and dyspnea.
- *Renal failure.* Chronic renal failure is more likely than acute renal failure to cause epistaxis and a tendency to bruise easily. More common signs and symptoms are oliguria or anuria, weight loss, anorexia, abdominal pain, diarrhea, nausea, vomiting, tissue wasting, dry mucous membranes, uremic breath, Kussmaul's respirations, deteriorating mental status, and tachycardia.

Skin changes include pruritus, pallor, yellow-bronze pigmentation, purpura, dry skin, excoriation, uremic frost, and brown arcs under the nail margins. Neurologic signs and symptoms may include muscle twitches, fasciculations, asterixis, paresthesia, and footdrop. Cardiovascular effects include hypertension, arrhythmias, signs of heart failure, signs of pericarditis, and peripheral edema.
- *Sarcoidosis.* Oozing epistaxis may occur in sarcoidosis, along with a nonproductive cough, substernal pain, malaise, and weight loss. Related findings include tachycardia, arrhythmias, parotid enlargement, cervical lymphadenopathy, skin lesions, hepatosplenomegaly, and arthritis in the ankles, knees, and wrists.
- *Scleroma.* With scleroma, oozing epistaxis occurs with a watery nasal discharge that becomes foul-smelling and crusty. Progressive anosmia and turbinate atrophy may also occur.
- *Sinusitis (acute).* With sinusitis, a bloody or blood-tinged nasal discharge may become purulent and copious after 24 to 48 hours. Associated signs and symptoms include nasal congestion, pain, tenderness, malaise, headache, low-grade fever, and red, edematous nasal mucosa.
- *Skull fracture.* Depending on the type of fracture, epistaxis can be direct (when blood flows directly down the nares) or indirect

Types of nasal packing

Nosebleeds may be controlled with anterior or posterior nasal packing.

Anterior nasal packing

The physician may treat an anterior nose-bleed by packing the anterior nasal cavity with a strip of antibiotic-impregnated petroleum gauze strip (shown at right) or with a nasal tampon.

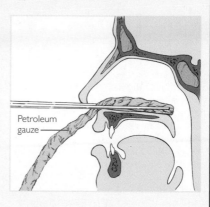

Petroleum gauze

A nasal tampon is made of tightly compressed absorbent material with or without a central breathing tube. The physician inserts a lubricated tampon along the floor of the nose and, with the patient's head tilted backward, instills 5 to 10 ml of antibiotic or normal saline solution. This causes the tampon to expand, stopping the bleeding. The tampon should be moistened periodically, and the central breathing tube should be suctioned regularly.

In a patient with blood dyscrasias, the physician may fashion an absorbable pack by moistening a gauzelike, regenerated cellulose material with a vasoconstrictor. Applied to a visible bleeding point, this substance will swell to form a clot. The packing is absorbable and doesn't need removal.

Posterior nasal packing

Posterior packing consists of a gauze roll shaped and secured by three sutures (one suture at each end and one in the middle) or a balloon-type catheter. To insert the packing, the physician advances one or two soft catheters into the patient's nostrils (shown at right). When the catheter tips appear in the nasopharynx, the physician grasps them with a Kelly clamp or bayonet forceps and pulls them forward through the mouth. He secures the two end sutures to the catheter tip and draws the catheter back through the nostrils.

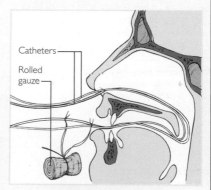

Catheters

Rolled gauze

This step brings the packing into place with the end sutures hanging from the patient's nostril. (The middle suture emerges from the patient's mouth to free the packing, when needed.)

The physician may weight the nose sutures with a clamp. Then he'll pull the packing securely into place behind the soft palate and against the posterior end of the septum (nasal choana).

After he examines the patient's throat (to ensure that the uvula hasn't been forced under the packing), he inserts anterior packing and secures the whole apparatus by tying the posterior pack strings around rolled gauze or a dental roll at the nostrils.

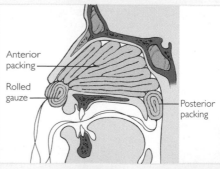

Anterior packing

Rolled gauze

Posterior packing

(when blood drains through the eustachian tube and into the nose). Abrasions, contusions, lacerations, or avulsions are common. A severe skull fracture may cause severe headache, decreased level of consciousness, hemiparesis, dizziness, seizures, projectile vomiting, and decreased pulse and respiratory rates.

A basilar fracture may also cause bleeding from the pharynx, ears, and conjunctiva as well as raccoon eyes and Battle's sign. Cerebrospinal fluid or even brain tissue may leak from the nose or ears. A sphenoid fracture may also cause blindness, whereas a temporal fracture may also cause unilateral deafness or facial paralysis.

● *Syphilis.* Epistaxis is most common in patients with tertiary syphilis, as posterior septum ulcerations produce a foul, bloody nasal discharge. It may be accompanied by a painful nasal obstruction and nasal deformity. Occasionally, primary syphilis causes painful nasal crusting and bleeding accompanied by the characteristic chancre sores.

● *Systemic lupus erythematosus (SLE).* Usually affecting females younger than age 50, SLE causes oozing epistaxis. More characteristic signs and symptoms include butterfly rash, lymphadenopathy, joint pain and stiffness, anorexia, nausea, vomiting, myalgia, and weight loss.

● *Typhoid fever.* Oozing epistaxis and dry cough are common. Typhoid fever may also cause abrupt onset of chills and high fever, vomiting, abdominal distention, constipation or diarrhea, splenomegaly, hepatomegaly, "rose-spot" rash, jaundice, anorexia, weight loss, and profound fatigue.

OTHER CAUSES

● *Chemical irritants.* Some chemicals — including phosphorus, sulfuric acid, hypochlorite, ammonia, printer's ink, and chromates — irritate the nasal mucosa, producing epistaxis.

● *Drugs.* Anticoagulants, such as warfarin, and anti-inflammatories, such as aspirin, can cause epistaxis. Cocaine use, especially if frequent, can also cause epistaxis.

● *Environment.* Dry environments, as occurs during winter use of heaters without humidity, may cause nosebleeds.

● *Surgery and procedures.* Rarely, epistaxis results from facial and nasal surgery, including septoplasty, rhinoplasty, antrostomy, endoscopic sinus procedures, orbital decompression, and dental extraction.

● *Vigorous nose blowing.* Vigorous nose blowing may rupture superficial blood vessels, especially in elderly people and young people, and cause nosebleeds.

NURSING CONSIDERATIONS

Until the bleeding is completely under control, continue to monitor the patient for signs of hypovolemic shock, such as tachycardia and clammy skin. If external pressure doesn't control the bleeding, insert cotton that has been impregnated with a vasoconstrictor and local anesthetic into the patient's nose.

If bleeding persists, expect to insert anterior or posterior nasal packing. (See *Types of nasal packing,* page 135.) Administer humidified oxygen by facemask to a patient with posterior packing.

A complete blood count may be ordered to evaluate blood loss and detect anemia. Clotting studies, such as prothrombin time and activated partial thromboplastin time, may be required to test coagulation time. Prepare the patient for X-rays if he has had a recent trauma.

PATIENT TEACHING

Advise the patient about proper pinching pressure techniques. For prevention, tell him to apply liberal amounts of petroleum jelly to nostrils to prevent drying, cracking, and avoid picking and to avoid bending and lifting. Instruct the patient to sneeze with his mouth open. Use of a humidifier at night and trimming fingernails are also recommended. Emphasize the need for follow-up care and periodic blood studies after an episode of epistaxis. Advise the patient to seek prompt medical treatment for nasal infections or irritation.

Erythema

Dilated or congested blood vessels produce red skin, or erythema, the most common sign of skin inflammation or irritation. Erythema may be localized or generalized and may occur suddenly or gradually. Skin color can range from bright red in patients with acute conditions to pale violet or brown in those with chronic problems. Erythema must be differentiated from purpura, which causes redness from bleeding into the skin. When pressure is applied directly to the skin, erythema blanches momentarily, but purpura doesn't.

Erythema usually results from changes in the arteries, veins, and small vessels that lead to increased small-vessel perfusion. Drugs and neurogenic mechanisms can allow extra blood to enter the small vessels. Erythema can also result from trauma and tissue damage and increased visibility of vessels due to changes in supporting tissues.

Act now If your patient has sudden progressive erythema with rapid pulse, dyspnea, hoarseness, and agitation, quickly take his vital signs. These may be indications of anaphylactic shock. Provide emergency respiratory support and give epinephrine.

ASSESSMENT
History
If erythema isn't associated with anaphylaxis, obtain a detailed health history. Find out how long the patient has had the erythema and where it first began. Has he had any associated pain or itching? Has he recently had a fever, upper respiratory tract infection, or joint pain? Does he have a history of skin disease or other illness? Does he or anyone in his family have allergies, asthma, or eczema? Find out if he has been exposed to someone who has had a similar rash or who is now ill. Did he have a recent fall or injury in the area of the erythema?

Obtain a complete drug history, including recent immunizations. Ask about food intake and exposure to chemicals.

Physical examination
Begin the physical examination by assessing the extent, distribution, and intensity of erythema. Look for edema and other skin lesions, such as hives, scales, papules, and purpura. Examine the affected area for warmth, and gently palpate it to check for tenderness or crepitus.

Pediatric pointers
Normally, newborn rash (erythema toxicum neonatorum), a pink papular rash, develops during the first 4 days after birth and spontaneously disappears by the 10th day. Neonates and infants can also develop erythema from infections and other disorders. For instance, candidiasis can produce thick white lesions over an erythematous base on the oral mucosa as well as diaper rash with beefy red erythema.

Roseola, rubeola, scarlet fever, granuloma annulare, and cutis marmorata also cause erythema in children.

Geriatric pointers
Elderly patients commonly have well-demarcated purple macules or patches, usually on the back of the hands and on the forearms. Known as *actinic purpura,* this condition results from blood leaking through fragile capillaries. The lesions disappear spontaneously.

MEDICAL CAUSES
- *Allergic reactions.* Foods, drugs, chemicals, and other allergens can cause an allergic reaction and erythema. A localized allergic reaction also produces hivelike eruptions and edema.

Anaphylaxis, a life-threatening condition, produces relatively sudden erythema in the form of urticaria. It also produces flushing; facial edema; diaphoresis; weakness; sneezing; bronchospasm with dyspnea and tachypnea; shock with hypotension and cool, clammy skin; and possibly airway edema with hoarseness and stridor.
- *Burns.* With thermal burns, erythema and swelling appear first, possibly followed by deep or superficial blisters and other signs of damage that vary with the severity of the burn. Burns from ultraviolet rays, such as sunburn, cause delayed erythema and tenderness on exposed areas of the skin.
- *Candidiasis.* When candidiasis—a fungal infection—affects the skin, it produces erythema and a scaly, papular rash under the breasts and at the axillae, neck, umbilicus, and groin, also known as *intertrigo.* Small pustules commonly occur at the periphery of the rash (satellite pustulosis).
- *Cellulitis.* Erythema, tenderness, and edema are a result of a bacterial infection of the skin (most commonly streptococcal and staphylococcal) and subcutaneous tissue.
- *Dermatitis.* Erythema commonly occurs in this family of inflammatory disorders. With atopic dermatitis, erythema and intense pruritus precede the development of small papules that may redden, weep, scale, and lichenify. These occur most commonly at skin folds of the extremities, neck, and eyelids.

Contact dermatitis occurs after exposure to an irritant. It quickly produces inflammation, erythema and vesicles, blisters, or ulcerations on exposed skin.

With seborrheic dermatitis, erythema appears with dull red or yellow lesions. Sharply marginated, these lesions are sometimes ring shaped and covered with greasy scales. They usually occur on the scalp, eyebrows, ears, and nasolabial folds, but they may form a butterfly rash on the face or move to the chest or to skin folds on the trunk. This disorder is common in patients infected with the human immunodeficiency virus and in infants (cradle cap).

- **Dermatomyositis.** Dermatomyositis, most common in females older than age 50, produces a dusky lilac rash on the face, neck, upper torso, and nail beds. Other symptoms include fever, malaise, and weakness. Gottron's papules (violet, flat-topped lesions) may appear on finger joints.

- **Erythema annulare centrifugum.** Small, pink, ring-shaped infiltrated papules appear on the trunk, buttocks, and inner thighs, slowly spreading at the margins and clearing in the center. Itching, scaling, and tissue hardening may occur.

- **Erythema marginatum rheumaticum.** Associated with rheumatic fever, erythema marginatum rheumaticum causes erythematous lesions that are superficial, flat, and slightly hardened. They shift, spread rapidly, and may last for hours or days, recurring after a time.

- **Erythema multiforme.** Erythema multiforme is an acute inflammatory skin disease that develops as a result of drug sensitivity after infection, most commonly herpes simplex and *Mycoplasma;* allergies; and pregnancy. One-half of the cases are of idiopathic origin.

Erythema multiforme minor has typical urticarial, red-pink, iris-shaped, localized lesions with little or no mucous membrane involvement. Most lesions occur on flexor surfaces of the extremities. Burning or itching may occur before or in conjunction with lesion development. Lesions appear in crops and last 2 to 3 weeks. After 1 week individual lesions become flat or hyperpigmented. Early signs and symptoms may include a mild fever, cough, and sore throat.

Erythema multiforme major usually occurs as a drug reaction; has widespread symmetrical, bullous lesions that may become confluent; and includes erosions of the mucous membranes. Erythema is characteristically preceded by blisters on the lips, tongue, and buccal mucosa and a sore throat. Additional signs and symptoms early in the course of the disease include cough, vomiting, diarrhea, coryza, and epistaxis. Later signs and symptoms include fever, prostration, difficulty with oral intake due to mouth and lip lesions, conjunctivitis due to ulceration, vulvitis, and balanitis.

The maximal variant of this disease is considered by many to be Stevens-Johnson syndrome. This is a multisystem disorder and can occasionally be fatal. In addition to all signs and symptoms mentioned above, patients develop exfoliation of the skin from disruptions of bullae, although less than 10% of the body surface area is affected. These areas resemble second-degree thermal burns and should be cared for as such. Fever may rise to 102° to 104° F (38.9° to 40° C). The patient may also experience tachypnea; weak, rapid pulse; chest pain; malaise; and muscle or joint pain.

- **Erythema nodosum.** Sudden bilateral eruption of tender erythematous nodules characterizes erythema nodosum. These firm, round, tender, protruding lesions usually appear in crops on the shins, knees, and ankles but may occur on the buttocks, arms, calves, and trunk as well. Other effects include mild fever, chills, malaise, muscle and joint pain and, possibly, swollen feet and ankles. Erythema nodosum is associated with various diseases, most notably inflammatory bowel disease, sarcoidosis, tuberculosis, and streptococcal and fungal infections.

- **Gout.** Gout, which generally affects males ages 40 to 60, is characterized by tight and erythematous skin over an inflamed, edematous joint.

- **Lupus erythematosus.** Both discoid and systemic lupus erythematosus (SLE) can produce a characteristic butterfly rash. This erythematous eruption may range from a blush with swelling to a scaly, sharply demarcated, macular rash with plaques that may spread to the forehead, chin, ears, chest, and other sun-exposed parts of the body.

With discoid lupus erythematosus, telangiectasia, hyperpigmentation, ear and nose deformity, and mouth, tongue, and eyelid lesions may occur.

With SLE, acute onset of erythema may also be accompanied by photosensitivity and mucous membrane ulcers, especially in the nose and mouth. Mottled erythema may occur on the hands, with edema around the nails and macular reddish purple lesions on the fingers. Telangiectasia occurs at the base of the nails or eyelids, along with purpura, petechiae, ecchymoses, and urticaria. Joint pain and stiffness are common. Other findings vary according to the body systems affected but typically include low-grade fever, malaise, weakness, headache, arthralgias, arthritis, depression, lymphadenopathy, fatigue, weight loss, anorexia, nausea, vomiting, diarrhea, and constipation.

- **Psoriasis.** Silvery white scales over a thickened erythematous base usually affect the elbows, knees, chest, scalp, and intergluteal folds. The fingernails may become thick and pitted.
- **Raynaud's disease.** Typically, the skin on the hands and feet blanches and cools after exposure to cold and stress. Later, it becomes warm and purplish red.
- **Rosacea.** Scattered erythema initially develops across the center of the face, followed by superficial telangiectases, papules, pustules, and nodules. Rhinophyma may occur on the lower half of the nose.
- **Rubella.** Typically, flat solitary lesions join to form a blotchy pink erythematous rash that spreads rapidly to the trunk and extremities in rubella. Occasionally, small red lesions (Forschheimer spots) occur on the soft palate. Lesions clear in 4 to 5 days. The rash usually follows fever (up to 102° F [38.9° C]), headache, malaise, sore throat, a gritty eye sensation, lymphadenopathy, pain in the joints, and coryza.

OTHER CAUSES

- **Drugs.** Many drugs commonly cause erythema. (See *Drugs associated with erythema.*)
- **Herbal remedies.** Ingestion of the fruit pulp of ginkgo biloba can cause severe erythema and edema of the mouth and rapid formation of vesicles. St. John's wort can cause heightened sun sensitivity, resulting in erythema or "sunburn."
- **Radiation and other treatments.** Radiation therapy may produce dull erythema and edema within 24 hours. As the erythema fades, the skin becomes light brown and mildly scaly. Any treatment that causes an allergic reaction can also cause erythema.

NURSING CONSIDERATIONS

Because erythema can cause fluid loss, closely monitor and replace fluids and electrolytes, especially in patients with burns or widespread erythema. Be sure to withhold all medications until the cause of the erythema has been identified. Then expect to administer an antibiotic and a topical or systemic corticosteroid.

For the patient with itching skin, expect to give soothing baths or apply open wet dressings containing starch, bran, or sodium bicarbonate; also administer an antihistamine and an analgesic as needed. Advise a patient with leg erythema to keep his legs elevated above heart level. For a burn patient with erythema, immerse the affected area in cold water, or apply a sheet soaked in cold water to reduce pain, edema, and erythema.

Prepare the patient for diagnostic tests, such as skin biopsy to detect cancerous lesions, cultures to identify infectious organisms, and sensitivity studies to confirm allergies.

PATIENT TEACHING

Teach the patient with a chronic disease, such as SLE or psoriasis, about the character of typical rashes so they can be alert to any flare-ups of the disease. Also, advise the patient to avoid sun exposure and to use sunblock when appropriate. Discuss measures to relieve itching.

Eye pain

Eye pain may be described as a burning, throbbing, itching, aching, or stabbing sensation in or around the eye. It may also be characterized as a foreign-body sensation. This sign varies from mild to severe; its duration and exact location provide clues to the causative disorder.

Eye pain usually results from corneal abrasion, but it may also be due to glaucoma or other eye disorders, trauma, and neurologic or systemic disorders. Any of these may stimulate nerve endings in the cornea or external eye, producing pain.

Act now If the patient's eye pain results from a chemical burn, remove contact lenses, if present, and irrigate the eye with at least 1 L of normal saline solution over 10 minutes. Evert the lids and wipe the fornices with a cotton-tipped applicator to remove any particles or chemicals. If the eye pain is the result of acute angle-closure glaucoma, immediate intervention is required to decrease intraocular pressure (IOP). If drug treatment doesn't reduce IOP, the patient needs laser iridotomy or surgical peripheral iridectomy to save his vision.

ASSESSMENT
History

If the patient's eye pain doesn't result from a chemical burn, take a complete history. Have the patient describe the pain fully. Is it an ache or a sharp pain? How long does it last? Is it accompanied by burning, itching, or discharge? Find out when it began. Is it worse in the morning or late in the evening? Ask about recent trauma or surgery, especially if the patient complains of sudden, severe pain. Does he have headaches? If so, find out how often and at what time of day they occur.

Physical examination

During the physical examination, *don't* manipulate the eye if you suspect trauma. Carefully assess the lids and conjunctiva for redness, inflammation, and swelling. Then examine the eyes for ptosis or exophthalmos. Finally, test visual acuity with and without correction, and assess extraocular movements. Characterize any discharge. (See *Examining the external eye.*)

Pediatric pointers

Trauma and infection are the most common causes of eye pain in children. Be alert for nonverbal clues to pain, such as tightly shutting or frequently rubbing the eyes.

Geriatric pointers

Glaucoma, which can cause eye pain, is usually a disease of older patients, becoming clinically significant after age 40. It usually occurs bilaterally and leads to slowly progressive vision loss, especially in peripheral visual fields.

MEDICAL CAUSES

See *Eye pain: causes and associated findings,* page 142.
- *Acute angle-closure glaucoma.* Blurred vision and sudden, excruciating pain in and around the eye characterize acute angle-closure glaucoma; the pain may be so severe that it causes nausea, vomiting, and abdominal pain. Other findings are halo vision, rapidly decreasing visual acuity, and a fixed, nonreactive, moderately dilated pupil.
- *Astigmatism.* Uncorrected astigmatism commonly causes headache and eye fatigue, aching, and redness. This disorder occurs in both older and younger people.
- *Blepharitis.* Burning pain in both eyelids is accompanied by itching, sticky discharge,

EXAMINING THE EXTERNAL EYE

For patients with eye pain or other ocular symptoms, examination of the external eye forms an important part of the ocular assessment. Here's how to examine the external eye.

First, inspect the eyelids for ptosis and incomplete closure. Also, observe the lids for edema, erythema, cyanosis, hematoma, and masses. Evaluate skin lesions, growths, swelling, and tenderness by gross palpation. Are the lids everted or inverted? Do the eyelashes turn inward? Have some been lost? Do the lashes adhere to one another or contain a discharge? Next, examine the lid margins, noting especially any debris, scaling, lesions, or unusual secretions. Also, watch for eyelid spasms.

Now gently retract the eyelid with your thumb and forefinger, and assess the conjunctiva for redness, cloudiness, follicles, and blisters or other lesions. Check for chemosis by pressing the lower lid against the eyeball and noting any bulging above this compression point. Observe the sclera, noting any change from its normal white color.

Next, shine a light across the cornea to detect scars, abrasions, or ulcers. Note any color changes, dots, or opaque or cloudy areas. Also, assess the anterior eye chamber, which should be clean, deep, shadow-free, and filled with clear aqueous humor.

Inspect the color, shape, texture, and pattern of the iris. Then assess the pupils' size, shape, and equality. Finally, evaluate their response to light. Are they sluggish, fixed, or unresponsive? Does pupil dilation or constriction occur only on one side?

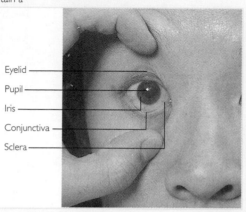

Eyelid
Pupil
Iris
Conjunctiva
Sclera

---

and conjunctival injection. Related findings include foreign-body sensation, lid ulcerations, and loss of eyelashes.

- *Burns.* With chemical burns, sudden and severe eye pain may occur with erythema and blistering of the face and lids, photophobia, miosis, conjunctival injection, blurring, and inability to keep the eyelids open. (See *Eye irrigation for chemical burns,* page 143.) With ultraviolet radiation burns, moderate to severe pain occurs about 12 hours after exposure along with photophobia and vision changes.
- *Chalazion.* A chalazion causes localized tenderness and swelling on the upper or lower eyelid. Eversion of the lid reveals conjunctival injection and a small red lump.
- *Conjunctivitis.* Some degree of eye pain and excessive tearing occurs with four types of conjunctivitis. Allergic conjunctivitis causes mild, burning, bilateral pain accompanied

by itching, conjunctival injection, and a characteristic ropey discharge.

Bacterial conjunctivitis causes pain only when it affects the cornea. Otherwise, it produces burning and a foreign-body sensation. A purulent discharge and conjunctival injection are also typical.

If the cornea is affected, fungal conjunctivitis may cause pain and photophobia. Even without corneal involvement, it produces itching, burning eyes; a thick, purulent discharge; and conjunctival injection.

Viral conjunctivitis produces itching, red eyes, foreign-body sensation, visible conjunctival follicles, and eyelid edema.

- *Corneal abrasions.* With corneal abrasions, eye pain is characterized by a foreign-body sensation. Excessive tearing, photophobia, and conjunctival injection are also common.

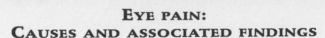

EYE PAIN:
CAUSES AND ASSOCIATED FINDINGS

COMMON CAUSES	Conjunctival injection	Corneal changes	Eye discharge	Eyelid edema	Foreign-body sensation	Pupillary changes	Tearing, increased	Vision changes	Visual floaters
Burns (chemical)	●	●			●	●	●	●	
Burns (ultraviolet)	●	●			●		●		
Conjunctivitis	●		●		●		●		
Corneal abrasion	●	●			●		●	●	
Corneal ulcer	●	●	●			●		●	
Dry eye syndrome	●		●		●				
Hordeolum (sty)				●					
Iritis (acute)	●					●		●	
Keratitis (interstitial)	●	●						●	
Scleritis	●						●		
Sclerokeratitis		●							
Trachoma		●	●	●			●	●	
Uveitis (anterior)	●					●			
Uveitis (posterior)	●					●		●	●

Major associated signs and symptoms

● *Corneal erosion (recurrent).* Severe pain occurs on waking and continues throughout the day. Accompanying the pain are conjunctival injection and photophobia.

● *Corneal ulcers.* Both bacterial and fungal corneal ulcers cause severe eye pain. They may also cause a purulent eye discharge, sticky eyelids, photophobia, and impaired visual acuity. In addition, bacterial corneal ulcers produce a grayish white, irregularly shaped ulcer on the cornea, unilateral pupil constriction, and conjunctival injection. Fungal corneal ulcers produce conjunctival injection, eyelid edema and erythema, and a dense, cloudy, central ulcer surrounded by progressively clearer rings.

● *Dacryoadenitis.* Temporal pain may affect both eyes in dacryoadenitis. Associated findings include exophthalmos, conjunctival injection, severe eyelid erythema and edema, and a purulent eye discharge.

● *Dacryocystitis.* Pain and tenderness near the tear sac characterize acute dacryocystitis. Additional signs include profuse tearing, a

EYE IRRIGATION FOR CHEMICAL BURNS

The patient's eye may be irrigated using either of these methods.

MORGAN LENS

Connected to irrigation tubing, a Morgan lens permits continuous lavage and also delivers medication to the eye. Use an adapter to connect the lens to the I.V. tubing and the solution container. Begin the irrigation at the prescribed flow rate. To insert the device, ask the patient to look down as you insert the lens under the upper eyelid. Then have her look up as you retract and release the lower eyelid over the lens.

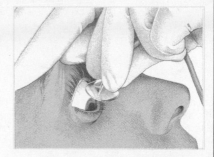

I.V. TUBE

If a Morgan lens isn't available, set up an I.V. bag and tubing without a needle. Direct a constant, gentle stream at the inner canthus so that the solution flows across the cornea to the outer canthus. Flush the eye for at least 15 minutes.

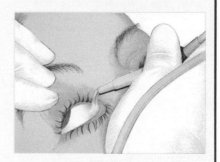

purulent discharge, eyelid erythema, and swelling in the lacrimal punctum area.

● *Episcleritis.* Deep eye pain occurs as tissues over sclera become inflamed. Related effects include photophobia, excessive tearing, conjunctival edema, and a red or purplish sclera.

● *Erythema multiforme major.* Erythema multiforme major commonly produces severe eye pain, entropion, trichiasis, purulent conjunctivitis, photophobia, and decreased tear formation.

● *Foreign bodies in the cornea and conjunctiva.* Sudden severe pain is common but vision usually remains intact. Other findings include excessive tearing, photophobia, miosis, a foreign-body sensation, a dark speck on the cornea, and dramatic conjunctival injection.

● *Glaucoma.* Open-angle glaucoma may cause mild aching in the eyes as well as loss of peripheral vision, halo vision, and reduced visual acuity that isn't corrected by glasses. Angle-closure glaucoma may cause pain and pressure over the eye, blurred vision, halo vision, decreased visual acuity, and nausea and vomiting.

● *Herpes zoster ophthalmicus.* Eye pain occurs with severe unilateral facial pain, usually several days before vesicles erupt. Other signs include red, swollen eyelids; excessive tearing; a serous eye discharge; conjunctival injection; and a white, cloudy cornea.

● *Hordeolum (stye).* Hordeolum is a lesion that usually produces localized eye pain that increases as the stye grows. Eyelid erythema and edema are also common.

● *Hyphema.* Occurring after eye injury or surgery, hyphema accompanies sudden pain in and around the eye. Orbital and lid edema, conjunctival injection, and visual impairment may occur.

- *Interstitial keratitis.* Associated with congenital syphilis, interstitial keratitis produces eye pain with photophobia, blurred vision, prominent conjunctival injection, and grayish pink corneas.
- *Iritis (acute).* Moderate to severe eye pain occurs with severe photophobia, dramatic conjunctival injection, and blurred vision. The constricted pupil may respond poorly to light.
- *Keratoconjunctivitis sicca.* Keratoconjunctivitis sicca — known as *dry eye syndrome* — causes chronic burning pain in both eyes, itching, a foreign-body sensation, photophobia, dramatic conjunctival injection, and difficulty moving the eyelids. Excessive mucoid discharge and inadequate tearing are typical.
- *Lacrimal gland tumor.* Lacrimal gland tumor is a neoplastic lesion that usually produces unilateral eye pain, impaired visual acuity, and some degree of exophthalmos.
- *Migraine headache.* Migraines can produce pain so severe that the eyes also ache. Additionally, nausea, vomiting, blurred vision, and light and noise sensitivity may occur.
- *Ocular laceration and intraocular foreign bodies.* Penetrating eye injuries usually cause mild to severe unilateral eye pain and impaired visual acuity. Eyelid edema, conjunctival injection, and an abnormal pupillary response may also occur.
- *Optic cellulitis.* Optic cellulitis causes dull, aching pain in the affected eye, some degree of exophthalmos, eyelid edema and erythema, purulent discharge, impaired extraocular movement and, occasionally, decreased visual acuity and fever.
- *Optic neuritis.* With optic neuritis, pain in and around the eye occurs with eye movement. Severe vision loss and tunnel vision develop but improve in 2 to 3 weeks. Pupils respond sluggishly to direct light but normally to consensual light.
- *Orbital floor fracture.* Sometimes called a *blowout fracture,* orbital floor fracture causes eye pain, dramatic eyelid edema and, possibly, enophthalmos and diplopia.
- *Orbital pseudotumor.* Orbital pseudotumor causes deep, boring eye pain and diplopia in about 50% of all patients. However, prominent exophthalmos and lateral ocular deviation are more characteristic. Eyelid edema and restricted extraocular movement may also occur.

- *Pemphigus.* With pemphigus, bilateral eye pain and irritation may be accompanied by blurred vision and a thick discharge. Blisters may develop on the conjunctiva alone or may extend to the nasal, oral, and vulvar mucous membranes as well as the skin.
- *Scleritis.* Scleritis is a inflammation that produces severe eye pain and tenderness, along with conjunctival injection, bluish purple sclera and, possibly, photophobia, loss of vision, and excessive tearing.
- *Sclerokeratitis.* Inflammation of the sclera and cornea causes pain, burning, irritation, and photophobia.
- *Subdural hematoma.* After head trauma, a subdural hematoma commonly causes severe eye ache and headache. Related neurologic signs depend on the hematoma's location and size.
- *Trachoma.* Along with pain in the affected eye, trachoma causes excessive tearing, photophobia, eye discharge, eyelid edema and redness, and visible conjunctival follicles.
- *Uveitis.* Anterior uveitis causes sudden onset of severe pain, dramatic conjunctival injection, photophobia, and a small, nonreactive pupil.

Posterior uveitis causes insidious onset of similar features, plus gradual blurring of vision and distorted pupil shape.

Lens-induced uveitis causes moderate eye pain, conjunctival injection, pupil constriction, and severely impaired visual acuity. In fact, the patient usually can perceive only light.

OTHER CAUSES
- *Medical treatments.* Contact lenses may cause eye pain and a foreign-body sensation. Ocular surgery may also produce eye pain, ranging from a mild ache to a severe pounding or stabbing sensation.

NURSING CONSIDERATIONS
To help ease eye pain, have the patient lie down in a darkened, quiet environment and close his eyes. Prepare him for diagnostic studies, including tonometry and orbital X-rays. Prepare to irrigate the eye, as ordered.

PATIENT TEACHING
Tell the patient that it's important to seek medical help for eye pain and stress the importance of meticulous compliance with drug therapy to prevent an increase in IOP.

Fasciculations

Fasciculations are local muscle contractions representing the spontaneous discharge of a muscle fiber bundle innervated by a single motor nerve filament. These contractions cause visible dimpling or wavelike twitching of the skin, but they aren't strong enough to cause a joint to move. They occur irregularly at frequencies ranging from once every several seconds to two or three times per second; infrequently, myokymia — continuous, rapid fasciculations that cause a rippling effect — may occur. Because fasciculations are brief and painless, they commonly go undetected or are ignored.

Benign, nonpathologic fasciculations are common and normal. They often occur in tense, anxious, or overtired people and typically affect the eyelid, thumb, or calf. However, fasciculations may also indicate a severe neurologic disorder, most notably a diffuse motor neuron disorder that causes loss of control over muscle fiber discharge. They're also an early sign of pesticide poisoning.

Act now Begin by asking the patient about the nature, onset, and duration of the fasciculations. If the onset was sudden, ask about any precipitating events, such as exposure to pesticides. Pesticide poisoning, although uncommon, is a medical emergency requiring prompt and vigorous intervention. You may need to maintain airway patency, monitor vital signs, give oxygen, and perform gastric lavage or induce vomiting.

ASSESSMENT
History
If the patient isn't in severe distress, find out if he has experienced any sensory changes, such as paresthesia, or any difficulty speaking, swallowing, breathing, or controlling bowel or bladder function. Ask him if he's in pain.

Explore the patient's medical history for neurologic disorders, cancer, and recent infections. Ask him about his lifestyle, especially stress at home, on the job, or at school.

Ask the patient about his dietary habits, especially recent intake of his foods and fluids, because electrolyte imbalances may also cause muscle twitching.

Physical examination
Perform a physical examination, looking for fasciculations while the affected muscle is at rest. Observe and test for motor and sensory abnormalities, particularly muscle atrophy and weakness, and decreased deep tendon reflexes. If you note these signs and symptoms, suspect motor neuron disease, and perform a comprehensive neurologic examination.

Pediatric pointers
Fasciculations, particularly of the tongue, are an important early sign of Werdnig-Hoffmann disease.

MEDICAL CAUSES
● *Amyotrophic lateral sclerosis.* Coarse fasciculations usually begin in the small muscles of the hands and feet, and then spread to the forearms and legs. Widespread, symmetrical

muscle atrophy and weakness may result in dysarthria; difficulty chewing, swallowing, and breathing; and, occasionally, choking and drooling.

● *Bulbar palsy.* Fasciculations of the face and tongue commonly appear early. Progressive signs and symptoms include dysarthria, dysphagia, hoarseness, and drooling. Eventually, weakness spreads to the respiratory muscles.

● *Guillain-Barré syndrome.* Fasciculations may occur, but the dominant neurologic symptom is muscle weakness, which typically begins in the legs and spreads quickly to the arms and face. Other findings include paresthesia, incontinence, footdrop, tachycardia, dysphagia, and respiratory insufficiency.

● *Herniated disk.* Fasciculations of the muscles innervated by compressed nerve roots may be widespread and profound, but the overriding symptom is severe low back pain that may radiate unilaterally to the leg. Coughing, sneezing, bending, and straining exacerbate the pain. Related effects include muscle weakness, atrophy, and spasms; paresthesia; footdrop; steppage gait; and hypoactive deep tendon reflexes in the leg.

● *Poliomyelitis (spinal paralytic).* Coarse fasciculations, usually transient but occasionally persistent, accompany progressive muscle weakness, spasms, and atrophy. The patient may also exhibit decreased reflexes, paresthesia, coldness and cyanosis in the affected limbs, bladder paralysis, dyspnea, elevated blood pressure, and tachycardia.

● *Spinal cord tumors.* Fasciculations may develop along with muscle atrophy and cramps, asymmetrically at first and then bilaterally as cord compression progresses. Motor and sensory changes distal to the tumor include weakness or paralysis, areflexia, paresthesia, and a tightening band of pain. Bowel and bladder control may be lost.

● *Syringomyelia.* Fasciculations may occur along with Charcot's joints, areflexia, muscle atrophy, and deep, aching pain. Additional findings include thoracic scoliosis and loss of pain and temperature sensation over the neck, shoulders, and arms.

OTHER CAUSES
● *Pesticide poisoning.* Ingestion of organophosphate or carbamate pesticides commonly produces acute onset of long, wavelike fasciculations and muscle weakness that

rapidly progresses to flaccid paralysis. Other common effects include nausea, vomiting, diarrhea, loss of bowel and bladder control, hyperactive bowel sounds, and abdominal cramping. Cardiopulmonary findings include bradycardia, dyspnea or bradypnea, and pallor or cyanosis. Seizures, vision disturbances (pupillary constriction or blurred vision), and increased secretions (tearing, salivation, pulmonary secretions, or diaphoresis) may also occur.

NURSING CONSIDERATIONS
Prepare the patient for diagnostic studies, such as spinal X-rays, myelography, computed tomography scan, magnetic resonance imaging, and electromyography (EMG) with nerve conduction velocity tests. Prepare the patient for laboratory tests such as serum electrolyte levels. Help the patient with progressive neuromuscular degeneration to cope with activities of daily living, and provide appropriate assistive devices.

PATIENT TEACHING
Teach the patient with stress-induced fasciculations effective stress management techniques. Refer him to physical therapy, occupational therapy, or home care services, as indicated.

Fever

Fever is a common sign that can arise from any one of several disorders. Because these disorders can affect virtually any body system, fever in the absence of other signs usually has little diagnostic significance. A persistent high fever, though, represents an emergency.

Fever can be classified as low (oral reading of 99° to 100.4° F [37.2° to 38° C]), moderate (100.5° to 104° F [38° to 40° C]), or high (above 104° F). Fever over 106° F (41.1° C) causes unconsciousness and, if sustained, leads to permanent brain damage.

Act now If you detect a fever higher than 106° F (41.1° C), take the patient's other vital signs and determine his level of consciousness. Administer an antipyretic and begin rapid cooling measures: Apply ice packs to the axillae and groin, give tepid sponge baths, or apply a cooling blanket. These methods may evoke a cooling response; to *prevent this, constantly monitor the patient's rectal temperature.*

Fever may also be classified as remittent, intermittent, sustained, relapsing, or undulant. *Remittent fever,* the most common type, is characterized by daily temperature fluctuations above the normal range. *Intermittent fever* is marked by a daily temperature drop into the normal range and then a rise back to above normal. An intermittent fever that fluctuates widely, typically producing chills and sweating, is called *hectic,* or *septic, fever.* *Sustained fever* involves persistent temperature elevation with little fluctuation. *Relapsing fever* consists of alternating feverish and afebrile periods. *Undulant fever* refers to a gradual increase in temperature that stays high for a few days and then decreases gradually.

Further classification involves duration — either brief (less than 3 weeks) or prolonged. Prolonged fevers include fever of unknown origin, a classification used when careful examination fails to detect an underlying cause.

ASSESSMENT
History
If the patient's fever is mild to moderate, ask him when it began and how high his temperature reached. Did the fever disappear, only to reappear later? Did he experience any other symptoms, such as chills, fatigue, or pain?

Obtain a complete medical history, noting immunosuppressive treatments or disorders, infection, trauma, surgery, diagnostic testing, and use of anesthesia or other medications. Ask about recent travel because certain diseases are endemic.

Physical examination
Let the history findings direct your physical examination. Because fever can accompany diverse disorders, the examination may range from a brief evaluation of one body system to a comprehensive review of all systems. (See *How fever develops,* pages 148.) Assess vital signs and evaluate the patient for complications related to the fever such as dehydration, body aches, fatigue, anorexia, and seizure activity.

Pediatric pointers
Infants and young children experience higher and more prolonged fevers, more rapid temperature increases, and greater temperature fluctuations than older children and adults.

Keep in mind that seizures commonly accompany extremely high fever, so take appropriate precautions. Also, instruct parents not to give aspirin to a child with varicella or flulike symptoms because of the risk of precipitating Reye's syndrome.

Common pediatric causes of fever include varicella, croup syndrome, dehydration, meningitis, mumps, otitis media, pertussis, roseola infantum, rubella, rubeola, and tonsillitis. Fever can also occur as a reaction to immunizations and antibiotics.

Geriatric pointers
Elderly people may have an altered sweating mechanism that predisposes them to heatstroke when exposed to high temperatures; they may also have an impaired thermoregulatory mechanism, making temperature change a much less reliable measure of disease severity.

MEDICAL CAUSES
● *Anthrax, cutaneous.* The patient may experience a fever along with lymphadenopathy, malaise, and headache. After the bacterium *Bacillus anthracis* enters a cut or abrasion on the skin, the infection begins as a small, painless or pruritic macular or papular lesion resembling an insect bite. Within 1 to 2 days, the lesion develops into a vesicle and then into a painless ulcer with a characteristic black, necrotic center.

● *Anthrax, GI.* Following the ingestion of contaminated meat from an animal infected with the bacterium *Bacillus anthracis,* the patient experiences fever, loss of appetite, nausea, and vomiting. The patient may also experience abdominal pain, severe bloody diarrhea, and hematemesis.

● *Anthrax, inhalation.* The initial signs and symptoms of inhalation anthrax are flulike ones, including fever, chills, weakness, cough, and chest pain. The disease generally occurs in two stages with a period of recovery after the initial symptoms. The second stage develops abruptly with rapid deterioration marked by fever, dyspnea, stridor, and hypotension, generally leading to death within 24 hours.

● *Escherichia coli O157:H7.* Fever, bloody diarrhea, nausea, vomiting, and abdominal cramps occur after eating undercooked beef or other foods contaminated with *E. coli* O157:H7. In children younger than age 5 and in elderly patients, hemolytic uremic

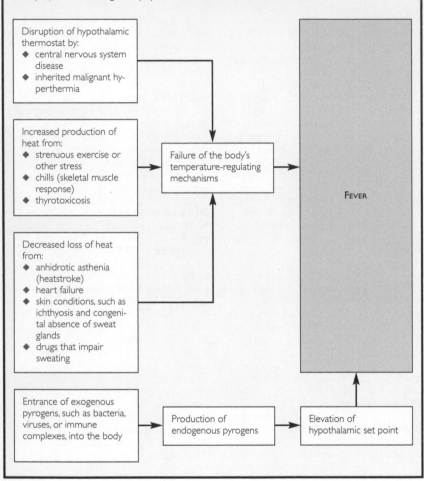

HOW FEVER DEVELOPS

Body temperature is regulated by the hypothalamic thermostat, which has a specific set point under normal conditions. Fever can result from a resetting of this set point or from an abnormality in the thermoregulatory system itself, as shown in this flowchart.

Disruption of hypothalamic thermostat by:
- central nervous system disease
- inherited malignant hyperthermia

Increased production of heat from:
- strenuous exercise or other stress
- chills (skeletal muscle response)
- thyrotoxicosis

Decreased loss of heat from:
- anhidrotic asthenia (heatstroke)
- heart failure
- skin conditions, such as ichthyosis and congenital absence of sweat glands
- drugs that impair sweating

Failure of the body's temperature-regulating mechanisms

Entrance of exogenous pyrogens, such as bacteria, viruses, or immune complexes, into the body

Production of endogenous pyrogens

Elevation of hypothalamic set point

FEVER

---

syndrome may develop (in which the red blood cells are destroyed), and this may ultimately lead to acute renal failure.

- *Immune complex dysfunction.* When present, fever usually remains low, although moderate elevations may accompany erythema multiforme. Fever may be remittent or intermittent, as in acquired immunodeficiency syndrome (AIDS) or systemic lupus erythematosus, or sustained, as in polyarteritis. As one of several vague, prodromal complaints (such as fatigue, anorexia, and weight loss), fever produces nocturnal diaphoresis and accompanies such associated signs and symptoms as diarrhea and a persistent cough (with AIDS) or morning stiffness (with rheumatoid arthritis). Other disease-specific findings include headache and vision loss (temporal arteritis); pain and stiffness in the neck, shoulders, back, or pelvis (ankylosing spondylitis and polymyalgia rheumatica); skin and mucous membrane lesions (erythema multiforme); and urethritis with urethral discharge and conjunctivitis (Reiter's syndrome).

- **Infectious and inflammatory disorders.** Fever ranges from low (in patients with Crohn's disease or ulcerative colitis) to extremely high (in those with bacterial pneumonia, necrotizing fasciitis, or Ebola or Hantavirus). It may be remittent, as in those with infectious mononucleosis or otitis media; hectic (recurring daily with sweating, chills, and flushing), as in those with lung abscess, influenza, or endocarditis; sustained, as in those with meningitis; or relapsing, as in those with malaria. Fever may arise abruptly, as in those with toxic shock syndrome or Rocky Mountain spotted fever, or insidiously, as in those with mycoplasmal pneumonia. In patients with hepatitis, fever may represent a disease prodrome; in those with appendicitis, it follows the acute stage. Its sudden late appearance with tachycardia, tachypnea, and confusion heralds life-threatening septic shock in patients with peritonitis or gram-negative bacteremia.

Associated signs and symptoms involve every system. The cyclic variations of hectic fever typically produce alternating chills and diaphoresis. General systemic complaints include weakness, anorexia, and malaise.

- **Listeriosis.** Signs and symptoms of listeriosis include fever, myalgias, abdominal pain, nausea, vomiting, and diarrhea. If the infection spreads to the nervous system, meningitis may develop; symptoms include fever, headache, nuchal rigidity, and change in level of consciousness.
- **Neoplasms.** Primary neoplasms and metastasis can produce prolonged fever of varying elevations. For instance, acute leukemia may present insidiously with low fever, pallor, and bleeding tendencies, or more abruptly with high fever, frank bleeding, and prostration. Occasionally, Hodgkin's disease produces undulant fever or Pel-Ebstein fever, an irregularly relapsing fever.

Besides fever and nocturnal diaphoresis, neoplastic disease often causes anorexia, fatigue, malaise, and weight loss. Examination may reveal lesions, lymphadenopathy, palpable masses, and hepatosplenomegaly.

- **Plague (Yersinia pestis).** The bubonic form of plague (transmitted to patient when bitten by infected fleas) causes fever, chills, and swollen, inflamed, and tender lymph nodes near the site of the bite. The sep-

ticemic form develops as a fulminant illness generally with the bubonic form. The pneumonic form manifests as a sudden onset of chills, fever, headache, and myalgias after person-to-person transmission via the respiratory tract. Other signs and symptoms of the pneumonic form include productive cough, chest pain, tachypnea, dyspnea, hemoptysis, increasing respiratory distress, and cardiopulmonary insufficiency.

- **Q fever.** Q fever is a rickettsial disease that's caused by the infection of *Coxiella burnetii* causes fever, chills, severe headache, malaise, chest pain, nausea, vomiting, and diarrhea. Fever may last up to 2 weeks. In severe cases, the patient may develop hepatitis or pneumonia.
- **Rhabdomyolysis.** Rhabdomyolysis results in muscle breakdown and release of the muscle cell contents (myoglobin) into the bloodstream, with signs and symptoms including fever, muscle weakness or pain, nausea, vomiting, malaise, or dark urine. Acute renal failure is the most frequently reported complication of the disorder. It results from renal structure obstruction and injury during the kidney's attempt to filter the myoglobin from the bloodstream.
- **Rift Valley fever.** Typical signs and symptoms of Rift Valley fever include fever, myalgia, weakness, dizziness, and back pain. A small percentage of patients may develop encephalitis or may progress to hemorrhagic fever that can lead to shock and hemorrhage. Inflammation of the retina may result in some permanent vision loss.
- **Severe acute respiratory syndrome (SARS).** SARS is an acute infectious disease caused by a coronavirus called SARS-associated coronavirus (SARS-CoV). Although most cases have been reported in Asia (China, Vietnam, Singapore, Thailand), cases have cropped up in Europe and North America. The incubation period is 2 to 7 days, and the illness generally begins with a fever (usually greater than 100.4° F [38° C]). Other symptoms include headache, malaise, a dry nonproductive cough, and dyspnea. The severity of the illness is highly variable, ranging from mild illness to pneumonia and, in some cases, progressing to respiratory failure and death.
- **Smallpox (variola major).** Initial signs and symptoms of smallpox include high fever, malaise, prostration, severe headache, backache, and abdominal pain. A maculopapular

rash develops on the mucosa of the mouth, pharynx, face, and forearms and then spreads to the trunk and legs. Within 2 days, the rash becomes vesicular and later pustular. The lesions develop at the same time, appear identical, and are more prominent on the face and extremities. The pustules are round, firm, and deeply embedded in the skin. After about 8 to 9 days, the pustules form a crust, and later the scab separates from the skin, leaving a pitted scar. In fatal cases, death results from encephalitis, extensive bleeding, or secondary infection.

● *Thermoregulatory dysfunction.* Sudden onset of fever that rises rapidly and remains as high as 107° F (41.7° C) occurs in life-threatening disorders, such as heatstroke, thyroid storm, neuroleptic malignant syndrome, and malignant hyperthermia, and in lesions of the central nervous system (CNS). Low or moderate fever appears in dehydrated patients.

Prolonged high fever commonly produces vomiting, anhidrosis, decreased level of consciousness (LOC), and hot, flushed skin. Related cardiovascular effects may include tachycardia, tachypnea, and hypotension. Other disease-specific findings include skin changes: dry skin and mucous membranes, poor skin turgor, and oliguria with dehydration; mottled cyanosis with malignant hyperthermia; diarrhea with thyroid storm; and ominous signs of increased intracranial pressure (decreased LOC with bradycardia, widened pulse pressure, and increased systolic pressure) with CNS tumor, trauma, or hemorrhage.

● *Tularemia.* Tularemia, also known as *rabbit fever,* is an infectious disease that causes abrupt onset of fever, chills, headache, generalized myalgias, nonproductive cough, dyspnea, pleuritic chest pain, and empyema.

● *Typhus.* With typhus — a rickettsial disease — the patient initially experiences headache, myalgia, arthralgia, and malaise. These signs and symptoms are followed by an abrupt onset of fever, chills, nausea, and vomiting. A maculopapular rash may be present in some cases.

● *West Nile encephalitis.* A brain infection caused by West Nile virus, the mosquito-borne flavivirus is commonly found in Africa, West Asia, the Middle East and, rarely, in North America. Mild infection is common; signs and symptoms include fever, headache, and body aches, often with skin rash and swollen lymph glands. More severe infection is marked by high fever, headache, neck stiffness, stupor, disorientation, coma, tremors, occasional convulsions, paralysis and, rarely, death.

OTHER CAUSES

● *Diagnostic tests.* Immediate or delayed fever infrequently follows radiographic tests that use contrast medium.

● *Drugs.* Fever and rash commonly result from hypersensitivity to antifungals, sulfonamides, penicillins, cephalosporins, tetracyclines, barbiturates, phenytoin, quinidine, iodides, phenolphthalein, methyldopa, procainamide, and some antitoxins. Fever can accompany chemotherapy, especially with bleomycin, vincristine, and asparaginase. It can result from drugs that impair sweating, such as anticholinergics, phenothiazines, and monoamine oxidase inhibitors. A drug-induced fever typically disappears after the involved drug is discontinued. Fever can also stem from toxic doses of salicylates, amphetamines, and tricyclic antidepressants.

Inhaled anesthetics and muscle relaxants can trigger malignant hyperthermia in patients with this inherited trait.

● *Medical treatments.* Remittent or intermittent low fever may occur for several days after surgery. Transfusion reactions characteristically produce abrupt onset of fever and chills.

NURSING CONSIDERATIONS

Regularly monitor the patient's temperature, and record it on a chart for easy follow-up of the temperature curve. Provide increased fluid and nutritional intake. When administering a prescribed antipyretic, minimize resultant chills and diaphoresis by following a regular dosage schedule. Promote patient comfort by maintaining a stable room temperature and providing frequent changes of bedding and clothing. Prepare the patient for laboratory tests, such as complete blood count and cultures of blood, urine, sputum, and wound drainage.

PATIENT TEACHING

If the patient hasn't been admitted to the facility, ask him to measure his oral temperature at home and record the time and value. Explain that fever is a response to an underlying condition that plays an important role in fighting infection. For this reason, advise him not to take an antipyretic until his body temperature reaches 101° F (38.3° C). Discuss signs and symptoms related to dehydration and when to notify the physician.

Flank pain

Pain in the flank, the area extending from the ribs to the ilium, is a leading indicator of renal and upper urinary tract disease or trauma. Depending on the cause, this symptom may vary from a dull ache to severe stabbing or throbbing pain, and may be unilateral or bilateral and constant or intermittent. It's aggravated by costovertebral angle (CVA) percussion and, in patients with renal or urinary tract obstruction, by increased fluid intake and ingestion of alcohol, caffeine, or diuretics. Unaffected by position changes, flank pain typically responds only to analgesics or, of course, to treatment of the underlying disorder.

Act now If the patient has suffered trauma, quickly look for a visible or palpable flank mass, associated injuries, CVA pain, hematuria, Turner's sign, and signs of shock (such as tachycardia and cool, clammy skin). If one or more is present, insert an I.V. line to allow fluid or drug infusion. Insert an indwelling urinary catheter to monitor urine output and evaluate hematuria. Obtain blood samples for typing and crossmatching, complete blood count, and electrolyte levels.

ASSESSMENT
History
If the patient's condition isn't critical, take a thorough history. Ask about the pain's onset and apparent precipitating events. Have him describe the pain's location, intensity, pattern, and duration. Find out if anything aggravates or alleviates it.

Ask the patient about any changes in his normal pattern of fluid intake and urine output. Explore his history for urinary tract infection (UTI) or obstruction, renal disease, or recent streptococcal infection.

Physical examination
During the physical examination, palpate the patient's flank area and percuss the CVA to determine the extent of pain.

Pediatric pointers
Assessment of flank pain can be difficult if a child can't describe the pain. In such cases, transillumination of the abdomen and flanks may help in assessment of bladder distention and identification of masses. Common causes of flank pain in children include obstructive uropathy, acute poststreptococcal glomerulonephritis, infantile polycystic kidney disease, and nephroblastoma.

MEDICAL CAUSES
See *Flank pain: Causes and associated findings,* pages 152 and 153.
- *Bladder cancer.* Dull, constant flank pain may be unilateral or bilateral and may radiate to the leg, back, and perineum. Commonly, the first sign of this cancer is gross, painless, intermittent hematuria, often with clots. Related effects may include urinary frequency and urgency, nocturia, dysuria, or pyuria; bladder distention; pain in the bladder, rectum, pelvis, back, or legs; diarrhea; vomiting; and sleep disturbances.
- *Calculi.* Renal and ureteral calculi produce intense unilateral, colicky flank pain. Typically, initial CVA pain radiates to the flank, suprapubic region, and perhaps the genitalia; abdominal and lower back pain are also possible. Nausea and vomiting often accompany severe pain. Associated findings include CVA tenderness, hematuria, hypoactive bowel sounds and, possibly, signs and symptoms of UTI (urinary frequency and urgency, dysuria, nocturia, fatigue, low-grade fever, and tenesmus).
- *Cortical necrosis (acute).* Unilateral flank pain is usually severe. Accompanying findings include gross hematuria, anuria, leukocytosis, and fever.
- *Cystitis (bacterial).* Unilateral or bilateral flank pain occurs secondarily to an ascending UTI. The patient may also report perineal, low back, and suprapubic pain. Other effects include dysuria, nocturia, hematuria, urinary frequency and urgency, tenesmus, fatigue, and low-grade fever.
- *Glomerulonephritis (acute).* Flank pain in patients with glomerulonephritis is bilateral, constant, and of moderate intensity. The most common findings are moderate facial and generalized edema, hematuria, oliguria or anuria, and fatigue. Other effects include slightly increased blood pressure, low-grade fever, malaise, headache, nausea, and vomiting. Accompanying signs of pulmonary con-

FLANK PAIN:
CAUSES AND ASSOCIATED FINDINGS

MAJOR ASSOCIATED SIGNS AND SYMPTOMS

COMMON CAUSES	Abdominal distention	Abdominal mass	Abdominal pain	Anuria	Back pain	Bladder distention	Blood pressure, decreased	Blood pressure, increased	Bowel sounds, hypoactive	Chills	Costovertebral angle tenderness	
Bladder cancer					●	●						
Calculi			●						●		●	
Cortical necrosis (acute)				●								
Cystitis (bacterial)					●							
Glomerulonephritis (acute)				●				●				
Obstructive uropathy	●	●	●	●		●			●		●	
Pancreatitis (acute)			●		●		●		●			
Papillary necrosis (acute)			●	●					●	●	●	
Perirenal abscess		●								●	●	
Polycystic kidney disease					●			●				
Pyelonephritis (acute)			●							●	●	
Renal cancer								●				
Renal infarction			●	●					●		●	
Renal trauma	●		●						●		●	
Renal vein thrombosis					●						●	

gestion include dyspnea, tachypnea, and crackles.

● *Obstructive uropathy.* With acute obstruction, flank pain may be excruciating; with gradual obstruction, it's typically a dull ache. With both, the pain may also localize in the upper abdomen and radiate to the groin. Nausea and vomiting, abdominal distention, anuria alternating with periods of oliguria and polyuria, and hypoactive bowel sounds may also occur. Additional findings — a pal-pable abdominal mass, CVA tenderness, and bladder distention — vary with the site and cause of the obstruction.

● *Pancreatitis (acute).* Bilateral flank pain may develop as severe epigastric or left-upper-quadrant pain radiates to the back. A severe attack causes extreme pain, nausea and persistent vomiting, abdominal tenderness and rigidity, hypoactive bowel sounds and, possibly, restlessness, low-grade fever,

	Dysuria	Edema, generalized	Fatigue	Fever	Flank mass	Groin pain	Hematuria	Leg pain	Nausea	Nocturia	Oliguria	Perineal pain	Polyuria	Pyuria	Suprapubic pain	Tenesmus	Urinary frequency	Urinary urgency	Urine retention	Vomiting
	•						•	•		•		•		•			•	•		•
	•		•	•		•	•		•	•					•	•	•	•		•
				•			•													
	•		•	•			•			•		•			•	•	•	•		
		•	•	•			•		•		•									•
					•		•		•			•								•
			•	•	•		•													•
				•			•				•			•						•
	•			•																
							•					•	•		•	•	•	•		
	•		•	•			•			•						•	•	•		
				•	•		•		•										•	•
				•			•		•		•									•
			•		•	•	•		•		•									•
			•				•		•		•									•

tachycardia, hypotension, and positive Turner's and Cullen's signs.
• *Papillary necrosis (acute).* Intense bilateral flank pain occurs along with renal colic, CVA tenderness, and abdominal pain and rigidity. Urinary signs and symptoms include oliguria or anuria, hematuria, and pyuria, with associated high fever, chills, vomiting, and hypoactive bowel sounds.
• *Perirenal abscess.* Intense unilateral flank pain and CVA tenderness accompany dy-

suria, persistent high fever, chills and, in some patients, a palpable abdominal mass.
• *Polycystic kidney disease.* Dull, aching, bilateral flank pain is commonly the earliest symptom of polycystic kidney disease—a renal disorder. The pain can become severe and colicky if cysts rupture and clots migrate or cause obstruction. Nonspecific early findings include polyuria, increased blood pressure, and signs of UTI. Later findings include

hematuria and perineal, low back, and suprapubic pain.

- **Pyelonephritis (acute).** Intense, constant, unilateral or bilateral flank pain develops over a few hours or days along with typical urinary features: dysuria, nocturia, hematuria, urgency, frequency, and tenesmus. Other common findings include persistent high fever, chills, anorexia, weakness, fatigue, generalized myalgia, abdominal pain, and marked CVA tenderness.
- **Renal cancer.** Unilateral flank pain, gross hematuria, and a palpable flank mass form the classic clinical triad. Flank pain is usually dull and vague, although severe colicky pain can occur during bleeding or passage of clots. Associated signs and symptoms include fever, increased blood pressure, and urine retention. Weight loss, leg edema, nausea, and vomiting are indications of advanced disease.
- **Renal infarction.** Unilateral, constant, severe flank pain and tenderness typically accompany persistent, severe upper abdominal pain. The patient may also develop CVA tenderness, anorexia, nausea and vomiting, fever, hypoactive bowel sounds, hematuria, and oliguria or anuria.
- **Renal trauma.** Variable bilateral or unilateral flank pain is a common symptom. A visible or palpable flank mass may also exist, along with CVA or abdominal pain—which may be severe and radiate to the groin. Other findings include hematuria, oliguria, abdominal distention, Turner's sign, hypoactive bowel sounds, and nausea or vomiting. Severe injury may produce signs of shock, such as tachycardia and cool, clammy skin.
- **Renal vein thrombosis.** Severe unilateral flank and low back pain with CVA and epigastric tenderness typify the rapid onset of venous obstruction. Other features include fever, hematuria, and leg edema. Bilateral flank pain, oliguria, and other uremic signs and symptoms (nausea, vomiting, and uremic fetor) typify bilateral obstruction.

NURSING CONSIDERATIONS

Administer pain medication. Continue to monitor the patient's vital signs, and maintain a precise record of the patient's intake and output.

Diagnostic evaluation may involve serial urine and serum analysis, excretory urography, flank ultrasonography, computed tomography scan, voiding cystourethrography, cystoscopy, and retrograde ureteropyelography, urethrography, and cystography.

PATIENT TEACHING

Provide information on the importance of increased fluid intake, unless contraindicated. Explain signs and symptoms that are imperative to report. Emphasize the importance of taking drugs as prescribed. Stress the importance of keeping follow-up appointments.

Gag reflex, abnormal

The gag reflex—a protective mechanism that prevents aspiration of food, fluid, and vomitus—normally can be elicited by touching the posterior wall of the oropharynx with a tongue depressor or by suctioning the throat. Prompt elevation of the palate, constriction of the pharyngeal musculature, and a sensation of gagging indicate a normal gag reflex. An abnormal gag reflex—either decreased or absent—interferes with the ability to swallow and, more important, increases susceptibility to life-threatening aspiration.

An impaired gag reflex can result from any lesion that affects its mediators—cranial nerves IX (glossopharyngeal) and X (vagus) or the pons or medulla. It can also occur during a coma, in muscle diseases such as severe myasthenia gravis, or as a temporary result of anesthesia.

Act now *If you detect an abnormal gag reflex, immediately stop the patient's oral intake to prevent aspiration. Quickly evaluate level of consciousness (LOC). If it's decreased, place him in a side-lying position to prevent aspiration; if not, place him in Fowler's position. Have suction equipment at hand.*

ASSESSMENT
History
Ask the patient (or a family member if the patient can't communicate) whether he has experienced swallowing difficulties. If so, determine onset and duration. Are liquids more difficult to swallow than solids? Is swallowing more difficult at certain times of the day (as occurs in the bulbar palsy associated with myasthenia gravis)? If the patient also has trouble chewing, suspect more widespread neurologic involvement because chewing involves different cranial nerves. Explore his history for vascular and degenerative disorders.

Physical examination
Assess the patient's respiratory status for evidence of aspiration, and perform a neurologic examination. Assess his gag reflex and determine whether other reflexes are also impaired.

Pediatric pointers
Brain stem glioma is an important cause of abnormal gag reflex in children.

MEDICAL CAUSES
● **Basilar artery occlusion.** Basilar artery occlusion may suddenly diminish or obliterate the gag reflex. It also causes diffuse sensory loss, dysarthria, facial weakness, extraocular muscle palsies, quadriplegia, and decreased LOC.
● **Brain stem glioma.** Brain stem glioma causes gradual loss of the gag reflex. Related symptoms reflect bilateral brain stem involvement and include diplopia and facial weakness. Common involvement of the corticospinal pathways causes spasticity and paresis of the arms and legs, as well as gait disturbances.
● **Bulbar palsy.** Loss of the gag reflex reflects temporary or permanent paralysis of

muscles supplied by cranial nerves IX and X. Other indicators of bulbar palsy include jaw and facial muscle weakness, dysphagia, loss of sensation at the base of the tongue, increased salivation, possible difficulty articulating and breathing, and fasciculations.

● *Myasthenia gravis.* In severe myasthenia, the motor limb of the gag reflex is reduced. Weakness worsens with repetitive use and may also involve other muscles.

● *Wallenberg's syndrome.* Paresis of the palate and an impaired gag reflex usually develop within hours to days of thrombosis. The patient may experience analgesia and thermanesthesia, occurring ipsilaterally on the face and contralaterally on the body, and vertigo. He may also display nystagmus, ipsilateral ataxia of the arm and leg, and signs of Horner's syndrome (unilateral ptosis and miosis, hemifacial anhidrosis).

OTHER CAUSES

● *Anesthesia.* General and local (throat) anesthesia can produce temporary loss of the gag reflex.

NURSING CONSIDERATIONS

Continually assess the patient's ability to swallow. If his gag reflex is absent, follow facility and state regulations regarding food texture or tube feeding options. Advise the patient to take small amounts and eat slowly while sitting or in high Fowler's position. Stay with him while he eats and observe for choking. Remember to keep suction equipment handy in case of aspiration. Keep accurate intake and output records, and assess the patient's nutritional status daily.

Refer the patient to a speech therapist to determine his aspiration risk and develop an exercise program to strengthen specific muscles. Other members of the interdisciplinary team who should be consulted include the dietitian, psychiatrist, social worker, pharmacist, nurse, and discharge planner.

Prepare the patient for diagnostic studies, such as swallow studies, computed tomography scan, magnetic resonance imaging, electroencephalography, lumbar puncture, and arteriography.

PATIENT TEACHING

Discuss diet and fluid restrictions and positioning requirements related to food and liquid consumption. Encourage the family to consider taking a course that will teach techniques to relieve an airway obstruction. If speech therapy is indicated, encourage the patient to begin as soon as possible and follow through with the suggestions and ongoing therapy. Teach the family about aspiration pneumonia and how to prevent it.

Gallop, atrial
[S$_4$]

An atrial or presystolic gallop is an extra heart sound (known as S$_4$) that's heard or often palpated immediately before the first heart sound, late in diastole. This low-pitched sound is heard best with the bell of the stethoscope pressed lightly against the cardiac apex. Some clinicians say that an S$_4$ has the cadence of the "Ten" in Tennessee (Ten = S$_3$; nes = S$_1$; see = S$_2$).

This gallop typically results from hypertension, conduction defects, valvular disorders, or other problems such as ischemia. Occasionally, it helps differentiate angina from other causes of chest pain. It results from abnormal forceful atrial contraction caused by augmented ventricular filling or by decreased left ventricular compliance. An atrial gallop usually originates from left atrial contraction, is heard at the apex, and doesn't vary with inspiration. A left-sided S$_4$ can occur in hypertensive heart disease, coronary artery disease, aortic stenosis, and cardiomyopathy. It may also originate from right atrial contraction. A right-sided S$_4$ is indicative of pulmonary hypertension and pulmonary stenosis. If so, it's heard best at the lower left sternal border and intensifies with inspiration.

An atrial gallop seldom occurs in normal hearts; however, it may occur in elderly people and in athletes with physiologic hypertrophy of the left ventricle.

Act now *Suspect myocardial ischemia if you auscultate an atrial gallop in a patient with chest pain. (See* Locating heart sounds. *See also* Interpreting heart sounds, *pages 158 and 159.) Take the patient's vital signs and quickly assess for signs of heart failure, such as dyspnea, crackles, and distended jugular veins. If you detect these signs, connect the patient to a cardiac monitor and obtain an electrocardiogram. Administer an antianginal and oxygen. If the patient has dyspnea, elevate the head of the bed. Then auscultate for ab-*

LOCATING HEART SOUNDS

When auscultating heart sounds, remember that certain sounds are heard best in specific areas. Use the auscultatory points shown at right to locate heart sounds quickly and accurately. Then expand your auscultation to nearby areas. Note that the numbers indicate pertinent intercostal spaces.

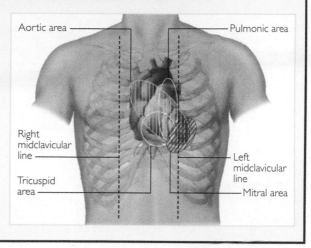

normal breath sounds. If you detect coarse crackles, ensure patent I.V. access and give oxygen and diuretics as needed. If the patient has bradycardia, he may require atropine and a pacemaker.

ASSESSMENT
History
When the patient's condition permits, ask about a history of hypertension, angina, valvular stenosis, or cardiomyopathy. If appropriate, have him describe the frequency and severity of anginal attacks.

Physical examination
Monitor the patient's vital signs and cardiac rhythm. Perform a complete cardiopulmonary examination, including the auscultation of heart sounds. Assess the patient's respiratory status, breath sounds, and oxygenation.

Pediatric pointers
An atrial gallop may occur normally in children, especially after exercise. However, it may also result from congenital heart diseases, such as atrial septal defect, ventricular septal defect, patent ductus arteriosus, and severe pulmonary valvular stenosis.

Geriatric pointers
Because the absolute intensity of an atrial gallop doesn't decrease with age, as it does

with an S_1, the relative intensity of S_4 increases compared with S_1. This explains the increased frequency of an audible S_4 in elderly patients and the reason this sound may be considered a normal finding in these patients.

MEDICAL CAUSES
- *Anemia.* In anemia, an atrial gallop may accompany increased cardiac output. Associated findings may include fatigue, pallor, dyspnea, tachycardia, bounding pulse, crackles, and a systolic bruit over the carotid arteries.
- *Angina.* An intermittent atrial gallop characteristically occurs during an anginal attack and disappears when angina subsides. This gallop may be accompanied by a paradoxical S_2 or a new murmur. Typically, the patient complains of anginal chest pain — a feeling of tightness, pressure, achiness, or burning that usually radiates from the retrosternal area to the neck, jaws, left shoulder, and arm. He may also exhibit dyspnea, tachycardia, palpitations, increased blood pressure, dizziness, diaphoresis, belching, nausea, and vomiting.
- *Aortic insufficiency (acute).* Aortic insufficiency causes an atrial gallop accompanied by a soft, short diastolic murmur along the left sternal border. S_2 may be soft or absent. Sometimes a soft, short midsystolic murmur may be heard over the second right inter-

INTERPRETING HEART SOUNDS

Detecting subtle variations in heart sounds requires both concentration and practice. Once you recognize normal heart sounds, the abnormal sounds become more obvious.

HEART SOUND AND CAUSE	TIMING AND CADENCE
First heart sound (S₁) Vibrations associated with mitral and tricuspid valve closure	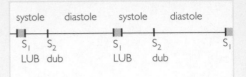
Second heart sound (S₂) Vibrations associated with aortic and pulmonic valve closure	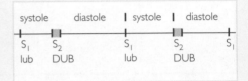
Ventricular gallop (S₃) Vibrations produced by rapid blood flow into the ventricles	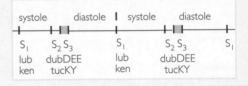
Atrial gallop (S₄) Vibrations produced by an increased resistance to sudden, forceful ejection of atrial blood	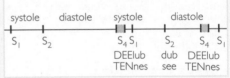
Summation gallop Vibrations produced in middiastole by simultaneous ventricular and atrial gallops, usually caused by tachycardia	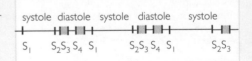

costal space. Related cardiopulmonary findings may include tachycardia, S₃, dyspnea, jugular vein distention, crackles and, possibly, angina. The patient may also be fatigued and have cool extremities.

● *Aortic stenosis.* Aortic stenosis usually causes an atrial gallop, especially when valvular obstruction is severe. Auscultation reveals a harsh, crescendo-decrescendo, sys-

tolic ejection murmur that's loudest at the right sternal border near the second intercostal space. Dyspnea, anginal chest pain, and syncope are cardinal associated findings. The patient may also display crackles, palpitations, fatigue, and diminished carotid pulses.

● *Atrioventricular (AV) block.* First-degree AV block may cause an atrial gallop accom-

Best heard with the diaphragm of the stethoscope at the apex (mitral area).

Best heard with the diaphragm of the stethoscope in the second or third right and left parasternal intercostal spaces with the patient sitting or in a supine position.

Best heard through the bell of the stethoscope at the apex with the patient in the left lateral position. May be visible and palpable during early diastole at the midclavicular line between the fourth and fifth intercostal spaces.

Best heard through the bell of the stethoscope at the apex with the patient in the left semilateral position. May be visible in late diastole at the midclavicular line between the fourth and fifth intercostal spaces. May also be palpable in the midclavicular area with the patient in the left lateral decubitus position.

Best heard through the bell of the stethoscope at the apex with the patient in the left lateral position. May be louder than S_1 or S_2. May be visible and palpable during diastole.

in intensity with S_1 and is loudest when atrial systole coincides with early, rapid ventricular filling during diastole. The patient may be asymptomatic or have hypotension, light-headedness, dizziness, or syncope, depending on the ventricular rate. Bradycardia may also aggravate or provoke angina or symptoms of heart failure such as dyspnea.

● *Cardiomyopathy.* An atrial gallop is a sign associated with cardiomyopathy, regardless of the type — dilated (most common), hypertrophic, or restrictive (least common). Additional findings may include dyspnea, orthopnea, crackles, fatigue, syncope, chest pain, palpitations, edema, jugular vein distention, S_3, and transient or sustained bradycardia usually associated with tachycardia.

● *Hypertension.* One of the earliest findings in systemic arterial hypertension is an atrial gallop. The patient may be asymptomatic, or he may experience headache, weakness, epistaxis, tinnitus, dizziness, and fatigue.

● *Mitral insufficiency.* In acute mitral insufficiency, auscultation may reveal an atrial gallop accompanied by an S_3, a harsh holosystolic murmur that's heard best at the apex or over the precordium. This murmur radiates to the axilla and back and along the left sternal border. Other features may include fatigue, dyspnea, tachypnea, orthopnea, tachycardia, crackles, and jugular vein distention.

● *Myocardial infarction (MI).* An atrial gallop is a classic sign of life-threatening MI; in fact, it may persist even after the infarction heals. Typically, the patient reports crushing substernal chest pain that may radiate to the back, neck, jaw, shoulder, and left arm. Associated signs and symptoms include dyspnea, restlessness, anxiety, a feeling of impending doom, diaphoresis, pallor, clammy skin, nausea, vomiting, and increased or decreased blood pressure.

● *Pulmonary embolism.* Pulmonary embolism is a life-threatening disorder that causes a right-sided atrial gallop that's usually heard along the lower left sternal border with a loud pulmonic closure sound. Other features include tachycardia, tachypnea, fever, chest pain, dyspnea, decreased breath sounds, crackles, a pleural chest rub, apprehension, diaphoresis, syncope, and cyanosis. The patient may have a productive cough with blood-tinged sputum, or a nonproductive cough.

panied by a faint first heart sound (S_1). Although the patient may have bradycardia, he's usually asymptomatic. In second-degree AV block, an atrial gallop is easily heard. If bradycardia develops, the patient may also experience hypotension, light-headedness, dizziness, and fatigue. An atrial gallop is also common in third-degree AV block. It varies

- *Thyrotoxicosis.* An atrial gallop and an S_3 may both be auscultated in thyroid hormone overproduction. Other cardinal features include tachycardia, bounding pulse, wide pulse pressure, palpitations, weight loss despite increased appetite, diarrhea, tremors, an enlarged thyroid, dyspnea, nervousness, difficulty concentrating, diaphoresis, heat intolerance, exophthalmos, weakness, fatigue, and muscle atrophy.

NURSING CONSIDERATIONS
Prepare the patient for diagnostic tests, such as electrocardiography, echocardiography, cardiac catheterization, laboratory tests such as CK-MB, troponin, and, possibly, a lung scan.

PATIENT TEACHING
Inform the patient about ways to reduce his cardiac risks. Teach him the correct way to measure his pulse rate. Emphasize conditions that require medical attention. Stress the importance of follow-up appointments.

Hematemesis

Hematemesis, the vomiting of blood, usually indicates GI bleeding above the ligament of Treitz, which suspends the duodenum at its junction with the jejunum. Bright red or blood-streaked vomitus indicates fresh or recent bleeding. Dark red, brown, or black vomitus (the color and consistency of coffee grounds) indicates that blood has been retained in the stomach and partially digested.

Although hematemesis usually results from a GI disorder, it may stem from a coagulation disorder or from a treatment that irritates the GI tract. Esophageal varices may also cause hematemesis. Swallowed blood from epistaxis or oropharyngeal erosion may also cause bloody vomitus. Hematemesis may be precipitated by straining, emotional stress, and the use of an anti-inflammatory or alcohol. In a patient with esophageal varices, hematemesis may be a result of trauma from swallowing hard or partially chewed food. (See *Rare causes of hematemesis,* page 162.)

Hematemesis is always an important sign, but its severity depends on the amount, source, and rapidity of the bleeding. Massive hematemesis (vomiting of 500 to 1,000 ml of blood) may be life-threatening.

Act now *If the patient has massive hematemesis, check his vital signs. If you detect signs of shock—such as tachypnea, hypotension, and tachycardia—place the patient in a supine position, and elevate his feet 20 to 30 degrees. Start a large-bore I.V. line for emergency fluid replacement. Also, send a blood sample for typing and crossmatching, hemoglobin level, hematocrit, serum amylase, and administer oxygen. Emergency endoscopy may be necessary to locate the source of bleeding. Prepare to insert a nasogastric (NG) tube for suction or iced lavage. A Sengstaken-Blakemore tube may be used to compress esophageal varices. (See* Managing hematemesis with intubation, *page 163.)*

ASSESSMENT
History
If the patient's hematemesis isn't immediately life-threatening, begin with a thorough history. First, have the patient describe the amount, color, and consistency of the vomitus. When did he first notice this sign? Has he ever had hematemesis before? Find out if he also has bloody or black, tarry stools. Note whether hematemesis is usually preceded by nausea, flatulence, diarrhea, or weakness. Has he recently had bouts of retching with or without vomiting?

Next, ask about a history of ulcers or of liver or coagulation disorders. Find out how much alcohol the patient drinks, if any. Does he regularly take aspirin or aspirin-containing medications, corticosteroids, anticoagulants, or nonsteroidal anti-inflammatory drugs (NSAIDs), such as phenylbutazone or indomethacin? These drugs may cause erosive gastritis or ulcers.

Physical examination
Begin the physical examination by checking for orthostatic hypotension, an early warning sign of hypovolemia. Take blood pressure and pulse with the patient in supine, sitting,

and standing positions. A decrease of 10 mm Hg or more in systolic pressure or an increase of 10 beats/minute or more in pulse rate indicates volume depletion. After obtaining other vital signs, inspect the mucous membranes, nasopharynx, and skin for any signs of bleeding or other abnormalities. Finally, palpate the abdomen for tenderness, pain, or masses. Note lymphadenopathy.

Pediatric pointers

Hematemesis is much less common in children than in adults and may be related to foreign-body ingestion. Occasionally, neonates develop hematemesis after swallowing maternal blood during delivery or breast-feeding from a cracked nipple. Hemorrhagic disease of the neonate and esophageal erosion may also cause hematemesis in infants; such cases require immediate fluid replacement.

Geriatric pointers

In elderly patients, hematemesis may be caused by a vascular anomaly, an aortoenteric fistula, or upper GI cancer. In addition, chronic obstructive pulmonary disease, chronic liver or renal failure, and chronic NSAID use all predispose elderly people to hemorrhage secondary to coexisting ulcerative disorders.

MEDICAL CAUSES

● *Achalasia.* Hematemesis is a rare effect of achalasia, which usually causes passive regurgitation. Achalasia also causes hoarseness or coughing that may be accompanied by aspiration and recurrent pulmonary infection. Usually painless, progressive dysphagia commonly occurs early.

● *Anthrax, GI.* Initial signs and symptoms after eating contaminated meat from an animal infected with the gram-positive, spore-forming bacterium *Bacillus anthracis* include loss of appetite, nausea, vomiting, and fever. Signs and symptoms may progress to hematemesis, abdominal pain, and severe bloody diarrhea.

● *Coagulation disorders.* Any disorder that disrupts normal clotting may result in GI bleeding and moderate to severe hematemesis. Bleeding may occur in other body systems as well, resulting in such signs as epistaxis and ecchymosis. Other associated effects vary, depending on the specific coagulation disorder, such as thrombocytopenia or hemophilia.

● *Esophageal cancer.* A late sign of esophageal cancer, hematemesis may be accompanied by steady chest pain that radiates to the back. Other features include substernal fullness, severe dysphagia, nausea, vomiting with nocturnal regurgitation and aspiration, hemoptysis, fever, hiccups, sore throat, melena, and halitosis.

● *Esophageal injury by caustic substances.* Ingestion of corrosive acids or alkalis produces esophageal injury associated with grossly bloody or coffee-ground vomitus. Hematemesis is accompanied by epigastric and anterior or retrosternal chest pain that's intensified by swallowing. With ingestion of alkaline agents, the oral and pharyngeal mucosa may produce a soapy white film. The mucosa becomes brown and edematous with time. Dysphagia, marked salivation, and fever may develop in 3 to 4 weeks and worsen as strictures form.

● *Esophageal rupture.* The severity of hematemesis depends on the cause of the rupture. When an instrument damages the esophagus, hematemesis is usually slight. However, rupture due to Boerhaave's syndrome (increased esophageal pressure from vomiting or retching) or other esophageal disorders typically causes more severe hematemesis. This life-threatening disorder may also produce severe retrosternal, epigas-

Managing hematemesis with intubation

A patient with hematemesis will need to have a GI tube inserted to allow blood drainage, to aspirate gastric contents, or to facilitate gastric lavage, if necessary. Here are the most common tubes and their uses.

Nasogastric tubes

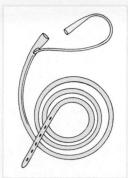

Wide-bore gastric tubes

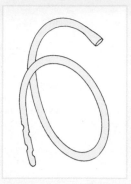

Esophageal tubes

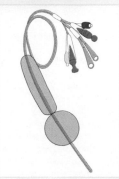

The Salem-Sump tube (above), a double-lumen nasogastric (NG) tube, is used to remove stomach fluid and gas, or to aspirate gastric contents. It may also be used for gastric lavage, drug administration, or feeding. Its main advantage over the Levin tube—a single-lumen NG device—is that it allows atmospheric air to enter the patient's stomach so the tube can float freely instead of risking adhesion and damage to the gastric mucosa.

The Edlich tube (above) has one wide-bore lumen with four openings near the closed distal tip. A funnel or syringe can be connected at the proximal end. Like the other tubes, the Edlich can aspirate a large volume of gastric contents quickly.

The Ewald tube, a wide-bore tube that allows quick passage of a large amount of fluid and clots, is especially useful for gastric lavage in patients with profuse GI bleeding and in those who have ingested poison. Another wide-bore tube, the double-lumen Levacuator, has a large lumen for evacuation of gastric contents and a small one for lavage.

The Sengstaken-Blakemore tube (above), a triple-lumen double-balloon esophageal tube, provides a gastric aspiration port that allows drainage from below the gastric balloon. It can also be used to instill medication. A similar tube, the Linton shunt, can aspirate esophageal and gastric contents without risking necrosis because it has no esophageal balloon. The Minnesota esophagogastric tamponade tube, which has four lumina and two balloons, provides pressure-monitoring ports for both balloons without the need for Y-connectors.

---

tric, neck, or scapular pain accompanied by chest and neck edema. Examination reveals subcutaneous crepitation in the chest wall, supraclavicular fossa, and neck. The patient may also show signs of respiratory distress, such as dyspnea and cyanosis.

• *Esophageal varices (ruptured).* Life-threatening rupture of esophageal varices may produce coffee-ground or massive, bright red vomitus. Signs of shock, such as hypotension or tachycardia, may follow or even precede hematemesis if the stomach fills with blood before vomiting occurs. Other symptoms may include abdominal distention and melena or painless hematochezia, ranging from slight oozing to massive rectal hemorrhage.

- *Gastric cancer.* Painless bright red or dark brown vomitus is a late sign of gastric cancer—an uncommon cancer—that usually begins insidiously with upper-abdominal discomfort. The patient then develops anorexia, mild nausea, and chronic dyspepsia unrelieved by antacids and exacerbated by food. Later symptoms may include fatigue, weakness, weight loss, feelings of fullness, melena, altered bowel habits, and signs of malnutrition, such as muscle wasting and dry skin.
- *Gastritis (acute).* Hematemesis and melena are the most common signs of acute gastritis. They may even be the only signs, although mild epigastric discomfort, nausea, fever, and malaise may also occur. Massive blood loss precipitates signs of shock. Typically, the patient has a history of alcohol abuse or has used aspirin or some other NSAID. Gastritis may also occur secondary to *Helicobacter pylori* infection.
- *Gastroesophageal reflux disease (GERD).* Although rare with GERD, hematemesis may produce significant blood loss. It's accompanied by pyrosis, flatulence, dyspepsia, and postural regurgitation that can be aggravated by lying down or stooping over. Related effects include dysphagia, retrosternal angina-like chest pain, weight loss, halitosis, and signs of aspiration, such as dyspnea and recurrent pulmonary infection.
- *GI leiomyoma.* GI leiomyoma is a benign tumor that occasionally involves the GI tract, eroding the mucosa or vascular supply to produce hematemesis. Other features vary with the tumor's size and location. For example, esophageal involvement may cause dysphagia and weight loss.
- *Mallory-Weiss syndrome.* Characterized by a mucosal tear of the mucous membrane at the junction of the esophagus and the stomach, Mallory-Weiss syndrome may produce hematemesis and melena. It's commonly triggered by severe vomiting, retching, or straining (as from coughing), most commonly in alcoholics or in people whose pylorus is obstructed. Severe bleeding may precipitate signs of shock, such as tachycardia, hypotension, dyspnea, and cool, clammy skin.
- *Peptic ulcer.* Hematemesis may occur when a peptic ulcer penetrates an artery, vein, or highly vascular tissue. Massive—and possibly life-threatening—hematemesis is typical when an artery is penetrated. Other features include melena or hematochezia,

chills, fever, and signs and symptoms of shock and dehydration, such as tachycardia, hypotension, poor skin turgor, and thirst. Most patients have a history of nausea, vomiting, epigastric tenderness, and epigastric pain that's relieved by foods or antacids. The patient may also have a history of habitual use of tobacco, alcohol, or NSAIDs.

OTHER CAUSES
- *Treatments.* Traumatic NG or endotracheal intubation may cause hematemesis associated with swallowed blood. Nose or throat surgery may also cause this sign in the same way.

NURSING CONSIDERATIONS
Closely monitor the patient's vital signs, and watch for signs of shock. Check the patient's stools regularly for occult blood, and keep accurate intake and output records. Place the patient on bed rest in a low or semi-Fowler's position to prevent aspiration of vomitus. Keep suctioning equipment nearby, and use it as needed. Provide frequent oral hygiene and emotional support—the sight of bloody vomitus can be very frightening. Administer a histamine-2 blocker I.V.; vasopressin may be required for variceal hemorrhage. As the bleeding tapers off, monitor the pH of gastric contents, and give hourly doses of antacids by NG tube as necessary.

PATIENT TEACHING
Explain diagnostic tests, such as endoscopy, barium swallow, and variceal banding. Explain laboratory tests, such as serum electrolyte levels and complete blood count. Provide information on medications that the patient should avoid, such as aspirin or anticoagulants, and instruct the patient on non-drug measures, such as relaxation and stress management, which help minimize symptoms. Stress the importance of avoiding alcohol.

Hematochezia

The passage of bloody stools, also known as *hematochezia,* usually indicates—and may be the first sign of—GI bleeding below the ligament of Treitz. However, this sign—usually preceded by hematemesis—may also accompany rapid hemorrhage of 1 L or more from the upper GI tract.

Hematochezia ranges from formed, blood-streaked stools to liquid, bloody stools that may be bright red, dark mahogany, or maroon in color. This sign usually develops abruptly and is heralded by abdominal pain.

Although hematochezia is commonly associated with GI disorders, it may also result from a coagulation disorder, exposure to toxins, or certain diagnostic tests. Always a significant sign, hematochezia may precipitate life-threatening hypovolemia.

Act now If the patient has severe hematochezia, check his vital signs. If you detect signs of shock, such as hypotension and tachycardia, place the patient in a supine position and elevate his feet 20 to 30 degrees. Prepare to administer oxygen, and start a large-bore I.V. line for emergency fluid replacement. Next, obtain a blood sample for typing and crossmatching, hemoglobin level, and hematocrit. Insert an NG tube. Iced lavage may be indicated to control bleeding. Endoscopy may be necessary to detect the source of the bleeding.

ASSESSMENT
History
If the hematochezia isn't immediately life-threatening, ask the patient to fully describe the amount, color, and consistency of the bloody stools. (If possible, also inspect and characterize the stools yourself.) How long have the stools been bloody? Do they always look the same, or does the amount of blood seem to vary? Ask about associated signs and symptoms.

Next, explore the patient's medical history, focusing on GI and coagulation disorders. Ask about use of GI irritants, such as alcohol, aspirin, and other NSAIDs.

Physical examination
Begin the physical examination by checking for orthostatic hypotension, an early sign of shock. Take the patient's blood pressure and pulse while he's lying down, sitting, and standing. If systolic pressure decreases by 10 mm Hg or more, or pulse rate increases by 10 beats/minute or more when he changes position, suspect volume depletion and impending shock.

Examine the skin for petechiae or spider angiomas. Palpate the abdomen for tenderness, pain, or masses. Also, note lym-phadenopathy. Finally, a digital rectal examination must be done to rule out any rectal masses or hemorrhoids.

Pediatric pointers
Hematochezia is much less common in children than in adults. It may result from structural disorders, such as intussusception and Meckel's diverticulum, and from inflammatory disorders, such as peptic ulcer disease and ulcerative colitis.

In children, ulcerative colitis typically produces chronic, rather than acute, signs and symptoms and may also cause slow growth and maturation related to malnutrition. Suspect sexual abuse in all cases of rectal bleeding in children.

Geriatric pointers
Because older people have an increased risk of colon cancer, hematochezia should be evaluated with colonoscopy after perirectal lesions have been ruled out as the cause of bleeding.

MEDICAL CAUSES
● *Amyloidosis.* Hematochezia occasionally occurs when amyloidosis affects the GI tract. Massive, rapid hematochezia may precipitate signs of shock, such as hypotension and tachycardia. Associated signs and symptoms include hypoactive or absent bowel sounds, abdominal pain, malabsorption, diarrhea, and renal disease. The patient may also have a stiff, enlarged tongue, resulting in dysarthria.
● *Anal fissure.* Slight hematochezia characterizes anal fissure; blood may streak the stools or appear on toilet tissue. Accompanying hematochezia is severe rectal pain that may make the patient reluctant to defecate, thereby causing constipation.
● *Angiodysplastic lesions.* Most common in elderly patients, angiodysplastic lesions of the ascending colon typically cause chronic, bright red rectal bleeding. Occasionally, this painless hematochezia may result in life-threatening blood loss and signs of shock, such as tachycardia and hypotension.
● *Anorectal fistula.* Blood, pus, mucus, and occasionally stools may drain from anorectal fistula. Other effects include rectal pain and pruritus.
● *Coagulation disorders.* Patients with a coagulation disorder (such as thrombocytopenia and disseminated intravascular coagula-

tion) may experience GI bleeding marked by moderate to severe hematochezia. Bleeding may also occur in other body systems, producing such signs as epistaxis and purpura. Associated findings vary with the specific coagulation disorder.

● **Colitis.** Ischemic colitis commonly causes bloody diarrhea, especially in elderly patients. The hematochezia may be slight or massive and is usually accompanied by severe, cramping lower abdominal pain and hypotension. Other effects include abdominal tenderness, distention, and absent bowel sounds. Severe colitis may cause life-threatening hypovolemic shock and peritonitis.

Ulcerative colitis typically causes bloody diarrhea that may also contain mucus. The hematochezia is preceded by mild to severe abdominal cramps and may cause slight to massive blood loss. Associated signs and symptoms include fever, tenesmus, anorexia, nausea, vomiting, hyperactive bowel sounds and, occasionally, tachycardia. Weight loss and weakness occur late.

● **Colon cancer.** Bright red rectal bleeding with or without pain is a telling sign, especially in cancer of the left colon.

Usually, a left colon tumor causes early signs of obstruction, such as rectal pressure, bleeding, and intermittent fullness or cramping. As the disease progresses, the patient also develops obstipation, diarrhea, or ribbon-shaped stools, and pain, which is typically relieved by passage of stools or flatus. Stools are grossly bloody.

Early tumor growth in the right colon may cause melena, abdominal aching, pressure, and dull cramps. As the disease progresses, the patient develops weakness and fatigue. Later, he may also experience diarrhea, anorexia, weight loss, anemia, vomiting, abdominal mass, and signs of obstruction, such as abdominal distention and abnormal bowel sounds.

● **Colorectal polyps.** Colorectal polyps are the most common cause of intermittent hematochezia in adults younger than age 60; however, sometimes such polyps produce no symptoms. When located high in the colon, polyps may cause blood-streaked stools. The stools yield a positive response when tested with guaiac. If the polyps are located closer to the rectum, they may bleed freely.

● **Crohn's disease.** Hematochezia isn't a common sign of Crohn's disease unless the perineum is involved. If rectal bleeding occurs, it's likely to be massive. The chief clinical features of Crohn's disease include fever, abdominal distention and pain with guarding, diarrhea, hyperactive bowel sounds, anorexia, nausea, and fatigue. A palpable mass in the colon area may be present.

● **Diverticulitis.** Most common in elderly patients, diverticulitis can suddenly cause mild to moderate rectal bleeding after the patient feels the urge to defecate. The bleeding may end abruptly or may progress to life-threatening blood loss with signs of shock. Associated signs and symptoms may include left-lower-quadrant pain that's relieved by defecation, alternating episodes of constipation and diarrhea, anorexia, nausea and vomiting, rebound tenderness, and a distended tympanic abdomen.

● **Dysentery.** Bloody diarrhea is common in infection with *Shigella, Amoeba,* and *Campylobacter,* but rare with *Salmonella.* Abdominal pain or cramps, tenesmus, fever, and nausea may also occur.

● **Esophageal varices (ruptured).** Ruptured esophageal varices are a life-threatening disorder, in which hematochezia may range from slight rectal oozing to grossly bloody stools and may be accompanied by mild to severe hematemesis or melena. This painless but massive hemorrhage may precipitate signs of shock, such as tachycardia and hypotension. In fact, signs of shock occasionally precede overt signs of bleeding. Typically, the patient has a history of chronic liver disease.

● **Food poisoning (staphylococcal).** The patient may have bloody diarrhea 1 to 6 hours after ingesting food toxins. Accompanying signs and symptoms include severe, cramping abdominal pain, nausea and vomiting, and prostration, all of which last a few hours.

● **Hemorrhoids.** Hematochezia may accompany external hemorrhoids, which typically cause painful defecation, resulting in constipation. Less painful internal hemorrhoids usually produce more chronic bleeding with bowel movements, which may eventually lead to signs of anemia, such as weakness and fatigue.

● **Leptospirosis.** The severe form of leptospirosis — Weil's syndrome — produces hematochezia or melena along with other signs of bleeding, such as epistaxis and hemoptysis. The bleeding is typically preceded by a sudden frontal headache and severe thigh and lumbar myalgia that may be accompanied by cutaneous hyperesthesia. Conjunctival suffusion is indicative. Bleeding is followed by chills, a rapidly rising fever, and perhaps nausea and vomiting. Fever, headache, and myalgia usually intensify and persist for weeks. Other findings may include right-upper-quadrant tenderness, hepatomegaly, and jaundice.

- *Peptic ulcer.* Upper GI bleeding is a common complication in peptic ulcer. The patient may display hematochezia, hematemesis, or melena, depending on the rapidity and amount of bleeding. If the peptic ulcer penetrates an artery or vein, massive bleeding may precipitate signs of shock, such as hypotension and tachycardia. Other findings may include chills, fever, nausea and vomiting, and signs of dehydration, such as dry mucous membranes, poor skin turgor, and thirst. The patient typically has a history of epigastric pain that's relieved by foods or antacids; he may also have a history of habitual use of tobacco, alcohol, or NSAIDs.
- *Rectal melanoma (malignant).* Rectal melanoma is a rare form of rectal cancer that typically causes recurrent rectal bleeding that arises from a painless, asymptomatic mass.
- *Small-intestine cancer.* Small-intestine cancer occasionally produces slight hematochezia or blood-streaked stools. Its characteristic features include colicky pain and postprandial vomiting. Other common signs and symptoms include weight loss, anorexia, and fever. Palpation may reveal abdominal masses.
- *Typhoid fever.* About 10% of patients with typhoid fever develop hematochezia, which is occasionally massive. However, melena is more common. Both signs of bleeding occur late and may be accompanied by mental dullness, marked abdominal distention, diarrhea, significant weight loss, and profound fatigue. Among earlier signs and symptoms are pathognomonic rose spots, headache, chills, fever, constipation, dry cough, conjunctivitis, and epistaxis.
- *Ulcerative proctitis.* Ulcerative proctitis typically causes an intense urge to defecate, but the patient passes only bright red blood, pus, or mucus. Other common signs and symptoms include acute constipation and tenesmus.

OTHER CAUSES
- *Diagnostic tests.* Certain procedures, especially colonoscopy, polypectomy, and proctosigmoidoscopy, may cause rectal bleeding. Bowel perforation is rare.
- *Heavy metal poisoning.* Bloody diarrhea is accompanied by cramping abdominal pain, nausea, and vomiting. Other signs may include tachycardia, hypotension, seizures, paresthesia, depressed or absent deep tendon reflexes, and an altered level of consciousness.

NURSING CONSIDERATIONS
Place the patient on bed rest and check his vital signs frequently, watching for signs of shock, such as hypotension, tachycardia, weak pulse, and tachypnea. Monitor the patient's intake and output hourly. Remember to provide emotional support because hematochezia may frighten the patient.

Prepare the patient for blood tests and GI procedures, such as endoscopy and GI X-rays. Visually examine the patient's stools and test them for occult blood. If necessary, send a stool sample to the laboratory to check for parasites.

PATIENT TEACHING
Provide information to the patient on signs and symptoms to report immediately. Teach the patient about ostomy self-care and consult the ostomy nurse or a home health care nurse to provide support to the patient upon discharge from the facility, as appropriate. Discuss proper bowel elimination habits. Explain dietary recommendations and restrictions.

Hemoptysis

Frightening to the patient and often ominous, hemoptysis is the expectoration of blood or bloody sputum from the lungs or tracheobronchial tree. It's sometimes confused with bleeding from the mouth, throat, nasopharynx, or GI tract. (See *Identifying hemoptysis,* page 168.) Expectoration of 200 ml of blood in a single episode suggests severe bleeding, whereas expectoration of 400 ml in 3 hours or more than 600 ml in 16 hours signals a life-threatening crisis.

Hemoptysis usually results from chronic bronchitis, lung cancer, or bronchiectasis. However, it may also result from inflammatory, infectious, cardiovascular, or coagulation disorders and, rarely, from a ruptured aortic aneurysm. In up to 15% of patients, the cause is unknown. The most common causes of *massive hemoptysis* are lung cancer, bronchiectasis, active tuberculosis, and cavitary pulmonary disease from necrotic infections or tuberculosis.

A number of pathophysiologic processes can cause hemoptysis. (See *What happens in hemoptysis.*)

Act now If the patient coughs up copious amounts of blood, endotracheal intubation may be required. Suction frequently to remove blood. Lavage may be necessary to loosen tenacious secretions or clots. Massive hemoptysis can cause airway obstruction and asphyxiation. Insert an I.V. line to allow fluid replacement, drug administration, and blood transfusions, if needed. An emergency bronchoscopy should be performed to identify the bleeding site. Monitor blood pressure and pulse to detect hypotension and tachycardia, and draw an arterial blood sample for laboratory analysis to monitor respiratory status.

ASSESSMENT
History

If the hemoptysis is mild, ask the patient when it began. Has he ever coughed up blood before? About how much blood is he coughing up now and about how often? Ask about a history of cardiac, pulmonary, or bleeding disorders. If he's receiving anticoagulant therapy, find out the drug, its dosage and schedule, and the duration of therapy. Is he taking other prescription drugs? Does he smoke? Ask the patient if he has had any recent infections. Has he been exposed to tuberculosis? When was his last tine test and what were the results?

Physical examination

Take the patient's vital signs and examine his nose, mouth, and pharynx for sources of bleeding. Inspect the configuration of his chest and look for abnormal movement during breathing, use of accessory muscles, and retractions. Observe his respiratory rate, depth, and rhythm. Finally, examine his skin for lesions.

Next, palpate the patient's chest for diaphragm level and for tenderness, respiratory excursion, fremitus, and abnormal pulsations; then percuss for flatness, dullness, resonance, hyperresonance, and tympany. Finally, auscultate the lungs, noting especially the quality and intensity of breath sounds. Also auscultate for heart murmurs, bruits, and pleural friction rubs.

Obtain a sputum sample and examine it for overall quantity, for the amount of blood it contains, and for its color, odor, and consistency.

Pediatric pointers

Hemoptysis in children may stem from Goodpasture's syndrome, cystic fibrosis, or (rarely) idiopathic primary pulmonary hemosiderosis. Sometimes no cause can be found for pulmonary hemorrhage occurring within the first 2 weeks of life; in such cases, the prognosis is poor.

Geriatric pointers

If the patient is receiving anticoagulants, determine any changes that need to be made in diet or medications (including over-the-counter and natural supplements) because these factors may affect clotting.

MEDICAL CAUSES

- *Aortic aneurysm (ruptured).* Rarely, an aortic aneurysm ruptures into the tracheobronchial tree, causing hemoptysis and sudden death.
- *Bronchial adenoma.* Bronchial adenoma is an insidious disorder that causes recurring hemoptysis in up to 30% of patients, along with a chronic cough and local wheezing.
- *Bronchiectasis.* Inflamed bronchial surfaces and eroded bronchial blood vessels cause hemoptysis, which can vary from blood-tinged sputum to blood (in about 20% of patients). The patient's sputum may also be copious, foul-smelling, and purulent. He may exhibit a chronic cough, coarse crackles, clubbing (a late sign), fever, weight loss, fatigue, weakness, malaise, and dyspnea on exertion.
- *Bronchitis (chronic).* The first sign of bronchitis is typically a productive cough that lasts at least 3 months. Eventually this leads to production of blood-streaked sputum; massive hemorrhage is unusual. Other respiratory effects include dyspnea, prolonged expirations, wheezing, scattered rhonchi, accessory muscle use, barrel chest, tachypnea, and clubbing (a late sign).
- *Coagulation disorders.* Such disorders as thrombocytopenia and disseminated intravascular coagulation can cause hemoptysis. Besides their specific related findings, coagulation disorders may share such general signs as multisystem hemorrhaging (for example, GI bleeding or epistaxis) and purpuric lesions.
- *Laryngeal cancer.* Hemoptysis occurs in laryngeal cancer, but hoarseness is the usual early sign. Other findings may include dysphagia, dyspnea, stridor, cervical lymphadenopathy, and neck pain.
- *Lung abscess.* In about 50% of patients, lung abscess produces blood-streaked sputum resulting from bronchial ulceration, necrosis, and granulation tissue. Common associated findings include a cough with large amounts of purulent, foul-smelling sputum; fever with chills; diaphoresis; anorexia; weight loss; headache; weakness; dyspnea; pleuritic or dull chest pain; and clubbing. Auscultation reveals tubular or cavernous breath sounds and crackles. Percussion reveals dullness on the affected side.
- *Lung cancer.* Ulceration of the bronchus commonly causes recurring hemoptysis (an early sign), which can vary from blood-streaked sputum to blood. Related findings

include a productive cough, dyspnea, fever, anorexia, weight loss, wheezing, and chest pain (a late symptom).

- **Plague (Yersinia pestis).** The pneumonic form of plague can produce hemoptysis, productive cough, chest pain, tachypnea, dyspnea, increasing respiratory distress, and cardiopulmonary insufficiency, along with the sudden onset of chills, fever, headache, and myalgias.
- **Pneumonia.** In up to 50% of patients, *Klebsiella* pneumonia produces dark brown or red (currant-jelly) sputum, which is so tenacious that the patient has difficulty expelling it from his mouth. This type of pneumonia begins abruptly with chills, fever, dyspnea, a productive cough, and severe pleuritic chest pain. Associated findings may include cyanosis, prostration, tachycardia, decreased breath sounds, and crackles.

  Pneumococcal pneumonia causes pinkish or rusty mucoid sputum. It begins with sudden shaking chills; a rapidly rising temperature; and, in more than 80% of patients, tachycardia and tachypnea. Within a few hours, the patient typically experiences a productive cough along with severe, stabbing, pleuritic pain. The agonizing chest pain leads to rapid, shallow, grunting respirations with splinting. Examination reveals respiratory distress with dyspnea and accessory muscle use, crackles, and dullness on percussion over the affected lung. Malaise, weakness, myalgia, and prostration accompany high fever.
- **Pulmonary arteriovenous fistula.** Occurring in young adults, pulmonary arteriovenous fistula causes intermittent hemoptysis. Associated signs and symptoms include cyanosis, clubbing, mild dyspnea, fatigue, vertigo, syncope, confusion, and speech and visual impairments. The patient may bleed from the nose, mouth, or lips. Ruby red patches appear on the face, tongue, skin, mucous membranes, or nail beds.
- **Pulmonary contusion.** Blunt chest trauma commonly causes a cough with hemoptysis. Other signs and symptoms appear gradually within several hours after the injury and include dyspnea, tachypnea, chest pain, tachycardia, hypotension, crackles, and decreased or absent breath sounds over the affected area. Severe respiratory distress — with oppressive dyspnea, nasal flaring, use of accessory muscles, extreme anxiety, cyanosis, and diaphoresis — may develop at any time.

- **Pulmonary edema.** Severe cardiogenic or noncardiogenic pulmonary edema commonly causes frothy, blood-tinged pink sputum, which accompanies severe dyspnea, orthopnea, gasping, anxiety, cyanosis, diffuse crackles, a ventricular gallop, and cold, clammy skin. This life-threatening condition may also cause tachycardia, lethargy, cardiac arrhythmias, tachypnea, hypotension, and a thready pulse.
- **Pulmonary embolism with infarction.** Hemoptysis is a common finding in pulmonary embolism with infarction — a life-threatening disorder — although massive hemoptysis is infrequent. Typical initial symptoms are dyspnea and anginal or pleuritic chest pain. Other common clinical features include tachycardia, tachypnea, low-grade fever, and diaphoresis. Less commonly, splinting of the chest, leg edema, and — with a large embolus — cyanosis, syncope, and distended jugular veins may occur. Examination reveals decreased breath sounds, pleural friction rub, crackles, diffuse wheezing, dullness on percussion, and signs of circulatory collapse (weak, rapid pulse; hypotension), cerebral ischemia (transient loss of consciousness, convulsions), and hypoxemia (restlessness and, particularly in elderly patients, hemiplegia and other focal neurologic deficits).
- **Pulmonary hypertension (primary).** Features generally develop late. Hemoptysis, exertional dyspnea, and fatigue are common. Angina-like pain usually occurs with exertion and may radiate to the neck but not to the arms. Other findings include arrhythmias, syncope, cough, and hoarseness.
- **Pulmonary tuberculosis.** Blood-streaked or blood-tinged sputum commonly occurs in pulmonary tuberculosis; massive hemoptysis may occur in advanced cavitary tuberculosis. Accompanying respiratory findings include a chronic productive cough, fine crackles after coughing, dyspnea, dullness to percussion, increased tactile fremitus, and possible amphoric breath sounds. The patient may also develop night sweats, malaise, fatigue, fever, anorexia, weight loss, and pleuritic chest pain.
- **Silicosis.** Initially, silicosis — a chronic disorder — causes a productive cough with mucopurulent sputum. Subsequently, the sputum becomes blood-streaked and, occasionally, massive hemoptysis may occur. Other findings include fine, end-inspiratory crackles

at lung bases, exertional dyspnea, tachypnea, weight loss, fatigue, and weakness.

- *Systemic lupus erythematosus (SLE).* In 50% of patients with SLE, pleuritis and pneumonitis cause hemoptysis, cough, dyspnea, pleuritic chest pain, and crackles. Related findings are a butterfly rash in the acute phase, nondeforming joint pain and stiffness, photosensitivity, Raynaud's phenomenon, convulsions or psychoses, anorexia with weight loss, and lymphadenopathy.
- *Tracheal trauma.* Torn tracheal mucosa may cause hemoptysis, hoarseness, dysphagia, neck pain, airway occlusion, and respiratory distress.
- *Wegener's granulomatosis.* Necrotizing, granulomatous vasculitis characterizes Wegener's granulomatosis — a multisystem disorder. Findings include hemoptysis, chest pain, cough, wheezing, dyspnea, epistaxis, severe sinusitis, and hemorrhagic skin lesions.

OTHER CAUSES
- *Diagnostic tests.* Lung or airway injury from bronchoscopy, laryngoscopy, mediastinoscopy, or lung biopsy can cause bleeding and hemoptysis.

NURSING CONSIDERATIONS
Comfort and reassure the patient, who may react to this alarming sign with anxiety and apprehension. If necessary, to protect the nonbleeding lung, place him in the lateral decubitus position, with the suspected bleeding lung facing down. Perform this maneuver with caution because hypoxemia may worsen with the healthy lung facing up.

Prepare the patient for diagnostic tests to determine the cause of bleeding. These may include a complete blood count, a sputum culture and smear, chest X-rays, coagulation studies, bronchoscopy, lung biopsy, pulmonary arteriography, and a lung scan.

PATIENT TEACHING
Explain that hemoptysis generally ceases (but not abruptly) during treatment of the causative disorder. Many chronic disorders, however, cause recurrent hemoptysis. Instruct the patient to report recurring episodes and to bring a sputum specimen containing blood if he returns for treatment or reevaluation.

Homans' sign is positive when deep calf pain results from strong and abrupt dorsiflexion of the ankle. This pain results from venous thrombosis or inflammation of the calf muscles. However, because a positive Homans' sign appears in only 35% of patients with these conditions, it's an unreliable indicator. (See *Eliciting Homans' sign,* page 172.) Even when accurate, a positive Homans' sign doesn't indicate the extent of the venous disorder.

This elicited sign may be confused with continuous calf pain, which can result from strains, contusions, cellulitis, or arterial occlusion, or with pain in the posterior ankle or Achilles' tendon (for example, in a female with Achilles' tendons shortened from wearing high heels).

ASSESSMENT
History
When you detect a positive Homans' sign, focus your patient history on signs and symptoms that can accompany deep vein thrombosis (DVT) or thrombophlebitis. These include throbbing, aching, heavy, or tight sensations in the calf, and leg pain during or after exercise or routine activity. Ask about shortness of breath or chest pain, which may indicate pulmonary embolism. Be sure to ask about predisposing events, such as leg injury, recent surgery, childbirth, use of hormonal contraceptives, associated diseases (cancer, nephrosis, hypercoagulable states), and prolonged inactivity or bed rest.

Physical examination
Inspect and palpate the patient's calf for warmth, tenderness, redness, swelling, and the presence of a palpable vein. If you strongly suspect DVT, elicit Homans' sign very carefully to avoid dislodging the clot, which could cause pulmonary embolism, a life-threatening condition.

In addition, measure the circumference of both the patient's calves. The calf with the positive Homans' sign may be larger because of edema and swelling.

ELICITING HOMANS' SIGN

To elicit Homans' sign, first support the patient's thigh with one hand and his foot with the other. Bend his leg slightly at the knee; then firmly and abruptly dorsiflex the ankle. Resulting deep calf pain indicates a positive Homans' sign. (The patient may also resist ankle dorsiflexion or flex the knee involuntarily if Homans' sign is positive.)

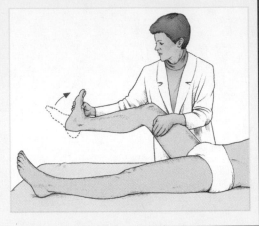

Pediatric pointers

Homans' sign is seldom assessed in children because DVT and thrombophlebitis are rare in pediatric patients.

MEDICAL CAUSES

- *Cellulitis (superficial).* Cellulitis typically affects the legs but can also affect the arms, producing pain, redness, tenderness, and edema. Some patients also experience fever, chills, tachycardia, headache, and hypotension.
- *Deep vein thrombophlebitis.* A positive Homans' sign and calf tenderness may be the only clinical features of deep vein thrombophlebitis. However, the patient may also have severe pain, heaviness, warmth, and swelling of the affected leg; visible, engorged superficial veins or palpable, cordlike veins; and fever, chills, and malaise.
- *Deep vein thrombosis.* DVT causes a positive Homans' sign along with tenderness over the deep calf veins, slight edema of the calves and thighs, a low-grade fever, and tachycardia. If DVT affects the femoral and iliac veins, you'll notice marked local swelling and tenderness. If DVT causes venous obstruction, you'll notice cyanosis and possibly cool skin in the affected leg.
- *Popliteal cyst (ruptured).* Rupture of this synovial cyst may produce a positive Homans' sign as well as sudden onset of calf tenderness, swelling, and redness.

NURSING CONSIDERATIONS

Be sure to place the patient on bed rest, with the affected leg elevated above the heart level. Apply warm, moist compresses to the affected area, and administer mild oral analgesics. In addition, prepare the patient for further diagnostic tests, such as Doppler studies and venograms.

Once the patient is ambulatory, advise him to wear elastic support stockings after his discomfort decreases (usually in 5 to 10 days) and to continue wearing them for at least 3 months. In addition, instruct the patient to keep the affected leg elevated while sitting and to avoid crossing his legs at the knees; this may impair circulation to the popliteal area. (Crossing at the ankles is acceptable.)

PATIENT TEACHING

Instruct the patient receiving long-term anticoagulant therapy to report any signs of prolonged clotting time, such as brown or red urine, bleeding gums, bruises, and black, tarry stools. Stress the importance of keeping follow-up appointments so that prothrombin time can be monitored.

Instruct the patient to avoid alcohol and restrict green leafy vegetables (spinach and parsley), which are high in vitamin K. Advise him to review all medications he's taking with his physician because some drugs may enhance or inhibit the effects of the anticoagulant. Remind the patient to ask his physician to confirm that any future prescriptions and over-the-counter medications are safe to take.

Hyperpnea

Hyperpnea indicates increased respiratory effort for a sustained period—a normal rate (at least 12 breaths/minute) with increased depth (a tidal volume greater than 7.5 ml/kg), an increased rate (more than 20 breaths/minute) with normal depth, or increased rate and depth. This sign differs from sighing (intermittent deep inspirations) and may or may not be associated with tachypnea (increased respiratory frequency).

The typical patient with hyperpnea breathes at a normal or increased rate and inhales deeply, displaying marked chest expansion. He may complain of shortness of breath if a respiratory disorder is causing hypoxemia, or he may not be aware of his breathing if a metabolic, psychiatric, or neurologic disorder is causing involuntary hyperpnea. Other causes of hyperpnea include profuse diarrhea or dehydration, loss of pancreatic juice or bile from GI drainage, and ureterosigmoidostomy. All these conditions and procedures cause a loss of bicarbonate ions, resulting in metabolic acidosis. Of course, hyperpnea may also accompany strenuous exercise, and voluntary hyperpnea can promote relaxation in patients experiencing stress or pain—for example, females in labor.

Hyperventilation, a consequence of hyperpnea, is characterized by alkalosis (arterial pH above 7.45 and $PaCO_2$ below 35 mm Hg). In central neurogenic hyperventilation, brain stem dysfunction (such as results from a severe cranial injury) increases the rate and depth of respirations. In acute intermittent hyperventilation, the respiratory pattern may be a response to hypoxemia, anxiety, fear, pain, or excitement. Hyperpnea may also be a compensatory mechanism to metabolic acidosis. Under these conditions, it's known as *Kussmaul's respirations.* (See *Kussmaul's respirations: A compensatory mechanism.*)

Act now Carefully examine the patient with hyperpnea for related signs of life-threatening conditions, such as increased intracra-

---

KUSSMAUL'S RESPIRATIONS: A COMPENSATORY MECHANISM

Kussmaul's respirations—fast, deep breathing without pauses—characteristically sound labored, with deep breaths that resemble sighs. This breathing pattern develops when respiratory centers in the medulla detect decreased blood pH, thereby triggering compensatory fast and deep breathing to remove excess carbon dioxide and restore pH balance.

> Disorders (such as diabetes mellitus and renal failure), drug effects, and other conditions cause metabolic acidosis (loss of bicarbonate ions and retention of acid).

↓

> Blood pH decreases.

↓

> Kussmaul's respirations develop to blow off excess carbon dioxide.

↓

> Blood pH increases.

↓

> Respiratory rate and depth decrease (corrected pH) in effective compensation.

---

nial pressure (ICP), metabolic acidosis, diabetic ketoacidosis, and uremia. Be prepared for rapid intervention. (See Managing hyperpnea, page 174.)

ASSESSMENT
History

If you've ruled out a life-threatening condition, confirmed that the patient's level of consciousness (LOC) permits, and determined that hyperpnea isn't interfering with his ability to speak, obtain his history. Has he experienced any recent illnesses or infections, such as severe diarrhea or an upper respiratory tract infection? Ask about ingestion of aspirin, other drugs, or chemicals, and

Managing hyperpnea

Carefully examine the patient with hyperpnea for related signs of life-threatening conditions, such as increased intracranial pressure (ICP), metabolic acidosis, diabetic ketoacidosis, and uremia. Be prepared for rapid intervention.

Increased ICP

If you observe hyperpnea in a patient who has signs of head trauma (soft-tissue injury, edema, or ecchymoses on the face or head) from a recent accident and has lost consciousness, act quickly to prevent further brain stem injury and irreversible deterioration. Then take the patient's vital signs, noting bradycardia, increased systolic blood pressure, and widening pulse pressure — signs of increased ICP.

Examine his pupillary reaction. Elevate the head of the bed 30 degrees (unless you sus-pect spinal cord injury), and insert an artificial airway. Connect the patient to a cardiac monitor, and continuously observe his respiratory pattern. (Irregular respirations signal deterioration.) Start an I.V. line at a slow infusion rate and prepare to administer an osmotic diuretic, such as mannitol, to decrease cerebral edema. Catheterize the patient to measure urine output, administer supplemental oxygen, and keep emergency resuscitation equipment close by. Obtain an arterial blood gas analysis to help guide treatments.

Metabolic acidosis

If the patient with hyperpnea doesn't have a head injury, his increased respiratory rate probably indicates metabolic acidosis. If the patient's level of consciousness is decreased, check his chart for history data to help you determine the cause of his metabolic acidosis, and intervene appropriately. Suspect shock if the patient has cold, clammy skin. Palpate for a rapid, thready pulse and take his blood pressure, noting hypotension. Elevate the patient's legs 30 degrees, apply pressure dressings to any obvious hemorrhage, start several large-bore I.V. lines, and prepare to administer fluids, vasopressors, and blood transfusions.

A patient with hyperpnea who has a history of alcohol abuse, is vomiting profusely, has diarrhea or profuse abdominal drainage, has ingested an overdose of aspirin, or is cachectic and has a history of starvation may also have metabolic acidosis. Inspect his skin for dryness and poor turgor, indicating dehydration. Take his vital signs, looking for low-grade fever and hypotension. Start an I.V. line for fluid replacement. Draw blood for electrolyte studies, and prepare to administer sodium bicarbonate.

Diabetic ketoacidosis

If the patient has a history of diabetes mellitus, is vomiting, and has a fruity breath odor (acetone breath), suspect diabetic ketoacidosis. Catheterize him to monitor increased urine output, and infuse saline solution. Perform a fingerstick to estimate blood glucose levels with a reagent strip. Obtain a urine specimen to test for glucose and acetone, and draw blood for glucose and ketone tests. Also, administer fluids, insulin, potassium, and sodium bicarbonate I.V.

Uremia

If the patient has a history of renal disease, an ammonia breath odor (uremic fetor), and a fine, white powder on his skin (uremic frost), suspect uremia. Start an I.V. line at a slow rate, and prepare to administer sodium bicarbon-ate. Monitor his electrocardiogram for arrhythmias due to hyperkalemia. Monitor his serum electrolyte, blood urea nitrogen, and creatinine levels as well until hemodialysis or peritoneal dialysis begins.

about inhalation of drugs or chemicals. Is he excessively thirsty or hungry? Does he have a history of diabetes mellitus, renal disease, or a pulmonary condition?

Physical examination

Observe the patient for clues to his abnormal breathing pattern. Is he unable to speak, or does he speak only in brief, choppy phrases? Is his breathing abnormally rapid? Examine him for cyanosis (especially of the mouth, lips, mucous membranes, and earlobes), restlessness, and anxiety — all signs of decreased tissue oxygenation, as occurs in shock. In addition, observe the patient for intercostal and abdominal retractions, use of accessory muscles, and diaphoresis, all of which may indicate deep breathing related to an insufficient supply of oxygen. Next, inspect for draining wounds or signs of infection, and ask about nausea and vomiting. Take the patient's vital signs, including oxygen saturation, noting fever, and examine his skin and mucous membranes for turgor, possibly indicating dehydration. Auscultate the patient's heart and lungs.

Pediatric pointers

Hyperpnea in children indicates the same metabolic or neurologic causes as in adults and requires the same prompt intervention. The most common cause of metabolic acidosis in children is diarrhea, which can cause a life-threatening crisis. In infants, Kussmaul's respirations may accompany acidosis due to inborn errors of metabolism.

MEDICAL CAUSES

● *Head injury.* Hyperpnea that results from a severe head injury is called *central neurogenic hyperventilation.* Whether its onset is acute or gradual, this type of hyperpnea indicates damage to the lower midbrain or upper pons. Accompanying signs reflect the site and extent of injury and can include loss of consciousness; soft-tissue injury or bony deformity of the face, head, or neck; facial edema; clear or bloody drainage from the mouth, nose, or ears; raccoon eyes; Battle's sign; an absent doll's eye sign; and motor and sensory disturbances.

Signs of increased ICP include decreased response to painful stimulation, loss of pupillary reaction, bradycardia, increased systolic pressure, and widening pulse pressure.

● *Hyperventilation syndrome.* Acute anxiety triggers episodic hyperpnea, resulting in respiratory alkalosis. Other findings may include agitation, vertigo, syncope, pallor, circumoral and peripheral paresthesia, muscle twitching, carpopedal spasm, weakness, and arrhythmias.

● *Hypoxemia.* Many pulmonary disorders that cause hypoxemia — for example, pneumonia, pulmonary edema, chronic obstructive pulmonary disease, and pneumothorax — may cause hyperpnea and episodes of hyperventilation with chest pain, dizziness, and paresthesia. Other effects include dyspnea, cough, crackles, rhonchi, wheezing, and decreased breath sounds.

● *Ketoacidosis.* Alcoholic ketoacidosis (occurring most commonly in females with a history of alcohol abuse) typically follows cessation of drinking after a marked increase in alcohol consumption has caused severe vomiting. Kussmaul's respirations begin abruptly and are accompanied by vomiting for several days, fruity breath odor, slight dehydration, abdominal pain and distention, and absent bowel sounds. The patient is alert and has a normal blood glucose level, unlike the patient with diabetic ketoacidosis.

Diabetic ketoacidosis is potentially life-threatening and typically produces Kussmaul's respirations. The patient usually experiences polydipsia, polyphagia, and polyuria before the onset of acidosis; he may or may not have a history of diabetes mellitus. Other clinical features include fruity breath odor; orthostatic hypotension; rapid, thready pulse; generalized weakness; decreased LOC (lethargy to coma); nausea; vomiting; anorexia; and abdominal pain.

Starvation ketoacidosis is also potentially life-threatening and can cause Kussmaul's respirations. Its onset is gradual; typical findings include signs of cachexia and dehydration, decreased LOC, bradycardia, and a history of severely limited food intake.

● *Renal failure.* Acute or chronic renal failure can cause life-threatening acidosis with Kussmaul's respirations. Signs and symptoms of severe renal failure include oliguria or anuria, uremic fetor, and yellow, dry, scaly skin. Other cutaneous signs include severe pruritus, uremic frost, purpura, and ecchymoses. The patient may complain of nausea and vomiting, weakness, burning pain in the legs and feet, and diarrhea or constipation.

As acidosis progresses, corresponding clinical features include frothy sputum, pleuritic chest pain, and signs of heart failure and pleural or pericardial effusion. Neurologic signs include altered LOC (lethargy to coma), twitching, and seizures. Hyperkalemia and hypertension, if present, require rapid intervention to prevent cardiovascular collapse.

- **Sepsis.** A severe infection may cause lactic acidosis, resulting in Kussmaul's respirations. Other findings include tachycardia, fever or a low temperature, chills, headache, lethargy, profuse diaphoresis, anorexia, cough, wound drainage, burning on urination, confusion or change in mental status, and other signs of local infection.
- **Shock.** Potentially life-threatening metabolic acidosis produces Kussmaul's respirations, hypotension, tachycardia, narrowed pulse pressure, weak pulse, dyspnea, oliguria, anxiety, restlessness, stupor that can progress to coma, and cool, clammy skin. Other clinical features may include external or internal bleeding (in hypovolemic shock); chest pain or arrhythmias and signs of heart failure (in cardiogenic shock); high fever, chills and, rarely, hypothermia (in septic shock); or stridor due to laryngeal edema (in anaphylactic shock). Onset is usually acute in hypovolemic, cardiogenic, or anaphylactic shock, but it may be gradual in septic shock.

OTHER CAUSES

- **Drugs.** Toxic levels of salicylates, ammonium chloride, acetazolamide, and other carbonic anhydrase inhibitors can cause Kussmaul's respirations. So can ingestion of methanol and ethylene glycol, found in antifreeze solutions.

NURSING CONSIDERATIONS

Monitor vital signs including oxygen saturation in all patients with hyperpnea, and observe for increasing respiratory distress or an irregular respiratory pattern signaling deterioration. Prepare for immediate intervention to prevent cardiovascular collapse: Start an I.V. line for administration of fluids, blood transfusions, and vasopressor drugs for hemodynamic stabilization, as ordered, and prepare to give ventilatory support. Prepare the patient for arterial blood gas analysis and blood chemistry studies.

PATIENT TEACHING

Teach the patient how to monitor his blood sugar level. Stress the importance of compliance with diabetes therapy, if applicable. Provide information on fluids and foods the patient should avoid. Discuss pulmonary hygiene and teach the patient ways to avoid respiratory infections. Emphasize the impor-

tance of abstinence from alcohol; refer to support groups or other resources that can assist, if indicated.

Hyperthermia

Hyperthermia, also known as *heat syndrome,* refers to an elevation of the core body temperature above normal. (See *Signs and symptoms of heat syndromes.*) It results when environmental and internal factors increase heat production or decrease heat loss beyond the body's ability to compensate. Hyperthermia affects males and females equally; however, incidence increases among elderly patients and neonates during excessively hot days. Risk factors for hyperthermia include obesity, salt and water depletion, alcohol use, poor physical condition, age, and socioeconomic status.

A temperature between 99° and 102° F (37.2° and 38.9° C) is considered mild hyperthermia; a temperature between 102° and 105° F (38.9° and 40.6° C) is considered moderate hyperthermia. A temperature of 105° F (40.6° C) or above is considered critical hyperthermia and represents an emergency—particularly if the temperature rises rapidly or stays elevated for a prolonged period.

Act now *For critical hyperthermia, immediate action should include providing supplemental oxygen and preparing the patient for endotracheal intubation and mechanical ventilation, if necessary. The goal is to reduce the patient's temperature, but not too rapidly; rapid reduction can lead to vasoconstriction, which can lead to shivering. Administer diazepam or chlorpromazine to control shivering. Shivering must be treated because it increases metabolic demands and oxygen consumption. Continuous cardiac monitoring will be instituted and the patient will be monitored for arrhythmias. Prepare the patient for pulmonary artery catheter insertion to monitor the body's core temperature. Closely observe the patient's vital signs and level of consciousness. Administer fluids and replace electrolytes, as ordered. Remove the patient's clothing and apply cool water to the skin, and then fan the patient with cool air.*

In mild and moderate hyperthermia, provide a cool, calm environment and allow the patient to rest. Encourage the oral intake and administration of I.V. fluids. Replace electrolytes, as necessary.

Signs and symptoms of heat syndromes

Hyperthermia, or heat syndrome, can be classified as mild (heat cramps), moderate (heat exhaustion), or critical (heatstroke). This table highlights assessment findings associated with each classification.

CLASSIFICATION	ASSESSMENT FINDINGS
Mild hyperthermia Heat cramps	◆ Mild agitation (central nervous system findings otherwise normal) ◆ Mild hypertension ◆ Moist, cool skin and muscle tenderness; involved muscle groups possibly hard and lumpy ◆ Muscle twitching and cramps ◆ Nausea and abdominal cramps ◆ Report of prolonged activity in a very warm or hot environment, without adequate salt intake ◆ Tachycardia ◆ Temperature ranging from 99° to 102° F (37.2° to 38.9° C)
Moderate hyperthermia Heat exhaustion	◆ Dizziness ◆ Headache ◆ Hypotension ◆ Muscle cramping ◆ Nausea and vomiting ◆ Oliguria ◆ Pale, moist skin ◆ Rapid, thready pulse ◆ Syncope or confusion ◆ Thirst ◆ Weakness ◆ Temperature elevated up to 105° F (40.6° C)
Critical hyperthermia Heatstroke	◆ Atrial or ventricular tachycardia ◆ Confusion, combativeness, and delirium ◆ Fixed, dilated pupils ◆ Hot, dry, reddened skin ◆ Loss of consciousness ◆ Seizures ◆ Tachypnea ◆ Temperature greater than 106° F (41.1° C)

ASSESSMENT
History

Ask the patient about the onset and duration of the fever. Ask the patient to describe the pattern of the fever. Did the temperature rise progressively or did it rise, disappear, and then reappear? Does he have accompanying symptoms, such as chills, headache, fatigue, diarrhea, or pain? Has the patient recently had an infection or exposure to an organism or someone else who was ill? Ask the patient whether he was exposed to high temperatures for a prolonged period of time. Ask about his work environment and water consumption while working. Has the patient experienced unusual physical or emotional stress recently? Ask if he has had any burns or trauma, undergone surgery under general anesthesia, or received a blood transfusion. Does the patient have a history of endocrine dysfunction or malignant hyperthermia? Is he taking thyroid medication? Ask the patient about other medications that disrupt thermoregulatory function such as salicylates as well as drugs that impair sweating, such as antibiotics, anticholinergics, monoamine oxidase inhibitors, or phenytoin.

Physical examination

Perform a physical examination based on the patient's health history. Note the rate and depth of the patient's breathing and any changes from normal respiratory patterns. Inspect the skin color and temperature. Check the skin turgor and monitor for diaphoresis. Assess for signs of trauma or needle marks on the arms or legs. Inspect for shivering of the body or flushing of the face. Assess his oral mucosa for lesions or signs of dehydration. Assess the patient's mental status and be alert for signs of malaise, fatigue, restlessness, or anxiety. Auscultate lung fields and the abdomen. Monitor vital signs and the cardiac rate, rhythm, and intensity. Keep in mind that palpating the thyroid gland of a patient with hyperthyroidism can induce thyrotoxicosis.

Pediatric pointers

Rarely, maternal thyrotoxicosis may be passed to the neonate, resulting in hyperthermia. More commonly, acquired thyrotoxicosis appears between ages 12 and 14, although this too is infrequent. Dehydration will also make a child sensitive to excessive heat.

MEDICAL CAUSES

● *Infection and inflammatory disorders.* Depending on the specific disorder, the temperature elevation may be insidious or abrupt. It can be a prodromal symptom and is often accompanied by chills, goose bumps, generalized symptoms of fatigue, headache, weakness, anorexia, malaise, and possibly, pain. If the temperature is high, you may find that the patient, particularly an elderly patient, is disoriented and confused. Other associated signs and symptoms depend on the disease and can involve any body system. The patient's history may include exposure to an infectious agent, travel to an endemic area, or exposure to the animal or insect vector of an infectious organism. Or his recent history may include a blood transfusion, surgery, trauma, or burns.

● *Malignant hyperthermia.* Rapid temperature increases occur at a rate of about 2° F (1.1° C) every 15 minutes to as high as 109.4° F (43° C). Usually the rise is preceded by skeletal muscle rigidity, cardiac arrhythmia, tachycardia, and tachypnea. The patient's history will include exposure to inhalant anesthesia, particularly halothane, or muscle relaxants, particularly succinylcholine, which can trigger malignant hyperthermia in patients with the inherited trait. Other predicting factors in susceptible persons include trauma, exercise, exposure to high environmental temperatures, and infection.

● *Neuroleptic malignant syndrome.* Neuroleptic malignant syndrome is marked by an explosive onset of hyperthermia accompanied by muscle rigidity, altered level of consciousness, cardiac arrhythmias, tachycardia, wide fluctuations in blood pressure, postural instability, dyspnea, and tachypnea. The patient history will include use of neuroleptic drugs such as haloperidol, chlorpromazine, thioridazine, or thiothixene.

● *Thermoregulatory dysfunction.* With thermoregulatory dysfunction, the patient's temperature rises suddenly and rapidly. The temperature then stays at 105° F to 107° F (40.6° C to 41.7° C). Assessment may reveal vomiting, hot flushed skin, and a decreased level of consciousness. The patient may also experience complications such as tachycardia, tachypnea, or hypotension. Other findings may include mottle cyanosis, if the patient has malignant hyperthermia; diarrhea if he is experiencing a thyroid storm; and signs of increased intracranial pressure when the problem is central nervous system trauma or hemorrhage. Heatstroke, brain stem compression, and thyroid storm are common causes of thermoregulatory dysfunction. Toxic doses of amphetamines and salicylates will also disrupt the thermoregulatory centers in the brain.

OTHER CAUSES

● *Drugs.* Hyperthermia can result from the use of tricyclic antidepressants and drugs that impair sweating, such as anticholinergics, phenothiazines, and monoamine oxidase inhibitors.

● *Impaired heat dissipation.* Impaired heat dissipation occurs with severe dehydration, in which sweat production decreases heat loss by evaporation. It also occurs when the environmental temperature is high, and the body can't rid itself of heat as fast as it's being received.

Nursing considerations

Treat mild to moderate hyperthermia by providing a cool, restful environment. Replace oral or I.V. fluid and electrolyte losses. If the patient is experiencing heatstroke, apply cool water to the skin and fan the patient. Apply a hyperthermia blanket or ice packs to the groin and axilla. Expect treatment to continue until the patient's body temperature drops to 102.2° F (39° C). Vital signs will require continuous monitoring, especially the core body temperature. Follow measures to avoid shivering. Employ additional external cooling measures, such as cool, wet sheets and tepid baths. Monitor hemodynamic parameters, fluid and electrolyte balance and laboratory and diagnostic studies. Monitor blood urea nitrogen and serum creatinine levels and assess for signs and symptoms associated with rhabdomyolysis.

Alert Don't reduce the patient's temperature too rapidly, as too rapid a reduction can lead to vasoconstriction, which can cause shivering.

Patient teaching

Caution the patient to reduce activity, especially outdoor activity, in the hot, humid weather. Advise him to wear light-colored, lightweight, loose-fitting clothing as well as a hat and sunglasses during hot weather. Instruct the patient to drink sufficient fluids, especially water, in hot weather and after vigorous physical activity. Warn him to avoid caffeine and alcohol in hot weather. Advise the patient to use air conditioning or to open windows and use a fan to help circulate air indoors.

Hypotension, orthostatic

In orthostatic hypotension, the patient's blood pressure drops 15 to 20 mm Hg or more — with or without an increase in the heart rate to at least 20 beats/minute — when he rises from a supine to a sitting or standing position. (Blood pressure should be measured 5 minutes after the patient has changed his position.) This common sign indicates failure of compensatory vasomotor responses to adjust to position changes. It's typically associated with light-headedness, syncope,

or blurred vision, and may occur in a hypotensive, normotensive, or hypertensive patient. Although commonly a nonpathologic sign in elderly patients, orthostatic hypotension may result from prolonged bed rest, fluid and electrolyte imbalance, endocrine or systemic disorders, and the effects of drugs.

To detect orthostatic hypotension, take and compare blood pressure readings and pulse rates with the patient supine, sitting, and then standing.

Act now If you detect orthostatic hypotension, quickly check for tachycardia, altered level of consciousness (LOC), and pale, clammy skin. If these signs are present, suspect hypovolemic shock. Insert a large-bore I.V. for fluid or blood replacement. Take the patient's vital signs every 15 minutes, and monitor his intake and output.

Assessment
History

If the patient's condition is stable, obtain his history. Ask whether he frequently experiences dizziness, weakness, or fainting when he stands. Ask whether he experienced associated symptoms, particularly fatigue, orthopnea, impotence, nausea, headache, abdominal or chest discomfort, and GI bleeding. Obtain a complete medication history, including his use of prescription, over-the-counter, herbal preparations, and other supplements. Also ask about his use of illicit drugs.

Physical examination

Begin the physical examination by checking the patient's skin turgor. Palpate peripheral pulses and auscultate the heart and lungs. Finally, test muscle strength and observe the patient's gait for unsteadiness.

Alert Assess the patient for signs and symptoms of hemorrhage and hypovolemic shock. Observe his skin color and check peripheral circulation and capillary refill time. Inspect the skin and mucous membranes for signs of bleeding.

Pediatric pointers

Because normal blood pressure is lower in children than in adults, familiarize yourself with normal age-specific values to detect orthostatic hypotension. From birth to age 3 months, normal systolic pressure is 40 to 80 mm Hg; from age 3 months to 1 year, 80 to 100 mm Hg; and from ages 1 to 12, 100 mm Hg plus 2 mm Hg for every year over age 1. Diastolic blood pressure is first heard at about age 4; it's normally 60 mm Hg at this age and gradually increases to 70 mm Hg by age 12.

The causes of orthostatic hypotension in children may be the same as those in adults.

Geriatric pointers

Elderly patients commonly experience autonomic dysfunction, which can present as orthostatic hypotension. Postprandial hypotension occurs 45 to 60 minutes after a meal and has been documented in up to one-third of nursing home residents.

MEDICAL CAUSES

- *Adrenal insufficiency.* Adrenal insufficiency typically begins insidiously, with progressively severe signs and symptoms. Orthostatic hypotension may be accompanied by fatigue, muscle weakness, poor coordination, anorexia, nausea and vomiting, fasting hypoglycemia, weight loss, abdominal pain, irritability, and a weak, irregular pulse. Another common feature is hyperpigmentation — bronze coloring of the skin — which is especially prominent on the face, lips, gums, tongue, buccal mucosa, elbows, palms, knuckles, waist, and knees. Diarrhea, constipation, decreased libido, amenorrhea, and syncope may also occur along with enhanced taste, smell, and hearing, and cravings for salty food.
- *Alcoholism.* Chronic alcoholism can lead to the development of peripheral neuropathy, which can present as orthostatic hypotension. Impotence is also a major issue in these patients. Other symptoms include numbness, tingling, nausea, vomiting, changes in bowel habits, and bizarre behavior.
- *Amyloidosis.* Orthostatic hypotension is commonly associated with amyloid infiltration of the autonomic nerves. Associated signs and symptoms vary widely and include angina, tachycardia, dyspnea, orthopnea, fatigue, and cough.
- *Diabetic autonomic neuropathy.* Here, orthostatic hypotension may be accompanied by syncope, dysphagia, constipation or diarrhea, painless bladder distention with overflow incontinence, impotence, and retrograde ejaculation.
- *Hyperaldosteronism.* Hyperaldosteronism typically produces orthostatic hypotension with sustained elevated blood pressure. Most other clinical effects of hyperaldostero-

nism result from hypokalemia, which increases neuromuscular irritability and produces muscle weakness, intermittent flaccid paralysis, fatigue, headache, paresthesia and, possibly, tetany with positive Trousseau's and Chvostek's signs. The patient may also exhibit vision disturbance, nocturia, polydipsia, and personality changes. Diabetes mellitus is a common finding.
- *Hyponatremia.* In hyponatremia, orthostatic hypotension is typically accompanied by headache, profound thirst, tachycardia, nausea and vomiting, abdominal cramps, muscle twitching and weakness, fatigue, oliguria or anuria, cold clammy skin, poor skin turgor, irritability, seizures, and decreased LOC. Cyanosis, thready pulse, and eventually vasomotor collapse may occur in severe sodium deficit. Common causes include adrenal insufficiency, hypothyroidism, syndrome of inappropriate antidiuretic hormone secretion, and use of thiazide diuretics.
- *Hypovolemia.* Mild to moderate hypovolemia may cause orthostatic hypotension associated with apathy, fatigue, muscle weakness, anorexia, nausea, and profound thirst. The patient may also develop dizziness, oliguria, sunken eyeballs, poor skin turgor, and dry mucous membranes.
- *Pheochromocytoma.* Although pheochromocytoma may produce orthostatic hypotension, its cardinal sign is paroxysmal or sustained hypertension. Typically, the patient is pale or flushed and diaphoretic, and his extreme anxiety makes him appear panicky. Associated signs and symptoms include tachycardia, palpitations, chest and abdominal pain, paresthesia, tremors, nausea and vomiting, low-grade fever, insomnia, and headache.
- *Shy-Drager syndrome.* Shy-Drager syndrome is a neurodegenerative disorder that's characterized by an insidious onset of multiple autonomic failure, manifested by orthostatic hypotension, urinary and fecal incontinence, decreased sweating, and impotence. This syndrome is most common in young and middle-aged adults.

OTHER CAUSES

- *Drugs.* Certain drugs may cause orthostatic hypotension by reducing circulating blood volume, causing blood vessel dilation, or depressing the sympathetic nervous system. These drugs include antihypertensives (especially guanethidine monosulfate and the

Performing preambulation exercises

Dear Patient:
To help minimize the effects of orthostatic hypotension, such as dizziness and blurred vision when you stand up, perform these leg exercises before getting out of bed.

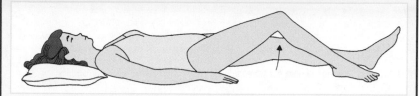

Lie flat on your back, and flex one knee slightly, keeping your heel on the bed.

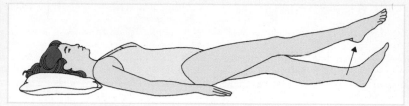

Straighten your leg.

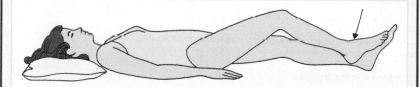

Flex your knee again, and lower your heel to the bed.

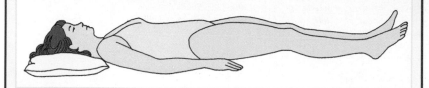

Repeat the procedure for the other leg. Alternating sides, perform the exercises six times for each leg.

initial dosage of prazosin hydrochloride), tricyclic antidepressants, phenothiazines, levodopa, nitrates, monoamine oxidase inhibitors, morphine, bretylium tosylate, and spinal anesthesia. Large doses of diuretics can also cause orthostatic hypotension.

● **Medical treatments.** Orthostatic hypotension is commonly associated with prolonged bed rest (24 hours or longer). It may also result from sympathectomy, which disrupts normal vasoconstrictive mechanisms.

NURSING CONSIDERATIONS

Monitor the patient's fluid balance by carefully recording his intake and output and weighing him daily. To help minimize orthostatic hypotension, advise the patient to change his position gradually. Elevate the head of the patient's bed, and help him to a sitting position with his feet dangling over the side of the bed. If he can tolerate this position, have him sit in a chair for brief periods. Immediately return him to bed if he becomes dizzy or pale, or displays other signs of hypotension.

Always keep the patient's safety in mind. Never leave him unattended while he's sitting or walking; evaluate his need for assistive devices, such as a cane or walker.

Prepare the patient for diagnostic tests, such as hematocrit, serum electrolyte and drug levels, urinalysis, 12-lead electrocardiogram, and chest X-ray.

PATIENT TEACHING

The patient with diabetes or another condition that can lead to autonomic dysfunction should be made aware of the acute drop in blood pressure that can occur with positional changes. Inform the patient that, should the problem occur, he'll need to avoid volume depletion and perform positional changes gradually instead of suddenly. (See *Performing preambulation exercises,* page 181.)

Hypothermia

Hypothermia refers to a core body temperature below 95° F (35° C) and affects chemical changes in the body. It may be classified as mild (89.6° to 95° F [32° to 35° C]), moderate (86° to 89.6° F [30° to 32° C]), or severe, which may be fatal (77° to 86° F [25° to 30° C]). Risk factors that contribute to serious cold injury, especially hypothermia, include lack of insulating body fat, wet or inadequate clothing, drug abuse, cardiac disease, smoking, fatigue, malnutrition and depletion of caloric reserves, and excessive alcohol intake. The incidence of hypothermia is highest in children and elderly people.

Hypothermia commonly results from cold-water near drowning and prolonged exposure to cold temperatures. It can also occur in normal temperatures, if disease or debility alters the patient's homeostasis. The administration of large amounts of cold blood or blood products can also cause hypothermia. A process such as hemodialysis, which circulates the blood outside of the body and then returns it to the body, will result in hypothermia.

Act now *Initiate cardiopulmonary resuscitation (CPR), if necessary. Hypothermia helps protect the brain from anoxia, which normally accompanies prolonged cardiopulmonary arrest. Therefore, even if the patient has been unresponsive for a long time, CPR may resuscitate him, especially after a cold-water near drowning.*

Institute continuous cardiac monitoring and administer supplemental oxygen. Prepare the patient for intubation and mechanical ventilation, if necessary. Institute rewarding measures. Prepare the patient for placement of a pulmonary artery catheter insertion to monitor core body temperatures. Monitor the patient's vital signs closely. Continue warming the patient until the core body temperature is within 1° to 2° F (0.6° to 1.1° C) of the desired body temperature. If the patient has been hypothermic for longer than 45 minutes, administer additional fluids, as ordered, to compensate for the expansion of the vascular space that occurs during vasodilation in warming.

Act now *If oxygen therapy is needed, be sure to use warm, humidified oxygen to prevent additional cooling.*

ASSESSMENT
History

Obtain the patient's history for clues to the causative factor. Was he exposed to cold and if so, what temperature and for what length of time? Ask whether he has recently undergone hemodialysis therapy. Has he had major surgery, especially a type of surgery that requires cooling of the patient's body? Has he recently received a blood transfusion that may have been administered while the blood was still cold? Does he have a history of thyroid, adrenal, liver, or cerebrovascular disease? Has the patient ingested any substances that result in a lowered body temperature, such as alcohol or barbiturates? If the exposure occurred indoors, determine whether the patient has adequate heat in his home. If the exposure occurred outdoors, determine whether he's homeless and sleeping outside.

Physical examination

Assess level of consciousness; a patient with mild hypothermia will have amnesia, a patient with moderate hypothermia is unresponsive, and the patient with severe hypothermia will be comatose. A patient with a body temperature below 86° F (30° C) is at risk for cardiopulmonary arrest. Assess for shivering, slurred speech, and peripheral cyanosis. Assess the patient's neurologic status and presence or absence of deep tendon reflexes. Assess for muscle rigidity that can produce a rigor-mortis-like state.

MEDICAL CAUSES

● *Prolonged exposure to extremely low temperatures.* The patient will have severe hypothermia, accompanied by lethargy or coma, depressed respiratory rate and depth, bradycardia, and muscle stiffness. The patient may have been exposed to an extremely low temperature with an excessive wind chill factor. If the patient is elderly or debilitated, he may have been exposed to a low room temperature. The patient may also have recently received a blood transfusion with cold blood or underwent a hemodialysis treatment.

OTHER CAUSES

● *Disorders.* Hypothermia may be a result of a certain disorder, but may not require immediate intervention. Endocrine disorders, such as hypothyroidism, hypoadrenalism, hypopituitarism, diabetes mellitus, cirrhosis, stroke, and renal failure, also affect the body's ability to regular temperature.
● *Drugs.* Alcohol ingestion and an overdose of barbiturates can induce mild to moderate hypothermia as a result of vasodilation, lowered metabolism, and central nervous system effects.

NURSING CONSIDERATIONS

Specific rewarming techniques include passive rewarming (the patient rewarms on his own); active rewarming (using heating blankets, warm-water immersion, heated objects such as water bottles, and radiant heat) and active core warming (using heated I.V. fluids, genitourinary tract irrigation, extracorporeal warming, and lavage). Arrhythmias that develop usually convert to a normal sinus rhythm with rewarming. Administration of oxygen, endotracheal intubation, controlled ventilation, I.V. fluids, and treatment of metabolic acidosis depends upon test results and careful patient monitoring.

✴ *Alert* Stay alert for signs and symptoms of hyperkalemia. If hyperkalemia occurs, administer calcium chloride, sodium bicarbonate, glucose, and insulin as ordered. Anticipate the need for sodium polystyrene sulfonate enemas.

PATIENT TEACHING

Advise the patient, especially if he's elderly, to maintain proper insulation in the home and keep the indoor temperature 70° F (21.1° C) or higher. Caution the patient to wear warm clothing and use warm bedding. Advise the patient of the importance of adequate nutrition, rest, and exercise. When the patient is expected to be out in the cold, especially for prolonged periods, advise him to wear loose-fitting clothing in layers and cover his hands, feet, and head; advise him to wear dry clothing and footwear and windand water-resistant outer garments and to avoid the intake of alcohol.

Intermittent claudication

Most common in the legs, intermittent claudication is cramping limb pain brought on by exercise and relieved by 1 to 2 minutes of rest. This pain may be acute or chronic; when acute, it may signal acute arterial occlusion. Intermittent claudication is most common in men ages 50 to 60 with a history of diabetes mellitus, hyperlipidemia, hypertension, or tobacco use. Without treatment, it may progress to pain at rest. With chronic arterial occlusion, limb loss is uncommon because collateral circulation usually develops.

With occlusive artery disease, intermittent claudication results from an inadequate blood supply. Pain in the calf (the most common area) or foot indicates disease of the femoral or popliteal arteries; pain in the buttocks and upper thigh, disease of the aortoiliac arteries. During exercise, the pain typically results from the release of lactic acid due to anaerobic metabolism in the ischemic segment, secondary to obstruction. When exercise stops, the lactic acid clears and the pain subsides.

Intermittent claudication may also have a neurologic cause: narrowing of the vertebral column at the level of the cauda equina. This condition creates pressure on the nerve roots to the lower extremities. Walking stimulates circulation to the cauda equina, causing increased pressure on those nerves and resultant pain.

Physical findings include pallor on elevation, rubor on dependency (especially the toes and soles), loss of hair on the toes, and diminished arterial pulses.

Act now If the patient has sudden intermittent claudication with severe or aching leg pain at rest, check the leg's temperature and color and palpate femoral, popliteal, posterior tibial, and dorsalis pedis pulses. Ask about numbness and tingling. Suspect acute arterial occlusion if pulses are absent; if the leg feels cold and looks pale, cyanotic, or mottled; and if paresthesia and pain are present. Mark the area of pallor, cyanosis, or mottling, and reassess it frequently, noting an increase in the area.

Don't elevate the leg. Protect it, allowing nothing to press on it. Prepare the patient for preoperative blood tests, urinalysis, electrocardiography, chest X-rays, lower-extremity Doppler studies, and angiography. Start an I.V. line, and administer an anticoagulant and analgesics.

ASSESSMENT
History

If the patient has chronic intermittent claudication, gather history data first. Ask how far he can walk before pain occurs and how long he must rest before it subsides. Can he walk less far now than before, or does he need to rest longer? Does the pain subside when the leg is hung downward? Does the pain-rest pattern vary? Has this symptom affected his lifestyle?

Obtain a history of risk factors for atherosclerosis, such as smoking, diabetes, hypertension, and hyperlipidemia. Next, ask about associated signs and symptoms, such as paresthesia in the affected limb and visible changes in the color of the fingers (white to blue to pink) when he's smoking, exposed to cold, or under stress. If the patient is male, does he experience impotence?

Physical examination

Focus the physical examination on the cardiovascular system. Palpate for femoral, popliteal, dorsalis pedis, and posterior tibial pulses. Note character, amplitude, and bilateral equality. Diminished or absent popliteal and pedal pulses with the femoral pulse present may indicate atherosclerotic disease of the femoral artery. Diminished femoral and distal pulses may indicate disease of the terminal aorta or iliac branches. Absent pedal pulses with normal femoral and popliteal pulses may indicate Buerger's disease.

Listen for bruits over the major arteries. Note color and temperature differences between his legs or compared with his arms; also note where on his leg the changes in temperature and color occur. Elevate the affected leg for 2 minutes; if it becomes pale or white, blood flow is severely decreased. When the leg hangs down, how long does it take for color to return? (Thirty seconds or longer indicates severe disease.) If possible, check the patient's deep tendon reflexes after exercise; note if they're diminished in his lower extremities.

Examine his feet, toes, and fingers for ulceration, and inspect his hands and lower legs for small, tender nodules and erythema along blood vessels. Note the quality of his nails and the location and amount of hair on his fingers, toes, and legs.

If the patient has arm pain, inspect his arms for a change in color (to white) on elevation. Next, palpate for changes in temperature, muscle wasting, and a pulsating mass in the subclavian area. Palpate and compare the radial, ulnar, brachial, axillary, and subclavian pulses to identify obstructed areas.

Pediatric pointers

Intermittent claudication rarely occurs in children. Although it sometimes develops in patients with coarctation of the aorta, extensive compensatory collateral circulation typically prevents manifestation of this sign. Muscle cramps from exercise and growing pains may be mistaken for intermittent claudication in children.

MEDICAL CAUSES

● *Aortic arteriosclerotic occlusive disease.* With aortic arteriosclerotic occlusive disease, intermittent claudication occurs in the buttock, hip, thigh, and calf, along with absent or diminished femoral pulses. Bruits can be auscultated over the femoral and iliac arteries. Examination reveals pallor of the affected limb on elevation and profound limb weakness. The leg may be cool to the touch.

● *Arterial occlusion (acute).* Arterial occlusion produces intense intermittent claudication. A saddle embolus may affect both legs. Associated findings include paresthesia, paresis, and a sensation of cold in the affected limb. The limb is cool, pale, and cyanotic (mottled) with absent pulses below the occlusion. Capillary refill time is increased.

● *Arteriosclerosis obliterans.* Arteriosclerosis obliterans usually affects the femoral and popliteal arteries, causing intermittent claudication (the most common symptom) in the calf. Typical associated findings include diminished or absent popliteal and pedal pulses, coolness in the affected limb, pallor on elevation, and profound limb weakness with continuing exercise. Other possible findings include numbness, paresthesia and, in severe disease, pain in the toes or foot while at rest, ulceration, and gangrene.

● *Buerger's disease.* Buerger's disease typically produces intermittent claudication of the instep. Males are affected more than females; most of the affected males smoke and are between ages 20 and 40. It's common in the Orient, southeast Asia, India, and the Middle East and rare in blacks. Early signs include migratory superficial nodules and erythema along extremity blood vessels (nodular phlebitis) as well as migratory venous phlebitis and easy leg fatigability. With exposure to cold, the feet initially become cold, cyanotic, and numb; later, they redden, become hot, and tingle. Occasionally, Buerger's disease also affects the hands and can cause painful ulcerations on the fingertips. Other characteristic findings include impaired peripheral pulses, paresthesia of the hands and feet, and migratory superficial thrombophlebitis. Ulcerations or moist gangrene may also occur.

● *Cauda equina syndrome.* Spinal stenosis causes pressure on nerve roots resulting in symptoms of claudication from the hip

IMPROVING CIRCULATION IN YOUR LEGS

Dear Patient:
To help stimulate circulation in your legs, perform these exercises (called Berger's exercises) as part of your regular exercise program. Do them four times each day or as often as your physician specifies.

Begin by lying flat on your back; then raise your legs straight up at a 90-degree angle, and hold this position for 2 minutes.

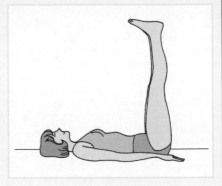

Now sit on the edge of a table or any flat surface that's high enough so that your legs don't touch the floor. Dangle your legs and swirl them in circles for 2 minutes.

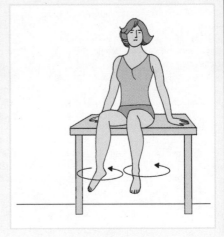

Finally, lie flat for 2 minutes; then repeat the sequence twice.

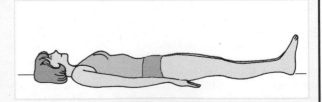

down as with Leriche's syndrome. Diagnosis can be determined by noninvasive exercise studies. With cauda equina syndrome, the pressure doesn't drop when the patient exercises on the treadmill.

- *Leriche's syndrome.* Arterial occlusion causes intermittent claudication of the hip, thigh, buttocks, and calf as well as impotence in men. Examination reveals bruits, global atrophy, absent or diminished pulses, and gangrene of the toes. The leg becomes cool and pale when elevated.

- *Neurogenic claudication.* Neurospinal disease causes pain from neurogenic intermittent claudication that requires a longer rest time than the 2 to 3 minutes needed in vascular claudication. Associated findings include paresthesia, weakness and clumsiness when walking, and hypoactive deep tendon reflexes after walking. Pulses are unaffected.

- *Thoracic outlet syndrome.* Activity that requires raising the hands above the shoulders, lifting a weight, or abducting the arm can cause intermittent pain along the ulnar distribution of the arm and forearm along with paresthesia and weakness. The pain isn't true claudication pain because it's related to position, not exercise. Signs and symptoms disappear when the arm is lowered. Other features include asymmetrical blood pressure and cool, pale skin.

NURSING CONSIDERATIONS

Encourage the patient to exercise to improve collateral circulation and increase venous return, and advise him to avoid prolonged sitting or standing as well as crossing his legs at the knees. (See *Improving circulation in your legs.*) If intermittent claudication interferes with the patient's lifestyle, he may require diagnostic tests (Doppler flow studies, arteriography, and digital subtraction angiography) to determine the location and degree of occlusion.

PATIENT TEACHING

Counsel the patient with intermittent claudication about risk factors. Encourage him to stop smoking, and refer him to a support group, if appropriate. Teach him to inspect his legs and feet for ulcers; to keep his extremities warm, clean, and dry; and to avoid injury.

Urge the patient to immediately report skin breakdown that doesn't heal. Also urge him to report any chest discomfort when circulation is restored to his legs. Increased exercise tolerance may lead to angina if the patient has coronary artery disease that was previously asymptomatic because of exercise limitations.

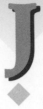

Jaw pain

Jaw pain may arise from either of the two bones that hold the teeth in the jaw—the maxilla (upper jaw) and the mandible (lower jaw). Jaw pain also includes pain in the temporomandibular joint (TMJ), where the mandible meets the temporal bone.

Jaw pain may develop gradually or abruptly and may range from barely noticeable to excruciating, depending on its cause. It usually results from disorders of the teeth, soft tissue, or glands of the mouth or throat or from local trauma or infection. Systemic causes include musculoskeletal, neurologic, cardiovascular, endocrine, immunologic, metabolic, and infectious disorders. Life-threatening disorders, such as myocardial infarction (MI) and tetany, also produce jaw pain, as do certain drugs and dental or surgical procedures.

Jaw pain is seldom a primary indicator of any one disorder; however, some causes are medical emergencies.

Act now Ask the patient when the jaw pain began. Did it arise suddenly or gradually? Is it more severe or frequent now than when it first occurred? Sudden severe jaw pain, especially when associated with chest pain, shortness of breath, or arm pain, requires prompt evaluation because it may herald a life-threatening disorder. Perform an electrocardiogram and obtain blood samples for cardiac enzyme levels. Administer oxygen, morphine sulfate, and a vasodilator as indicated.

ASSESSMENT
History

Begin the patient history by asking the patient to describe the pain's character, intensity, and frequency. When did he first notice the jaw pain? Where on the jaw does he feel pain? Does the pain radiate to other areas? Sharp or burning pain arises from the skin or subcutaneous tissues. Causalgia, an intense burning sensation, usually results from damage to the fifth cranial, or trigeminal, nerve. This type of superficial pain is easily localized, unlike dull, aching, boring, or throbbing pain, which originates in muscle, bone, or joints. Also ask about aggravating or alleviating factors.

Ask about recent trauma, surgery, or procedures, especially dental work. Ask about associated signs and symptoms, such as joint or chest pain, dyspnea, palpitations, fatigue, headache, malaise, anorexia, weight loss, intermittent claudication, diplopia, and hearing loss. (Keep in mind that jaw pain may accompany more characteristic signs and symptoms of life-threatening disorders, such as chest pain in a patient with an MI.)

Physical examination

Focus your physical examination on the jaw. Inspect the painful area for redness, and palpate for edema or warmth. Facing the patient directly, look for facial asymmetry indicating swelling. Check the TMJs by placing your fingertips just anterior to the external auditory meatus and asking the patient to open and close, and to thrust out and retract his jaw. Note the presence of crepitus, an abnormal scraping or grinding sensation in the joint. (Clicks heard when the jaw is widely spread apart are normal.) How wide can the patient open his mouth? Less than 1⅛″ (3 cm) or more than 2⅜″ (6 cm) between upper and lower teeth is abnormal. Next, palpate the parotid area for pain and swelling, and inspect and palpate the oral cavity for lesions, elevation of the tongue, or masses.

Pediatric pointers

Be alert for nonverbal signs of jaw pain, such as rubbing the affected area or wincing while talking or swallowing. In infants, initial signs of tetany from hypocalcemia include episodes of apnea and generalized jitteriness progressing to facial grimaces and generalized rigidity. Finally, seizures may occur.

Jaw pain in children sometimes stems from disorders uncommon in adults. Mumps, for example, causes unilateral or bilateral swelling from the lower mandible to the zygomatic arch. Parotiditis due to cystic fibrosis also causes jaw pain. When trauma causes jaw pain in children, always consider the possibility of abuse.

MEDICAL CAUSES

- *Angina pectoris.* Angina may produce jaw pain (usually radiating from the substernal area) and left arm pain. Angina is less severe than the pain of an MI. It's commonly triggered by exertion, emotional stress, or ingestion of a heavy meal and usually subsides with rest and the administration of nitroglycerin. Other signs and symptoms include shortness of breath, nausea and vomiting, tachycardia, dizziness, diaphoresis, belching, and palpitations.
- *Arthritis.* With osteoarthritis, which usually affects the small joints of the hand, aching jaw pain increases with activity (talking, eating) and subsides with rest. Other features are crepitus heard and felt over the TMJ, enlarged joints with a restricted range of motion, and stiffness on awakening that improves with a few minutes of activity. Redness and warmth are usually absent.

Rheumatoid arthritis causes symmetrical pain in all joints (commonly affecting proximal finger joints first), including the jaw. The joints display limited range of motion and are tender, warm, swollen, and stiff after inactivity, especially in the morning. Myalgia is common. Systemic signs and symptoms include fatigue, weight loss, malaise, anorexia, lymphadenopathy, and mild fever. Painless, movable rheumatoid nodules may appear on

the elbows, knees, and knuckles. Progressive disease causes deformities, crepitation with joint rotation, muscle weakness and atrophy around the involved joint, and multiple systemic complications.

- *Head and neck cancer.* Many types of head and neck cancer, especially of the oral cavity and nasopharynx, produce aching jaw pain of insidious onset. Other findings include a history of leukoplakia ulcers of the mucous membranes; palpable masses in the jaw, mouth, and neck; dysphagia; bloody discharge; drooling; lymphadenopathy; and trismus.
- *Hypocalcemic tetany.* Besides painful muscle contractions of the jaw and mouth, hypocalcemic tetany — a life-threatening disorder — produces paresthesia and carpopedal spasms. The patient may complain of weakness, fatigue, and palpitations. Examination reveals hyperreflexia and positive Chvostek's and Trousseau's signs. Muscle twitching, choreiform movements, and muscle cramps may also occur. With severe hypocalcemia, laryngeal spasm may occur with stridor, cyanosis, seizures, and cardiac arrhythmias.
- *Ludwig's angina.* An acute streptococcal infection of the sublingual and submandibular spaces that produces severe jaw pain in the mandibular area with tongue elevation, sublingual edema, and drooling. Fever is a common sign. Progressive disease produces dysphagia, dysphonia, and stridor and dyspnea due to laryngeal edema and obstruction by an elevated tongue.
- *Myocardial infarction.* Initially, MI — a life-threatening disorder — causes intense, crushing substernal pain that's unrelieved by rest or nitroglycerin. The pain may radiate to the lower jaw, left arm, neck, back, or shoulder blades. (Rarely, jaw pain occurs without chest pain.) Other findings include pallor, clammy skin, dyspnea, excessive diaphoresis, nausea and vomiting, anxiety, restlessness, a feeling of impending doom, low-grade fever, decreased or increased blood pressure, arrhythmias, an atrial gallop, new murmurs (in many cases from mitral insufficiency), and crackles.
- *Osteomyelitis.* Bone infection after trauma, sinus infection, dental injury, or surgery (dental or facial) may produce diffuse, aching jaw pain along with warmth, swelling, tenderness, erythema, and restricted jaw movement. Acute osteomyelitis may also cause tachycardia, sudden fever, nausea, and

malaise. Chronic osteomyelitis may recur after minor trauma.

- **Sialolithiasis.** With sialolithiasis, stones form in the salivary glands, causing painful swelling that makes chewing uncomfortable. Jaw pain occurs in the lower jaw, floor of the mouth, and TMJ. It may also radiate to the ear or neck.
- **Sinusitis.** Maxillary sinusitis produces intense boring pain in the maxilla and cheek that may radiate to the eye. This type of sinusitis also causes a feeling of fullness, increased pain on percussion of the first and second molars and, in those with nasal obstruction, the loss of the sense of smell. Sphenoid sinusitis causes scanty nasal discharge and chronic pain at the mandibular ramus and vertex of the head and in the temporal area. Other signs and symptoms of both types of sinusitis include fever, halitosis, headache, malaise, cough, sore throat, and fever.
- **Suppurative parotitis.** Bacterial infection of the parotid gland by *Staphylococcus aureus* tends to develop in debilitated patients with dry mouth or poor oral hygiene. Besides the abrupt onset of jaw pain, high fever, and chills, findings include erythema and edema of the overlying skin; a tender, swollen gland; and pus at the second top molar (Stensen's ducts). Infection may lead to disorientation; shock and death are common.
- **Temporal arteritis.** Most common in females older than age 60, temporal arteritis produces sharp jaw pain after chewing or talking. Nonspecific signs and symptoms include low-grade fever, generalized muscle pain, malaise, fatigue, anorexia, and weight loss. Vascular lesions produce jaw pain; throbbing, unilateral headache in the frontotemporal region; swollen, nodular, tender and, possibly, pulseless temporal arteries; and, at times, erythema of the overlying skin.
- **Temporomandibular joint syndrome.** Temporomandibular joint syndrome produces jaw pain at the TMJ; spasm and pain of the masticating muscle; clicking, popping, or crepitus of the TMJ; and restricted jaw movement. Unilateral, localized pain may radiate to other head and neck areas. The patient typically reports teeth clenching, bruxism, and emotional stress. He may also experience ear pain, headache, deviation of the jaw to the affected side upon opening the mouth, and jaw subluxation or dislocation, especially after yawning.

- **Tetanus.** A rare, acute life-threatening disorder caused by a bacterial toxin, tetanus produces stiffness and pain in the jaw and difficulty opening the mouth. Early nonspecific signs and symptoms (commonly unnoticed or mistaken for influenza) include headache, irritability, restlessness, low-grade fever, and chills. Examination reveals tachycardia, profuse diaphoresis, and hyperreflexia. Progressive disease leads to painful, involuntary muscle spasms that spread to the abdomen, back, or face. The slightest stimulus may produce reflex spasms of any muscle group. Ultimately, laryngospasm, respiratory distress, and seizures may occur.
- **Trauma.** Injury to the face, head, or neck — particularly fracture of the maxilla or mandible — may produce jaw pain and swelling and decreased jaw mobility. Associated findings include hypotension and tachycardia (indicating shock), lacerations, ecchymoses, and hematomas. Rhinorrhea or otorrhea indicates the leakage of cerebrospinal fluid; blurred vision indicates orbital involvement.
- **Trigeminal neuralgia.** Trigeminal neuralgia is marked by paroxysmal attacks of intense unilateral jaw pain (stopping at the facial midline) or rapid-fire shooting sensations in one division of the trigeminal nerve (usually the mandibular or maxillary division). This superficial pain, felt mainly over the lips and chin and in the teeth, lasts from 1 to 15 minutes. Mouth and nose areas may be hypersensitive. Involvement of the ophthalmic branch of the trigeminal nerve causes a diminished or absent corneal reflex on the same side. Attacks can be triggered by mild stimulation of the nerve (for example, lightly touching the cheeks), exposure to heat or cold, or consumption of hot or cold foods or beverages.

OTHER CAUSES
- **Drugs.** Some drugs, such as phenothiazines, affect the extrapyramidal tract, causing dyskinesias; others cause tetany of the jaw secondary to hypocalcemia.

NURSING CONSIDERATIONS
If the patient is in severe pain, withhold food, liquids, and oral medications until the diagnosis is confirmed. Administer an analgesic. Prepare the patient for diagnostic tests such as jaw X-rays. Apply an ice pack if the

jaw is swollen, and discourage the patient from talking or moving his jaw.

PATIENT TEACHING

Instruct the patient on measures to relieve jaw discomfort depending on the source of the pain. Inform patients of the link between sudden severe jaw pain and cardiac dysfunction and to seek medical assistance immediately.

Jugular vein distention

Jugular vein distention is the abnormal fullness and height of the pulse waves in the internal or external jugular veins. For a patient in a supine position with his head elevated 45 degrees, a pulse wave height greater than 1¼" to 1½" (3 to 4 cm) above the angle of Louis indicates distention. Engorged, distended veins reflect increased venous pressure in the right side of the heart, which in turn, indicates an increased central venous pressure. This common sign characteristically occurs in heart failure and other cardiovascular disorders, such as constrictive pericarditis, tricuspid stenosis, and obstruction of the superior vena cava.

Act now *Evaluating jugular vein distention involves visualizing and assessing venous pulsations. (See* Evaluating jugular vein distention, page 192.) *If you detect jugular vein distention in a patient with pale, clammy skin who suddenly appears anxious and dyspneic, take his blood pressure. If you note hypotension and paradoxical pulse, suspect cardiac tamponade. Elevate the foot of the bed 20 to 30 degrees, give supplemental oxygen, and monitor cardiac status and rhythm, oxygen saturation, and mental status. Start an I.V. line for medication administration, and keep cardiopulmonary resuscitation equipment close by. Assemble the needed equipment for emergency pericardiocentesis (to relieve pressure on the heart.) Throughout the procedure, monitor the patient's blood pressure, heart rhythm, and respirations.*

ASSESSMENT
History

If the patient isn't in severe distress, obtain a personal history. Has he recently gained weight? Does he have difficulty putting on shoes? Are his ankles swollen? Ask about chest pain, shortness of breath, paroxysmal nocturnal dyspnea, anorexia, nausea or vomiting, and a history of cancer or cardiac, pulmonary, hepatic, or renal disease. Obtain a drug history noting diuretic use and dosage. Is the patient taking drugs as prescribed? Ask the patient about his regular diet patterns, noting a high sodium intake.

Physical examination

Next, perform a physical examination, beginning with vital signs. Tachycardia, tachypnea, and increased blood pressure indicate fluid overload that's stressing the heart. Inspect and palpate the patient's extremities and face for edema. Then weigh the patient and compare that weight to his baseline.

Auscultate his lungs for crackles and his heart for gallops, a pericardial friction rub, and muffled heart sounds. Inspect his abdomen for distention, and palpate and percuss for an enlarged liver. Finally monitor urine output and note any decrease.

Pediatric pointers

Jugular vein distention is difficult (sometimes impossible) to evaluate in most infants and toddlers because of their short, thick necks. Even in school-age children, measurement of jugular vein distention can be unreliable because the sternal angle may not be the same distance (2" to 2¾" [5 to 7 cm]) above the right atrium as it is in adults.

MEDICAL CAUSES

- *Cardiac tamponade.* Cardiac tamponade is a life-threatening condition that produces jugular vein distention along with anxiety, restlessness, cyanosis, chest pain, dyspnea, hypotension, and clammy skin. It also causes tachycardia, tachypnea, muffled heart sounds, a pericardial friction rub, weak or absent peripheral pulses or pulses that decrease during inspiration (pulsus paradoxus), and hepatomegaly. The patient may sit upright or lean forward to ease breathing.
- *Heart failure.* Sudden or gradual development of right-sided heart failure commonly causes jugular vein distention, along with weakness and anxiety, cyanosis, dependent edema of the legs and sacrum, steady weight gain, confusion, and hepatomegaly. Other findings include nausea and vomiting, abdominal discomfort, and anorexia due to visceral edema. Ascites is a late sign. Massive

EVALUATING JUGULAR VEIN DISTENTION

With the patient in a supine position, position him so that you can visualize jugular vein pulsations reflected from the right atrium. Elevate the head of the bed 45 to 90 degrees. (In the normal patient, veins distend only when the patient lies flat.) Next, locate the angle of Louis (sternal notch) — the reference point for measuring venous pressure. To do so, palpate the clavicles where they join the sternum (the suprasternal notch). Place your first two fingers on the suprasternal notch. Then without lifting them from the skin, slide them down the sternum until you feel a bony protuberance — this is the angle of Louis.

Find the internal jugular vein (which indicates venous pressure more reliably than the external jugular vein). Shine a flashlight across the patient's neck to create shadows that highlight his venous pulse. Be sure to distinguish jugular vein pulsations from carotid artery pulsations. One way to do this is to palpate the vessel: Arterial pulsations continue, whereas venous pulsations disappear with light finger pressure. Also, venous pulsations increase or decrease with changes in body position; arterial pulsations remain constant.

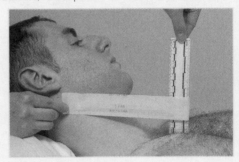

Next, locate the highest point along the vein where you can see pulsations. Using a centimeter ruler, measure the distance between that high point and the sternal notch. Record this finding as well as the angle at which the patient was lying. A finding greater than 1¼" to 1½" (3 to 4 cm) above the sternal notch, with the head of the bed at a 45-degree angle, indicates jugular vein distention.

right-sided heart failure may produce anasarca and oliguria.

If left-sided heart failure precedes right-sided heart failure, jugular vein distention is a late sign. Other signs and symptoms include fatigue, dyspnea, orthopnea, paroxysmal nocturnal dyspnea, tachypnea, tachycardia, and arrhythmias. Auscultation reveals crackles and a ventricular gallop.

● *Hypervolemia.* Markedly increased intravascular fluid volume causes jugular vein distention, along with rapid weight gain, elevated blood pressure, bounding pulse, peripheral edema, dyspnea, and crackles.

● *Pericarditis (chronic constrictive).* Progressive signs and symptoms of restricted heart filling include jugular vein distention that's more prominent on inspiration (Kussmaul's sign). The patient usually complains of chest pain. Other signs and symptoms include fluid retention with dependent edema, fever, hepatomegaly, ascites, and an audible pericardial friction rub.

● *Superior vena cava obstruction.* A tumor or, rarely, thrombosis may gradually lead to jugular vein distention when the veins of the head, neck, and arms fail to empty effectively, causing facial, neck, and upper arm edema. Metastasis of a malignant tumor to the mediastinum may cause dyspnea, cough, substernal chest pain, and hoarseness.

NURSING CONSIDERATIONS

If the patient has cardiac tamponade, prepare him for pericardiocentesis. If he doesn't have cardiac tamponade, restrict fluids and monitor his intake and output. Insert an indwelling urinary catheter if necessary. If the patient has heart failure, administer a diuretic. Routinely change his position to avoid skin breakdown from peripheral edema. Prepare the patient for a central venous or Swan-Ganz catheter insertion in order to measure right-sided and left-sided heart pressure.

PATIENT TEACHING

Teach the patient with heart failure about appropriate treatments, including dietary restrictions (such as a low-sodium diet).

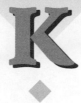

Kernig's sign

A reliable early indicator and tool used to diagnose meningeal irritation, Kernig's sign elicits both resistance and hamstring muscle pain when the examiner attempts to extend the knee while the hip and knee are both flexed 90 degrees. However, when the patient's thigh isn't flexed on the abdomen, he's usually able to completely extend his leg. (See *Eliciting Kernig's sign,* page 194.) This sign is usually elicited in meningitis or subarachnoid hemorrhage. With these potentially life-threatening disorders, hamstring muscle resistance results from stretching the blood- or exudate-irritated meninges surrounding spinal nerve roots.

Kernig's sign can also indicate a herniated disk or spinal tumor. With these disorders, sciatic pain results from disk or tumor pressure on spinal nerve roots.

Act now Because Kernig's sign may signal meningitis or subarachnoid hemorrhage, both life-threatening central nervous system disorders, take the patient's vital signs at once to obtain baseline information. Then test for Brudzinski's sign to obtain further evidence of meningeal irritation. Next, ask the patient or his family to describe the onset of illness. Typically, the progressive onset of headache, fever, nuchal rigidity, and confusion suggests meningitis. Conversely, the sudden onset of a severe headache, nuchal rigidity, photophobia and, possibly, loss of consciousness usually indicates subarachnoid hemorrhage.

If you elicit a positive Kernig's sign and suspect life-threatening meningitis or sub-arachnoid hemorrhage, immediately prepare for emergency intervention.

ASSESSMENT
History

If you suspect meningitis, ask the patient about recent infections, especially tooth abscesses. Ask about exposure to infected persons or places where meningitis is endemic. Meningitis is usually a complication of another bacterial infection, so blood cultures are needed to determine the causative organism. If subarachnoid hemorrhage is the suspected diagnosis, ask about a history of hypertension, cerebral aneurysm, head trauma, or arteriovenous malformation. Check the patient's pupils for dilation, and assess him for signs of increasing intracranial pressure, such as bradycardia, increased systolic blood pressure, and widening pulse pressure.

If you don't suspect meningeal irritation, ask the patient if he feels any back pain that radiates down one or both legs. Does he also feel leg numbness, tingling, or weakness? Ask about other signs and symptoms, and find out if he has a history of cancer or back injury.

Physical examination

Perform a physical examination, concentrating on motor and sensory function. Assess motor function by inspecting the muscles and testing muscle tone and strength. Perform cerebellar testing. Cerebellar deficits affect the patient's voluntary movements, equilibrium, integration of sensations, and sense of position. Assess sensory function by checking the patient's sensitivity to pain,

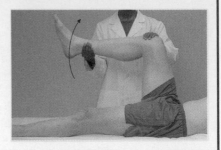

ELICITING KERNIG'S SIGN

To elicit Kernig's sign, place the patient in a supine position. Flex his leg at the hip and knee, as shown here. Then try to extend the leg while you keep the hip flexed. If the patient experiences pain and possibly spasm in the hamstring muscle and resists further extension, you can assume that meningeal irritation has occurred.

light touch, vibration, position, and discrimination.

Pediatric pointers
Kernig's sign is considered ominous in children because of their greater potential for rapid deterioration.

MEDICAL CAUSES
● *Lumbosacral herniated disk.* A positive Kernig's sign may be elicited in patients with lumbosacral herniated disk, but the cardinal and earliest feature is sciatic pain on the affected side or on both sides. Associated findings include postural deformity (lumbar lordosis or scoliosis), paresthesia, hypoactive deep tendon reflexes in the involved leg, and dorsiflexor muscle weakness.
● *Meningitis.* A positive Kernig's sign usually occurs early with meningitis, along with fever and, possibly, chills. Other signs and symptoms of meningeal irritation include nuchal rigidity, hyperreflexia, Brudzinski's sign, and opisthotonos. As intracranial pressure (ICP) increases, headache and vomiting may occur. In severe meningitis, the patient may experience stupor, coma, and seizures. Cranial nerve involvement may produce ocular palsies, facial weakness, deafness, and photophobia. An erythematous maculopapular rash may occur in viral meningitis; a purpuric rash may be seen in those with meningococcal meningitis.
● *Spinal cord tumor.* Kernig's sign can be elicited occasionally, but the earliest symptom is typically pain felt locally or along the spinal nerve, commonly in the leg. Associated findings include weakness or paralysis distal to the tumor, paresthesia, urine reten-

tion, urinary or fecal incontinence, and sexual dysfunction.
● *Subarachnoid hemorrhage.* Kernig's sign and Brudzinski's sign can both be elicited within minutes after the initial bleed. The patient experiences a sudden onset of severe headache that begins in a localized area and then spreads, pupillary inequality, nuchal rigidity, and decreased level of consciousness. Photophobia, fever, nausea and vomiting, dizziness, and seizures are possible. Focal signs include hemiparesis or hemiplegia, aphasia, and sensory or vision disturbances. Increasing ICP may produce bradycardia, increased blood pressure, respiratory pattern change, and rapid progression to coma.

NURSING CONSIDERATIONS
Prepare the patient for diagnostic tests, such as a computed tomography scan, magnetic resonance imaging, spinal X-ray, myelography, and lumbar puncture. Closely monitor his vital signs, ICP, and cardiopulmonary and neurologic status. Ensure bed rest, quiet, and minimal stress.

If the patient has a subarachnoid hemorrhage, darken the room and elevate the head of the bed at least 30 degrees to reduce ICP. If he has a herniated disk or spinal tumor, he may require pelvic traction.

PATIENT TEACHING
Teach the patient the signs and symptoms of meningitis. Discuss measures to prevent meningitis. Explain the activities that a patient with a herniated disk should avoid. Teach the patient how to apply a back brace or cervical collar, as needed.

Level of consciousness, decreased

A decrease in level of consciousness (LOC), from lethargy to stupor to coma, usually results from a neurologic disorder and may signal a life-threatening complication, such as hemorrhage, trauma, or cerebral edema. However, this sign can also result from a metabolic, GI, musculoskeletal, urologic, or cardiopulmonary disorder; severe nutritional deficiency; the effects of toxins; or drug use. LOC can deteriorate suddenly or gradually and can remain altered temporarily or permanently.

Consciousness is affected by the reticular activating system (RAS), an intricate network of neurons with axons extending from the brain stem, thalamus, and hypothalamus to the cerebral cortex. A disturbance in any part of this integrated system prevents the intercommunication that makes consciousness possible. Loss of consciousness can result from a bilateral cerebral disturbance, an RAS disturbance, or both. Cerebral dysfunction characteristically produces the least dramatic decrease in a patient's LOC. In contrast, dysfunction of the RAS produces the most dramatic decrease in LOC—coma.

The most sensitive indicator of decreased LOC is a change in the patient's mental status. The Glasgow Coma Scale, which measures a patient's ability to respond to verbal, sensory, and motor stimulation, can be used to evaluate and monitor trends in the patient's LOC. (See *Glasgow Coma Scale,* page 196.)

Act now *After evaluating the patient's airway, breathing, and circulation, use the Glasgow Coma Scale to quickly determine his LOC and to obtain baseline data. If the patient's score is 13 or less, emergency surgery may be necessary. Insert an artificial airway, elevate the head of the bed 30 degrees and, if spinal cord injury has been ruled out, turn the patient's head to the side. Prepare to suction the patient if necessary. You may need to hyperventilate him to reduce carbon dioxide levels and decrease intracranial pressure (ICP). Then determine the rate, rhythm, and depth of spontaneous respirations. Support his breathing with a handheld resuscitation bag, if necessary. If the patient's Glasgow Coma Scale score is 7 or less, intubation and resuscitation may be necessary.*

Continue to monitor the patient's vital signs, being alert for signs of increasing ICP, such as bradycardia and widening pulse pressure. When his airway, breathing, and circulation are stabilized, perform a neurologic examination.

ASSESSMENT
History

Try to obtain history information from the patient, if he's lucid, and from his family. Did the patient complain of headache, dizziness, nausea, visual or hearing disturbances, weakness, fatigue, or any other problems before his LOC decreased? Has his family noticed any changes in the patient's behavior, personality, memory, or temperament? Also ask about a history of neurologic disease, cancer, or recent trauma or infections; drug and alcohol use; and the development of other signs and symptoms.

GLASGOW COMA SCALE

You've probably heard such terms as *lethargic, obtunded,* and *stuporous* used to describe a progressive decrease in a patient's level of consciousness (LOC). However, the Glasgow Coma Scale provides a more accurate, less subjective method of recording such changes, grading consciousness in relation to eye opening and motor and verbal responses.

To use the Glasgow Coma Scale, test the patient's ability to respond to verbal, motor, and sensory stimulation. The scoring system doesn't determine exact LOC, but it does provide an easy way to describe the patient's basic status and helps to detect and interpret changes from baseline findings. A decreased reaction score in one or more categories may signal an impending neurologic crisis. A score of 7 or less indicates severe neurologic damage.

TEST	REACTION	SCORE
Eyes	Open spontaneously	4
	Open to verbal command	3
	Open to pain	2
	No response	1
Best motor response	Obeys verbal command	6
	Localizes painful stimulus	5
	Flexion — withdrawal	4
	Flexion — abnormal (decorticate rigidity)	3
	Extension (decerebrate rigidity)	2
	No response	1
Best verbal response	Oriented and converses	5
	Disoriented and converses	4
	Inappropriate words	3
	Incomprehensible sounds	2
	No response	1
Total		3 to 15

Physical examination

Because decreased LOC can result from a disorder affecting virtually any body system, tailor the remainder of your evaluation according to the patient's associated symptoms. Perform a complete neurologic assessment and a physical assessment. Determine the patient's baseline Glasgow Coma Scale score and evaluate on an ongoing basis.

Pediatric pointers

The primary cause of decreased LOC in children is head trauma, which often results from physical abuse or a motor vehicle accident. Other causes include accidental poisoning, hydrocephalus, and meningitis or brain abscess following an ear or respiratory infection. To reduce the parents' anxiety, include them in the child's care. Offer them support and realistic explanations of their child's condition.

MEDICAL CAUSES

● **Adrenal crisis.** Decreased LOC, ranging from lethargy to coma, may develop within 8 to 12 hours of onset. Early associated findings include progressive weakness, irritability, anorexia, headache, nausea and vomiting, diarrhea, abdominal pain, and fever. Later signs and symptoms include hypotension; rapid, thready pulse; oliguria; cool, clammy skin; and flaccid extremities. The patient with chronic adrenocortical hypofunction may have hyperpigmented skin and mucous membranes.

● **Brain abscess.** Decreased LOC varies from drowsiness to deep stupor, depending on abscess size and site. Early signs and symptoms — constant intractable headache, nausea, vomiting, and seizures — reflect increasing ICP. Typical later features include ocular disturbances (nystagmus, vision loss, and pupillary inequality) and signs of infection such as fever. Other findings may include personality changes, confusion, abnormal behavior, dizziness, facial weakness, aphasia, ataxia, tremor, and hemiparesis.

- *Brain tumor.* LOC decreases slowly, from lethargy to coma. The patient may also experience apathy, behavior changes, memory loss, decreased attention span, morning headache, dizziness, vision loss, ataxia, and sensorimotor disturbances. Aphasia and seizures are possible, along with signs of hormonal imbalance, such as fluid retention or amenorrhea. Signs and symptoms vary according to the location and size of the tumor. In later stages, papilledema, vomiting, bradycardia, and widening pulse pressure also appear. In the final stages, the patient may exhibit decorticate or decerebrate posture.

- *Cerebral aneurysm (ruptured).* Somnolence, confusion and, at times, stupor characterize a moderate bleed; deep coma occurs with severe bleeding, which can be fatal. Onset is usually abrupt, with sudden, severe headache, nausea, and vomiting. Nuchal rigidity, back and leg pain, fever, restlessness, irritability, occasional seizures, and blurred vision point to meningeal irritation. The type and severity of other findings vary with the site and severity of the hemorrhage and may include hemiparesis, hemisensory defects, dysphagia, and visual defects.

- *Cerebral contusion.* Usually unconscious for a prolonged period, the patient may develop dilated, nonreactive pupils and decorticate or decerebrate posture. If he's conscious or recovers consciousness, he may be drowsy, confused, disoriented, agitated, or even violent. Associated findings include blurred or double vision, fever, headache, pallor, diaphoresis, tachycardia, altered respirations, aphasia, and hemiparesis. Residual effects include seizures, impaired mental status, slight hemiparesis, and vertigo.

- *Diabetic ketoacidosis.* Diabetic ketoacidosis produces a rapid decrease in LOC, ranging from lethargy to coma, commonly preceded by polydipsia, polyphagia, and polyuria. The patient may complain of weakness, anorexia, abdominal pain, nausea, and vomiting. He may also exhibit orthostatic hypotension, fruity breath odor, and Kussmaul's respirations, as well as warm, dry skin and a rapid, thready pulse. Untreated, this condition invariably leads to coma and death.

- *Encephalitis.* Within 24 to 48 hours after onset, the patient may develop LOC changes ranging from lethargy to coma. Other possible findings include abrupt onset of fever, headache, nuchal rigidity, nausea, vomiting, irritability, personality changes, seizures, aphasia, ataxia, hemiparesis, nystagmus, photophobia, myoclonus, and cranial nerve palsies.

- *Encephalomyelitis (postvaccinal).* Encephalomyelitis is a life-threatening disorder that produces rapid LOC deterioration from drowsiness to coma. The patient also experiences rapid onset of fever, headache, nuchal rigidity, back pain, vomiting, and seizures.

- *Encephalopathy.* With hepatic encephalopathy, signs and symptoms develop in four stages: in the prodromal stage, slight personality changes (disorientation, forgetfulness, slurred speech) and slight tremor; in the impending stage, tremor progressing to asterixis (the hallmark of hepatic encephalopathy), lethargy, aberrant behavior, and apraxia; in the stuporous stage, stupor and hyperventilation, with the patient noisy and abusive when aroused; in the comatose stage, coma with decerebrate posture, hyperactive reflexes, positive Babinski's reflex, and fetor hepaticus.

With life-threatening hypertensive encephalopathy, LOC progressively decreases from lethargy to stupor to coma. Besides markedly elevated blood pressure, the patient may experience severe headache, vomiting, seizures, vision disturbances, transient paralysis, and eventually Cheyne-Stokes respirations.

With hypoglycemic encephalopathy, LOC rapidly deteriorates from lethargy to coma. Early signs and symptoms include nervousness, restlessness, agitation, and confusion accompanied by hunger, alternate flushing and cold sweats, and headache, trembling, and palpitations. Blurred vision progresses to motor weakness, hemiplegia, dilated pupils, pallor, decreased pulse rate, shallow respirations, and seizures. Flaccidity and decerebrate posture appear late.

Depending on its severity, hypoxic encephalopathy produces a sudden or gradual decrease in LOC, leading to coma and brain death. Early on, the patient appears confused and restless, with cyanosis and increased heart and respiratory rates and blood pressure. Later, his respiratory pattern becomes abnormal, and assessment reveals decreased pulse, blood pressure, and deep tendon reflexes (DTRs); Babinski's reflex; and fixed pupils.

With uremic encephalopathy, LOC decreases gradually from lethargy to coma. Early on, the patient may appear apathetic, inattentive, confused, and irritable and may complain of headache, nausea, fatigue, and anorexia. Other findings include vomiting, tremors, edema, papilledema, hypertension, cardiac arrhythmias, dyspnea, crackles, oliguria, and Kussmaul's and Cheyne-Stokes respirations.

● *Epidural hemorrhage (acute).* Epidural hemorrhage is a life-threatening posttraumatic disorder that produces momentary loss of consciousness, sometimes followed by a lucid interval. While lucid, the patient has a severe headache, nausea, vomiting, and bladder distention. Rapid deterioration in consciousness follows, possibly leading to coma. Other findings include irregular respirations, seizures, decreased and bounding pulse, increased pulse pressure, hypertension, unilateral or bilateral fixed and dilated pupils, unilateral hemiparesis or hemiplegia, decerebrate posture, and Babinski's reflex.

● *Heatstroke.* As body temperature increases, LOC gradually decreases from lethargy to coma. Early signs and symptoms include malaise, tachycardia, tachypnea, orthostatic hypotension, muscle cramps, rigidity, and syncope. The patient may be irritable, anxious, and dizzy and may report a severe headache. At the onset of heatstroke, the patient's skin is hot, flushed, and diaphoretic with blotchy cyanosis; later, when his fever exceeds 105° F (40.5° C), his skin becomes hot, flushed, and anhidrotic. Pulse and respiratory rate increase markedly, and blood pressure drops precipitously. Other findings include vomiting, diarrhea, dilated pupils, and Cheyne-Stokes respirations.

● *Hypercapnia with pulmonary syndrome.* LOC decreases gradually from lethargy to coma (usually not prolonged). The patient becomes confused or drowsy and develops asterixis and muscle twitching. He may complain of headache and exhibit mental dullness, papilledema, and small, reactive pupils.

● *Hypernatremia.* Hypernatremia, life-threatening if acute, causes LOC to deteriorate from lethargy to coma. The patient is irritable and exhibits twitches progressing to seizures. Other associated signs and symptoms include a weak, thready pulse, possibly

accompanied by nausea, malaise, fever, thirst, flushed skin, and dry mucous membranes.

● *Hyperosmolar hyperglycemic nonketotic syndrome.* LOC decreases rapidly from lethargy to coma. Early findings include polyuria, polydipsia, hyperglycemia, hyperkalemia, weight loss, and weakness. Later, the patient may develop hypotension, poor skin turgor, dry skin and mucous membranes, tachycardia, tachypnea, oliguria, and seizures.

● *Hyperventilation syndrome.* Brief episodes of unconsciousness follow stress-induced deep, rapid breathing associated with anxiety and agitation. Associated findings include dizziness, circumoral and peripheral paresthesia, twitching, carpopedal spasm, and arrhythmias.

● *Hypokalemia.* LOC gradually decreases to lethargy; coma is rare. Other findings include confusion, nausea, vomiting, diarrhea, and polyuria. The patient may also exhibit weakness, decreased reflexes, and malaise, along with dizziness, hypotension, arrhythmias, and abnormal electrocardiogram results.

● *Hyponatremia.* Hyponatremia, life-threatening if acute, produces decreased LOC in late stages. Early nausea and malaise may progress to behavior changes, confusion, lethargy, incoordination and, eventually, seizures and coma.

● *Hypothermia.* With severe hypothermia (temperature below 90° F [32.2° C]), LOC decreases from lethargy to coma. DTRs disappear, and ventricular fibrillation occurs, possibly followed by cardiopulmonary arrest. With mild to moderate hypothermia, the patient may experience memory loss and slurred speech as well as shivering, weakness, fatigue, and apathy. Other early signs and symptoms include ataxia, muscle stiffness, and hyperactive DTRs; diuresis; tachycardia and decreased respiratory rate and blood pressure; and cold, pale skin. Later, muscle rigidity and decreased reflexes may develop, along with peripheral cyanosis, bradycardia, arrhythmias, severe hypotension, decreased respiratory rate with shallow respirations, and oliguria.

● *Intracerebral hemorrhage.* Intracerebral hemorrhage is a life-threatening disorder that produces a rapid, steady loss of consciousness within hours, commonly accompanied by severe headache, dizziness, nausea, and vomiting. Associated signs and symptoms vary and may include increased blood pressure, irregular respirations, Babinski's reflex, seizures, aphasia, decreased sensations, hemiplegia, decorticate or decerebrate posture, and dilated pupils.

● *Listeriosis.* If this serious infection spreads to the nervous system and causes meningitis, signs and symptoms include decreased LOC, fever, headache, and nuchal rigidity. Early signs and symptoms of listeriosis include fever, myalgias, abdominal pain, nausea, vomiting, and diarrhea.

● *Meningitis.* Confusion and irritability are expected; however, stupor, coma, and seizures may occur in those with severe meningitis. Fever develops early, possibly accompanied by chills. Associated findings include severe headache, nuchal rigidity, hyperreflexia and, possibly, opisthotonos. The patient exhibits Kernig's and Brudzinski's signs and, possibly, ocular palsies, photophobia, facial weakness, and hearing loss.

● *Myxedema crisis.* The patient may exhibit a swift decline in LOC. Other findings include severe hypothermia, hypoventilation, hypotension, bradycardia, hypoactive reflexes, periorbital and peripheral edema, impaired hearing and balance, and seizures.

● *Pontine hemorrhage.* A sudden, rapid decrease in LOC to the point of coma occurs within minutes and death within hours. The patient may also exhibit total paralysis, decerebrate posture, Babinski's reflex, absent doll's eye sign, and bilateral miosis (however, the pupils remain reactive to light).

● *Seizure disorders.* A complex partial seizure produces decreased LOC, manifested as a blank stare, purposeless behavior (picking at clothing, wandering, lip smacking or chewing motions), and unintelligible speech. The seizure may be heralded by an aura and followed by several minutes of mental confusion.

An absence seizure usually involves a brief change in LOC, indicated by blinking or eye rolling, blank stare, and slight mouth movements.

A generalized tonic-clonic seizure typically begins with a loud cry and sudden loss of consciousness. Muscle spasm alternates with relaxation. Tongue biting, incontinence, labored breathing, apnea, and cyanosis may also occur. Consciousness returns after the seizure, but the patient remains confused and may have difficulty talking. He may

complain of drowsiness, fatigue, headache, muscle aching, and weakness and may fall into deep sleep.

An atonic seizure produces sudden unconsciousness for a few seconds.

Status epilepticus, rapidly recurring seizures without intervening periods of physiologic recovery and return of consciousness, can be life-threatening.

● *Shock.* Decreased LOC—lethargy progressing to stupor and coma—occurs late in shock. Associated findings include confusion, anxiety, and restlessness; hypotension; tachycardia; weak pulse with narrowing pulse pressure; dyspnea; oliguria; and cool, clammy skin.

Hypovolemic shock is generally the result of massive or insidious bleeding, either internally or externally. Cardiogenic shock may produce chest pain or arrhythmias and signs of heart failure, such as dyspnea, cough, edema, jugular vein distention, and weight gain. Septic shock may be accompanied by high fever and chills. Anaphylactic shock usually involves stridor.

● *Stroke.* LOC changes vary in degree and onset, depending on the lesion's size and location and the presence of edema. A thrombotic stroke usually follows multiple transient ischemic attacks (TIAs). LOC changes may be abrupt or take several minutes, hours, or days. An embolic stroke occurs suddenly, and deficits reach their peak almost at once. Deficits associated with a hemorrhagic stroke usually develop over minutes or hours.

Associated findings vary with stroke type and severity and may include disorientation; intellectual deficits, such as memory loss and poor judgment; personality changes; and emotional lability. Other possible findings include dysarthria, dysphagia, ataxia, aphasia, apraxia, agnosia, unilateral sensorimotor loss, and vision disturbances. In addition, urine retention, incontinence, constipation, headache, vomiting, and seizures may occur.

● *Subdural hematoma (chronic).* LOC deteriorates slowly. Other signs and symptoms include confusion, decreased ability to concentrate, and personality changes accompanied by headache, light-headedness, seizures, and a dilated ipsilateral pupil with ptosis.

● *Subdural hemorrhage (acute).* With subdural hemorrhage—a potentially life-threatening disorder—agitation and confusion are followed by progressively decreasing LOC from somnolence to coma. The patient may also experience headache, fever, unilateral pupil dilation, decreased pulse and respiratory rates, widening pulse pressure, seizures, hemiparesis, and Babinski's reflex.

- **Thyroid storm.** LOC decreases suddenly and can progress to coma. Irritability, restlessness, confusion, and psychotic behavior precede the deterioration. Associated signs and symptoms include tremors and weakness; vision disturbances; tachycardia, arrhythmias, angina, and acute respiratory distress; warm, moist, flushed skin; and vomiting, diarrhea, and fever to 105°F (40.5° C).

- **Transient ischemic attack (TIA).** LOC decreases abruptly (with varying severity) and gradually returns to normal within 24 hours. Site-specific findings may include vision loss, nystagmus, aphasia, dizziness, dysarthria, unilateral hemiparesis or hemiplegia, tinnitus, paresthesia, dysphagia, or staggering or incoordinated gait.

- **West Nile encephalitis.** This brain infection is caused by the West Nile virus, a mosquito-borne flavivirus commonly found in Africa, West Asia, and the Middle East and, less commonly, in the United States. Mild infection is common. Signs and symptoms include fever, headache, and body aches, commonly with skin rash and swollen lymph glands. More severe infection is marked by high fever, headache, neck stiffness, stupor, disorientation, coma, tremors, occasional convulsions, paralysis and, rarely, death.

OTHER CAUSES

- **Alcohol.** Alcohol use causes varying degrees of sedation, irritability, and incoordination; intoxication commonly causes stupor.

- **Drugs.** Sedation and other degrees of decreased LOC can result from an overdose of a barbiturate, another central nervous system depressant, or aspirin.

- **Poisoning.** Toxins, such as lead, carbon monoxide, and snake venom, can cause varying degrees of decreased LOC. Confusion is common, as are headache, nausea, and vomiting. Other general features include hypotension, cardiac arrhythmias, dyspnea, sensorimotor loss, and seizures.

NURSING CONSIDERATIONS

Reassess the patient's LOC and neurologic status at least hourly. Carefully monitor ICP and intake and output. Ensure airway patency and proper nutrition. Take precautions to help ensure the patient's safety. Keep him on bed rest with the side rails up and maintain seizure precautions. Keep emergency resuscitation equipment at the patient's bedside. Prepare the patient for a computed tomography scan of the head, magnetic resonance imaging of the brain, EEG, and lumbar puncture. Maintain an elevation of the head of the bed to at least 30 degrees. Don't administer an opioid or sedative because either may further decrease the patient's LOC and hinder an accurate, meaningful neurologic examination. Apply restraints only if necessary because their use may increase his agitation and confusion. Talk to the patient even if he appears comatose; your voice may help reorient him to reality.

PATIENT TEACHING

Explain the treatments and procedures the patient needs. Teach safety and seizure precautions. Provide referrals to sources of support. Discuss quality of life issues with the patient and his family, as indicated.

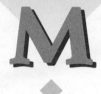

Melena

A common sign of upper GI bleeding, melena is the passage of black, tarry stools containing digested blood. Characteristic color results from bacterial degradation and hydrochloric acid acting on the blood as it travels through the GI tract. At least 100 ml of blood is needed to produce this sign. (See *Comparing melena to hematochezia,* page 202.)

Severe melena can signal acute bleeding and life-threatening hypovolemic shock. Usually, melena indicates bleeding from the esophagus, stomach, or duodenum, although it can also indicate bleeding from the jejunum, ileum, or ascending colon. This sign can also result from swallowing blood, as in epistaxis; from taking certain drugs; or from ingesting alcohol. Because false melena may be caused by ingestion of lead, iron, bismuth, or licorice (which produces black stools without the presence of blood), all black stools should be tested for occult blood.

Act now If the patient is experiencing severe melena, quickly take orthostatic vital signs to detect hypovolemic shock. A decline of 10 mm Hg or more in systolic pressure or an increase of 10 beats/minute or more in pulse rate indicates volume depletion. Quickly examine the patient for other signs of shock, such as tachycardia, tachypnea, and cool, clammy skin. Insert a large-bore I.V. line to administer replacement fluids and allow blood transfusion. Obtain a hematocrit, prothrombin time, international normalized ratio, and partial thromboplastin time. Place the patient flat with his head turned to the side and his feet elevated. Administer supplemental oxygen as needed.

ASSESSMENT
History
If the patient's condition permits, ask when he discovered his stools were black and tarry. Ask about the frequency and quantity of bowel movements. Has he had melena before? Ask about other signs and symptoms, notably hematemesis or hematochezia, and about use of anti-inflammatories, alcohol, or other GI irritants. Also, find out if he has a history of GI lesions. Ask if the patient takes iron supplements, which may also cause black stools; also ask if the patient has ingested black licorice, lead, Pepto-Bismol, or blueberries. Obtain a drug history, noting the use of warfarin or other anticoagulants.

Physical examination
Next, inspect the patient's mouth and nasopharynx for evidence of bleeding. Perform an abdominal examination that includes auscultation, palpation, and percussion. Perform a cardiovascular assessment to detect signs and symptoms of shock.

Pediatric pointers
Neonates may experience melena neonatorum due to extravasation of blood into the alimentary canal. In older children, melena usually results from peptic ulcer, gastritis, or Meckel's diverticulum.

Geriatric pointers
In elderly patients with recurrent intermittent GI bleeding without a clear etiology, angiog-

COMPARING MELENA TO HEMATOCHEZIA

With GI bleeding, the site, amount, and rate of blood flow through the GI tract determine if a patient will develop melena (black, tarry stools) or hematochezia (bright red, bloody stools). Usually, melena indicates *upper* GI bleeding, and hematochezia indicates *lower* GI bleeding. However, with some disorders, melena may alternate with hematochezia. This chart helps differentiate these two commonly related signs.

SIGN	SITES	CHARACTERISTICS
Melena	Esophagus, stomach, duodenum; rarely, jejunum, ileum, ascending colon.	Black, loose, tarry stools. Delayed or minimal passage of blood through GI tract.
Hematochezia	Usually distal to or affecting the colon; rapid hemorrhage of 1 L or more is associated with esophageal, stomach, or duodenal bleeding.	Bright red or dark, mahogany-colored stools; pure blood; blood mixed with formed stool; or bloody diarrhea. Reflects lower GI bleeding or rapid blood loss and passage of undigested blood through GI tract.

raphy or exploratory laparotomy should be considered once the risk from continued anemia is deemed to outweigh the risk associated with the procedures.

MEDICAL CAUSES

● *Colon cancer.* On the right side of the colon, early tumor growth may cause melena accompanied by abdominal aching, pressure, or cramps. As the disease progresses, the patient develops weakness, fatigue, and anemia. Eventually, he also experiences diarrhea or obstipation, anorexia, weight loss, vomiting, and other signs and symptoms of intestinal obstruction.

With a tumor on the left side, melena is a rare sign until late in the disease. Early tumor growth commonly causes rectal bleeding with intermittent abdominal fullness or cramping and rectal pressure. As the disease progresses, the patient may develop obstipation, diarrhea, or pencil-shaped stools. At this stage, bleeding from the colon is signaled by melena or bloody stools.

● *Ebola virus.* Melena, hematemesis, and bleeding from the nose, gums, and vagina may occur later with Ebola virus. Patients usually report abrupt onset of headache, malaise, myalgia, high fever, diarrhea, abdominal pain, dehydration, and lethargy on the fifth day of illness. Pleuritic chest pain, dry hacking cough, and pharyngitis have also been noted. A maculopapular rash develops between days 5 and 7 of the illness.

● *Esophageal cancer.* Melena is a late sign of esophageal cancer that's three times more common in males than females. Increasing obstruction first produces painless dysphagia, then rapid weight loss. The patient may experience steady chest pain with substernal fullness, nausea, vomiting, and hematemesis. Other findings include hoarseness, persistent cough (possibly hemoptysis), hiccups, sore throat, and halitosis. In the later stages, signs and symptoms include painful dysphagia, anorexia, and regurgitation.

● *Esophageal varices (ruptured).* Esophageal varices is a life-threatening disorder that can produce melena, hematochezia, and hematemesis. Melena is preceded by signs of shock, such as tachycardia, tachypnea, hypotension, and cool, clammy skin. Agitation or confusion signals developing hepatic encephalopathy.

- **Gastric cancer.** Melena and altered bowel habits may occur late with gastric cancer. More common findings include insidious onset of upper abdominal or retrosternal discomfort and chronic dyspepsia, which are unrelieved by antacids and exacerbated by food. Anorexia and slight nausea often occur, along with hematemesis, pallor, fatigue, weight loss, and a feeling of abdominal fullness.

- **Gastritis.** Melena and hematemesis are common. The patient may also experience mild epigastric or abdominal discomfort that's exacerbated by eating; belching; nausea; vomiting; and malaise.

- **Malaria.** Melena may accompany persistent high fever and orthostatic hypotension in severe malaria. Other features include hemoptysis, vomiting, abdominal pain, diarrhea, oliguria, and headache, seizures, delirium, or coma. These findings are interspersed throughout the malarial paroxysm—chills, then high fever, and then profuse diaphoresis.

- **Mallory-Weiss syndrome.** Mallory-Weiss syndrome is characterized by massive bleeding from the upper GI tract due to a tear in the mucous membrane of the esophagus or the junction of the esophagus and the stomach. Melena and hematemesis follow vomiting. Severe upper abdominal bleeding leads to signs and symptoms of shock, such as tachycardia, tachypnea, hypotension, and cool, clammy skin. The patient may also report epigastric or back pain.

- **Mesenteric vascular occlusion.** Mesenteric vascular occlusion is a life-threatening disorder that produces slight melena with 2 to 3 days of persistent, mild abdominal pain. Later, abdominal pain becomes severe and may be accompanied by tenderness, distention, guarding, and rigidity. The patient may also experience anorexia, vomiting, fever, and profound shock.

- **Peptic ulcer.** Melena may signal life-threatening hemorrhage from vascular penetration. The patient may also develop decreased appetite, nausea, vomiting, hematemesis, hematochezia, and left epigastric pain that's gnawing, burning, or sharp and may be described as heartburn or indigestion. With hypovolemic shock comes tachycardia, tachypnea, hypotension, dizziness, syncope, and cool, clammy skin.

- **Small-bowel tumors.** Small-bowel tumors may bleed and produce melena. Other signs and symptoms include abdominal pain, distention, and increasing frequency and pitch of bowel sounds.

- **Thrombocytopenia.** Melena or hematochezia may accompany other manifestations of bleeding tendency: hematemesis, epistaxis, petechiae, ecchymoses, hematuria, vaginal bleeding, and characteristic blood-filled oral bullae. Typically, the patient displays malaise, fatigue, weakness, and lethargy.

- **Typhoid fever.** Melena or hematochezia occurs late in typhoid fever and may occur with hypotension and hypothermia. Other late findings include mental dullness or delirium, marked abdominal distention and diarrhea, marked weight loss, and profound fatigue.

- **Yellow fever.** Melena, hematochezia, and hematemesis are ominous signs of hemorrhage, a classic feature, which occurs along with jaundice. Other findings include fever, headache, nausea, vomiting, epistaxis, albuminuria, petechiae and mucosal hemorrhage, and dizziness.

OTHER CAUSES

- **Drugs and alcohol.** Aspirin, other nonsteroidal anti-inflammatory drugs (NSAIDs), or alcohol can cause melena as a result of gastric irritation.

NURSING CONSIDERATIONS

Monitor vital signs, and look closely for signs of hypovolemic shock. For general comfort, encourage bed rest, and keep the patient's perianal area clean and dry to prevent skin irritation and breakdown. A nasogastric tube may be necessary to assist with drainage of gastric contents and decompression. Prepare him for diagnostic tests, including blood studies, gastroscopy or other endoscopic studies, barium swallow, and upper GI series. Prepare the patient for blood transfusions as indicated by his hematocrit.

Alert *If the patient requires large volumes of blood, be alert for changes in calcium levels because calcium binds to citrate in the stored blood, thereby decreasing the body's free calcium levels. Monitor serum calcium levels, and anticipate replacement if levels are low. Also be alert for coagulation problems, because transfusions of large amounts of blood can cause coagulopathy.*

PATIENT TEACHING

Explain the changes in bowel elimination that are important for the patient to recognize and report. Stress the importance of undergoing colorectal cancer screening. Explain to the patient the need to avoid aspirin, other NSAIDS, anticoagulants, and alcohol. Instruct the patient on a diet rich in natural fiber, which may decrease the incidence of constipation; provide consultation to a dietitian if necessary.

Murmurs

Murmurs are auscultatory sounds heard within the heart chambers or major arteries. They're classified by their timing and duration in the cardiac cycle, auscultatory location, loudness, configuration, pitch, and quality.

Timing can be characterized as systolic (between S_1 and S_2), holosystolic (continuous throughout systole), diastolic (between S_2 and S_1), or continuous throughout systole and diastole; systolic and diastolic murmurs can be further characterized as early, middle, or late.

Location refers to the area of maximum loudness, such as the apex, the lower left sternal border, or an intercostal space. *Loudness* is graded on a scale of 1 to 6. A grade 1 murmur is very faint, only detected after careful auscultation. A grade 2 murmur is a soft, evident murmur. A grade 3 murmur is moderately loud. A grade 4 murmur is a loud murmur with a possible intermittent thrill. Grade 5 murmurs are loud and associated with a palpable precordial thrill. Grade 6 murmurs are loud (audible even when the stethoscope is lifted from the thoracic wall) and, like grade 5 murmurs, are associated with a thrill.

Configuration, or shape, refers to the nature of loudness — crescendo (grows louder), decrescendo (grows softer), crescendo-decrescendo (first rises, then falls), decrescendo-crescendo (first falls, then rises), plateau (even intensity), or variable (uneven intensity). The murmur's *pitch* may be high or low. Its *quality* may be described as harsh, rumbling, blowing, scratching, buzzing, musical, or squeaking.

Murmurs can reflect accelerated blood flow through normal or abnormal valves; forward blood flow through a narrowed or irregular valve or into a dilated vessel; blood backflow through an incompetent valve, septal defect, or patent ductus arteriosus; or decreased blood viscosity. Commonly the result of organic heart disease, murmurs occasionally may signal an emergency situation — for example, a loud holosystolic murmur after an acute myocardial infarction (MI) may signal papillary muscle rupture or ventricular septal defect. Murmurs may also result from surgical implantation of a prosthetic valve. Some murmurs are innocent, or functional. An *innocent systolic murmur* is generally soft, medium-pitched, and loudest along the left sternal border at the second or third intercostal space. It's exacerbated by physical activity, excitement, fever, pregnancy, anemia, or thyrotoxicosis. Examples include Still's murmur in children and mammary souffle, often heard over either breast during late pregnancy and early postpartum. (See *Detecting congenital murmurs.*)

Act now *Although, not normally a sign of an emergency, murmurs — especially newly developed ones — may signal a serious complication in patients with bacterial endocarditis or a recent acute MI. When caring for a patient with known or suspected bacterial endocarditis, carefully auscultate for any new murmurs. Their development along with crackles, distended jugular veins, or orthopnea, and dyspnea may signal heart failure. Regular and ongoing auscultation is also important in a patient who has experienced an acute MI. A loud decrescendo holosystolic murmur at the apex that radiates to the axilla and left sternal border or throughout the chest is significant, particularly in association with a widely split S_2 and an atrial gallop (S_4). This murmur, when accompanied by signs of acute pulmonary edema, usually indicates the development of acute mitral regurgitation due to rupture of the chordae tendineae — a medical emergency.*

ASSESSMENT
History

Obtain a patient history. Ask if the murmur is a new discovery, or if it has been known since birth or childhood. Find out if the patient has experienced any associated symptoms, particularly palpitations, dizziness, syncope, chest pain, dyspnea, and fatigue. Explore the patient's medical history, noting especially any incidence of rheumatic fever,

DETECTING CONGENITAL MURMURS

HEART DEFECT	TYPE OF MURMUR
Aortopulmonary septal defect	*Small defect:* a continuous rough or crackling murmur best heard at the upper left sternal border and below the left clavicle, possibly accompanied by a systolic ejection click. *Large defect:* a harsh systolic murmur heard at the left sternal border.
Atrial septal defect	A midsystolic, spindle-shaped murmur of grade II or III intensity heard at the upper left sternal border, with a fixed splitting of S_2. Large shunts may also produce a low- to medium-pitched early diastolic murmur over the lower left sternal border.
Bicuspid aortic valve	An early systolic, loud, high-pitched ejection sound or click that's best heard at the apex and is commonly accompanied by a soft, early or midsystolic murmur at the upper right sternal border. The aortic component of S_2 is usually accentuated at the apex. This murmur may not be recognized until early childhood.
Coarctation of the aorta	Usually a systolic ejection click at the base of the heart, at the apex, and occasionally over the carotid arteries, often accompanied by a systolic ejection murmur at the base. This disorder may also produce a blowing diastolic murmur of aortic insufficiency or an apical pansystolic murmur of unknown origin.
Common atrioventricular canal defects (endocardial cushion defect)	*With a competent mitral valve:* a midsystolic, spindle-shaped murmur of grade II or III intensity heard at the upper left sternal border, with a fixed splitting of S_2; may be accompanied by a low- to medium-pitched early diastolic murmur over the lower left sternal border. *With an incompetent mitral valve:* an early systolic or holosystolic decrescendo murmur at the apex, along with a widely split S_2 and frequently an S_4.
Ebstein's anomaly	A soft, high-pitched holosystolic blowing murmur that increases with inspiration (Carvallo's sign); best heard over the lower left sternal border and the xiphoid area; possibly accompanied by a low-pitched diastolic rumbling murmur at the apex. Fixed splitting of S_2 and a loud split S_4 also occur.
Left ventricular-right atrial communication	A holosystolic, decrescendo murmur of grades II to IV intensity heard along the lower left sternal border, accompanied by a normal S_2; large shunts also produce a diastolic rumbling murmur over the apex.
Mitral atresia	A nonspecific systolic murmur and a diastolic flow rumble at the lower left sternal border, with one loud S_2.
Partial anomalous pulmonary venous connection	A midsystolic, spindle-shaped grade II to III murmur at the upper left sternal border, possibly accompanied by a low- to medium-pitched early diastolic murmur over the lower left sternal border.
Patent ductus arteriosus	A continuous rough or crackling murmur best heard at the upper left sternal border and below the left clavicle. The murmur is accentuated late in systole.
Pulmonic insufficiency	An early to middiastolic, soft, medium-pitched crescendo-decrescendo murmur best heard at the second or third right intercostal space.
Pulmonic stenosis	An early systolic, harsh, crescendo-decrescendo murmur of grades IV to VI intensity heard at the second left intercostal space, possibly radiating along the left sternal border.

(continued)

HEART DEFECT	TYPE OF MURMUR
Single atrium	A holosystolic regurgitant murmur at the apex, accompanied by a fixed splitting of S_2.
Supravalvular aortic stenosis	A systolic ejection murmur best heard over the second right intercostal space or higher in the episternal notch or over the lower right side of the neck. The aortic closure sound is usually preserved, and no ejection clicks are heard.
Tetralogy of Fallot	A midsystolic murmur with a systolic thrill palpable at the left midsternal border; softer murmurs occurring earlier in systole generally indicate a more severe obstruction.
Tricuspid atresia	Variable, depending on associated defects.
Trilogy of Fallot	A systolic, harsh, crescendo-decrescendo murmur, best heard at the upper left sternal border with radiation toward the left clavicle. The pulmonic component of S_2 becomes progressively softer with increasing degrees of obstruction.
Ventricular septal defect	*Small defect:* usually a holosystolic (but may be limited to early or midsystole), grades II to IV decrescendo murmur heard along the lower left sternal border, accompanied by a normal S_2.
	Large defect: a holosystolic murmur at the lower left sternal border and a midsystolic rumbling murmur at the apex, accompanied by an increased S_1 at the lower left sternal border and an increased pulmonic component of S_2.

recent dental work, heart disease, or heart surgery, particularly prosthetic valve replacement.

Physical examination

If you discover a murmur, try to determine its type through careful auscultation. (See *Identifying common murmurs*.) Use the bell of your stethoscope for low-pitched murmurs; the diaphragm for high-pitched murmurs.

Perform a systematic physical examination. Note especially the presence of cardiac arrhythmias, jugular vein distention, and such pulmonary signs and symptoms as dyspnea, orthopnea, and crackles. Is the patient's liver tender or palpable? Does he have peripheral edema?

Pediatric pointers

Innocent murmurs, such as Still's murmur, are commonly heard in young children and typically disappear in puberty. Pathognomonic heart murmurs in infants and young children usually result from congenital heart disease, such as atrial and ventricular septal defects. Other murmurs can be acquired, as with rheumatic heart disease.

MEDICAL CAUSES

● *Aortic insufficiency.* Acute aortic insufficiency typically produces a soft, short diastolic murmur over the left sternal border that's best heard when the patient sits and leans forward and at the end of a forced held expiration. S_2 may be soft or absent. Sometimes, a soft, short midsystolic murmur may also be heard over the second right intercostal space. Associated findings include tachycardia, dyspnea, jugular vein distention, crackles, increased fatigue, and pale, cool extremities.

Chronic aortic insufficiency causes a high-pitched, blowing, decrescendo diastolic murmur that's best heard over the second or third right intercostal space or the left sternal border with the patient sitting, leaning forward, and holding his breath after deep expiration. An Austin Flint murmur — a rumbling, mid-to-late diastolic murmur best heard at the apex — may also occur. Compli-

IDENTIFYING COMMON MURMURS

The timing and configuration of a murmur can help you identify its underlying cause. Learn to recognize the characteristics of these common murmurs.

AORTIC INSUFFICIENCY (CHRONIC)

Thickened valve leaflets fail to close correctly, permitting backflow of blood into the left ventricle.

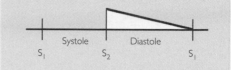

AORTIC STENOSIS

Thickened, scarred, or calcified valve leaflets impede ventricular systolic ejection.

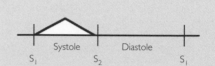

MITRAL PROLAPSE

Incompetent mitral valve bulges into the left atrium because of an enlarged posterior leaflet and elongated chordae tendineae.

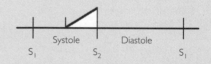

MITRAL INSUFFICIENCY (CHRONIC)

Incomplete mitral valve closure permits backflow of blood into the left atrium.

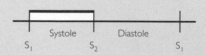

MITRAL STENOSIS

Thickened or scarred valve leaflets cause valve stenosis and restrict blood flow.

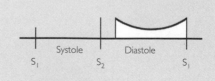

cations may not develop until ages 40 to 50; then, typical findings include palpitations, tachycardia, angina, increased fatigue, dyspnea, orthopnea, and crackles.

- **Aortic stenosis.** With aortic stenosis — a valvular disorder — the murmur is systolic, beginning after S_1 and ending at or before aortic valve closure. It's harsh and grating, medium-pitched, and crescendo-decrescendo. Loudest over the second right intercostal space when the patient is sitting and leaning forward, this murmur may also be heard at the apex, at the suprasternal notch (Erb's point), and over the carotid arteries.

  If the patient has advanced disease, S_2 may be heard as a single sound, with inaudible aortic closure. An early systolic ejection click at the apex is typical but is absent when the valve is severely calcified. Associated signs and symptoms usually don't appear until age 30 in congenital aortic stenosis, ages 30 to 65 in stenosis due to rheumatic disease, and after age 65 in calcific aortic stenosis. They may include dizziness, syncope, dyspnea on exertion, paroxysmal nocturnal dyspnea, fatigue, and angina.

- **Cardiomyopathy (hypertrophic).** Cardiomyopathy generates a harsh late systolic murmur, ending at S_2. Best heard over the left sternal border and at the apex, the murmur is commonly accompanied by an audible S_3 or S_4. The murmur decreases with squatting and increases with sitting down. Major associated symptoms are dyspnea and chest pain; palpitations, dizziness, and syncope may also occur.

- **Mitral insufficiency.** Acute mitral insufficiency is characterized by a medium-pitched blowing, early systolic or holosystolic decrescendo murmur at the apex, along with a widely split S_2 and commonly an S_4. This murmur doesn't get louder on inspiration as with tricuspid insufficiency. Associated findings typically include tachycardia and signs of acute pulmonary edema.

  Chronic mitral insufficiency produces a high-pitched, blowing, holosystolic plateau murmur that's loudest at the apex and usually radiates to the axilla or back. Fatigue, dyspnea, and palpitations may also occur.

- **Mitral prolapse.** Mitral prolapse generates a midsystolic to late-systolic click with a high-pitched late-systolic crescendo murmur, best heard at the apex and left sternal border. Occasionally, multiple clicks may be heard, with or without a systolic murmur. Associated findings include cardiac awareness, migraine headaches, dizziness, weakness, syncope, palpitations, chest pain, dyspnea, severe episodic fatigue, mood swings, and anxiety.

- **Mitral stenosis.** With mitral stenosis, the murmur is soft, low-pitched, rumbling, crescendo-decrescendo, and diastolic, accompanied by a loud S_1 or an opening snap — a cardinal sign. It's best heard at the apex with the patient in the left lateral position. Mild exercise will help make this murmur audible.

  With severe stenosis, the murmur of mitral regurgitation may also be heard. Other findings include hemoptysis, exertional dyspnea and fatigue, and signs of acute pulmonary edema.

- **Myxomas.** A left atrial myxoma (most common) usually produces a middiastolic murmur and a holosystolic murmur that's loudest at the apex, with an S_4, an early diastolic thudding sound (tumor plop), and a loud, widely split S_1. Related features include dyspnea, orthopnea, chest pain, fatigue, weight loss, and syncope.

  A right atrial myxoma causes a late diastolic rumbling murmur, a holosystolic crescendo murmur, and tumor plop, best heard at the lower left sternal border. Other findings include fatigue, peripheral edema, ascites, and hepatomegaly.

  A left ventricular myxoma (rare) produces a systolic murmur, best heard at the lower left sternal border, arrhythmias, dyspnea, and syncope.

  A right ventricular myxoma commonly generates a systolic ejection murmur with delayed S_2 and a tumor plop, best heard at the left sternal border. It's accompanied by peripheral edema, hepatomegaly, ascites, dyspnea, and syncope.

- **Papillary muscle rupture.** Papillary muscle rupture is a life-threatening complication of an acute MI, in which a loud holosystolic murmur can be auscultated at the apex. Related findings include severe dyspnea, chest pain, syncope, hemoptysis, tachycardia, and hypotension.

- **Rheumatic fever with pericarditis.** A pericardial friction rub along with murmurs and gallops are heard best with the patient leaning forward on his hands and knees during forced expiration. The most common murmurs heard are the systolic murmur of mitral regurgitation, a midsystolic murmur due to swelling of the leaflet of the mitral valve, and the diastolic murmur of aortic regurgitation. Other signs and symptoms include fever, joint and sternal pain, edema, and tachypnea.

● *Tricuspid insufficiency.* Tricuspid insufficiency is a valvular abnormality that's characterized by a soft, high-pitched, holosystolic blowing murmur that increases with inspiration (Carvallo's sign), decreases with exhalation and Valsalva's maneuver, and is best heard over the lower left sternal border and the xiphoid area. Following a lengthy asymptomatic period, exertional dyspnea and orthopnea may develop, along with jugular vein distention, ascites, peripheral cyanosis and edema, muscle wasting, fatigue, weakness, and syncope.

● *Tricuspid stenosis.* Tricuspid stenosis is a valvular disorder that produces a diastolic murmur similar to that of mitral stenosis, but louder with inspiration and decreased with exhalation and Valsalva's maneuver. S_1 may also be louder. Associated signs and symptoms include fatigue, syncope, peripheral edema, jugular vein distention, ascites, hepatomegaly, and dyspnea.

OTHER CAUSES

● *Medical treatments.* Prosthetic valve replacement may cause variable murmurs, depending on the location, valve composition, and method of operation.

NURSING CONSIDERATIONS

Prepare the patient for diagnostic tests, such as electrocardiography, echocardiography, and angiography. Administer an antibiotic and an anticoagulant as appropriate. Because any cardiac abnormality is frightening to the patient, provide emotional support.

PATIENT TEACHING

Instruct the patient to contact his physician before undergoing invasive procedures or dental work because prophylactic antibiotics may be necessary. Explain the signs and symptoms the patient should report.

Muscle spasms

Muscle spasms are strong, painful contractions. They can occur in virtually any muscle but are most common in the calf and foot. Muscle spasms typically occur from simple muscle fatigue, after exercise, and during pregnancy. However, they may also develop in electrolyte imbalances and neuromuscular disorders, or as the result of certain drugs. They're typically precipitated by movement, especially a quick or jerking movement, and can usually be relieved by slow stretching.

Act now *If the patient complains of frequent or unrelieved spasms in many muscles, accompanied by paresthesia in his hands and feet, quickly attempt to elicit Chvostek's and Trousseau's signs. If these signs are present, suspect hypocalcemia. Evaluate respiratory function, watching for the development of laryngospasm; provide supplemental oxygen as necessary, and prepare to intubate the patient and provide mechanical ventilation. Draw blood for calcium and electrolyte levels and arterial blood gas analysis, and insert an I.V. line for administration of a calcium supplement. Monitor cardiac status, and prepare to begin resuscitation if necessary.*

ASSESSMENT
History

If the patient isn't in distress, ask when the spasms began. Is there any particular activity that precipitates them? How long do they last? How painful are they? Does anything worsen or lessen the pain? Ask about other symptoms, such as weakness, sensory loss, or paresthesia.

Physical examination

Evaluate muscle strength and tone. Then, check all major muscle groups and note whether any movements precipitate spasms. Test the presence and quality of all peripheral pulses, and examine the limbs for color and temperature changes. Test capillary refill time (normal is less than 3 seconds), and inspect for edema, especially in the involved area. Observe for signs and symptoms of dehydration such as dry mucous membranes. Obtain a thorough drug and diet history. Ask the patient if he has had recent vomiting or diarrhea. Finally, test reflexes and sensory function in all extremities.

Pediatric pointers

Muscle spasms rarely occur in children. However, their presence may indicate hypoparathyroidism, osteomalacia, rickets or, rarely, congenital torticollis.

MEDICAL CAUSES

● *Amyotrophic lateral sclerosis (ALS).* With ALS, muscle spasms may accompany progressive muscle weakness and atrophy that typically begin in one hand, spread to the arm, and then spread to the other hand and arm. Eventually, muscle weakness and atrophy affect the trunk, neck, tongue, larynx, pharynx, and legs; progressive respiratory muscle weakness leads to respiratory insufficiency. Other findings include muscle flaccidity progressing to spasticity, coarse fasciculations, hyperactive deep tendon reflexes, dysphagia, impaired speech, excessive drooling, and depression.

- *Arterial occlusive disease.* Arterial occlusion typically produces spasms and intermittent claudication in the leg, with residual pain. Associated findings are usually localized to the legs and feet and include loss of peripheral pulses, pallor or cyanosis, decreased sensation, hair loss, dry or scaling skin, edema, and ulcerations.
- *Cholera.* Muscle spasms, severe water and electrolyte loss, thirst, weakness, decreased skin turgor, oliguria, tachycardia, and hypotension occur along with abrupt watery diarrhea and vomiting.
- *Dehydration.* Sodium loss may produce limb and abdominal cramps. Other findings include a slight fever, decreased skin turgor, dry mucous membranes, tachycardia, orthostatic hypotension, muscle twitching, seizures, nausea, vomiting, and oliguria.
- *Fracture.* Localized spasms and pain are mild if the fracture is nondisplaced, intense if it's severely displaced. Other findings include swelling, limited mobility and, possibly, bony crepitation.
- *Hypocalcemia.* The classic feature is tetany—a syndrome of muscle cramps and twitching, carpopedal and facial muscle spasms, and seizures, possibly with stridor. Both Chvostek's and Trousseau's signs may be elicited. Related findings include paresthesia of the lips, fingers, and toes; choreiform movements; hyperactive deep tendon reflexes; fatigue; palpitations; and cardiac arrhythmias.
- *Hypothyroidism.* Muscle involvement may produce spasms and stiffness, along with leg muscle hypertrophy or proximal limb weakness and atrophy. Other findings include forgetfulness and mental instability; fatigue; cold intolerance; dry, pale, cool, doughy skin; puffy face, hands, and feet; periorbital edema; dry, sparse, brittle hair; bradycardia; and weight gain despite anorexia.

- *Muscle trauma.* Excessive muscle strain may cause mild to severe spasms. The injured area may be painful, swollen, reddened, or warm.
- *Respiratory alkalosis.* Acute onset of muscle spasms may be accompanied by twitching and weakness, carpopedal spasms, circumoral and peripheral paresthesia, vertigo, syncope, pallor, and extreme anxiety. With severe alkalosis, cardiac arrhythmias may occur.
- *Spinal injury or disease.* Muscle spasms can result from spinal injury, such as cervical extension injury or spinous process fracture, or from spinal disease such as infection.

OTHER CAUSES
- *Drugs.* Common spasm-producing drugs include diuretics, corticosteroids, and estrogens.

NURSING CONSIDERATIONS
Depending on the cause, help alleviate your patient's spasms by slowly stretching the affected muscle in the direction opposite the contraction. If necessary, administer a mild analgesic.

Administer antibiotics and an anticoagulant, as appropriate. Prepare the patient for diagnostic tests, such as electrocardiography, endocardiography, echocardiography, and angiography. Diagnostic studies may include serum calcium, sodium and carbon dioxide levels, thyroid function tests, and blood flow studies or arteriography.

Because a cardiac abnormality is frightening to the patient and family, provide emotional support.

PATIENT TEACHING
Explain the use of prophylactic antibiotics. Also explain the signs and symptoms the patient should report immediately. Provide information on the importance of follow-up care and monitoring.

Myoclonus

Myoclonus—sudden, shocklike contractions of a single muscle or muscle group—occurs with various neurologic disorders and may herald onset of a seizure. These contractions may be isolated or repetitive, rhythmic or arrhythmic, symmetrical or asymmetrical, synchronous or asynchronous, and generalized or focal. They may be precipitated by bright flickering lights, a loud sound, or unexpected physical contact. One type, intention myoclonus, is evoked by intentional muscle movement.

Myoclonus occurs normally just before falling asleep and as a part of the natural startle reaction. It also occurs with some poisonings and, rarely, as a complication of hemodialysis.

Act now *If you observe myoclonus, check for seizure activity. Take vital signs to rule out arrhythmias or a blocked airway. Have resuscitation equipment on hand.*

If the patient has a seizure, gently help him lie down. Place a pillow or a rolled-up towel under his head to prevent concussion. Loosen constrictive clothing, especially around the neck, and turn his head (gently, if possible) to one side to prevent airway occlusion or aspiration of secretions.

ASSESSMENT
History

If the patient is stable, evaluate his level of consciousness and mental status. Ask about the frequency, severity, location, and circumstances of the myoclonus. Has he ever had a seizure? If so, did myoclonus precede it? Is the myoclonus ever precipitated by a sensory stimulus?

Physical examination

During the physical examination, check for muscle rigidity and wasting, and test deep tendon reflexes. Evaluate level of consciousness and mental condition. Perform a complete neurologic and musculoskeletal assessment.

Pediatric pointers

Although myoclonus is relatively uncommon in infants and children, it can result from subacute sclerosing panencephalitis, severe meningitis, progressive poliodystrophy, childhood myoclonic epilepsy, and encephalopathies, such as Reye's syndrome.

MEDICAL CAUSES
● *Alzheimer's disease.* Generalized myoclonus may occur in advanced stages of Alzheimer's disease, which is a slowly progressive dementia. Other late findings include mild choreoathetoid movements, mus-

cle rigidity, bowel and bladder incontinence, delusions, and hallucinations.
● *Creutzfeldt-Jakob disease.* Diffuse myoclonic jerks appear early in Creutzfeldt-Jakob disease—a rapidly progressive dementia. Initially random, they gradually become more rhythmic and symmetrical, often occurring in response to sensory stimuli. Associated effects include ataxia, aphasia, hearing loss, muscle rigidity and wasting, fasciculations, hemiplegia, and vision disturbance, or possibly, blindness.
● *Encephalitis (viral).* With encephalitis, myoclonus is usually intermittent and either localized or generalized. Associated findings vary but may include rapidly decreasing level of consciousness, fever, headache, irritability, nuchal rigidity, vomiting, seizures, aphasia, ataxia, hemiparesis, facial muscle weakness, nystagmus, ocular palsies, and dysphagia.
● *Encephalopathy.* Hepatic encephalopathy occasionally produces myoclonic jerks in association with asterixis and focal or generalized seizures.

Hypoxic encephalopathy may produce generalized myoclonus or seizures almost immediately after restoration of cardiopulmonary function. The patient may also have a residual intention myoclonus.

Uremic encephalopathy commonly produces myoclonic jerks and seizures. Other signs and symptoms include apathy, fatigue, irritability, headache, confusion, gradually decreasing level of consciousness, nausea, vomiting, oliguria, edema, and papilledema. The patient may also exhibit elevated blood pressure, dyspnea, arrhythmias, and abnormal respirations.
● *Epilepsy.* With idiopathic epilepsy, localized myoclonus is usually confined to an arm or leg and occurs singly or in short bursts, usually upon awakening. It's usually more frequent and severe during the prodromal stage of a major generalized seizure, after which it diminishes in frequency and intensity.

Myoclonic jerks are usually the first signs of myoclonic epilepsy, the most common cause of progressive myoclonus. At first, myoclonus is infrequent and localized, but over a period of months, it becomes more frequent and involves the entire body, disrupting voluntary movement (intention myoclonus). As the disease progresses, myoclonus is accompanied by generalized seizures and dementia.

OTHER CAUSES
- *Drug withdrawal.* Myoclonus may be seen in patients with alcohol, opioid, or sedative withdrawal, or delirium tremens.
- *Poisoning.* Acute intoxication with methyl bromide, bismuth, or strychnine may produce an acute onset of myoclonus and confusion.

NURSING CONSIDERATIONS
If your patient's myoclonus is progressive, institute seizure precautions. Keep oral airway and suction equipment at his bedside, and pad the side rails of the bed. As needed, administer drugs that suppress myoclonus: ethosuximide, L-5-hydroxytryptophan, phenobarbital, clonazepam, or carbidopa. An electroencephalogram may be needed to evaluate myoclonus and related brain activity.

Because myoclonus may cause falls, remove potentially harmful objects from the patient's environment, and remain with him while he walks. Be sure to instruct the patient and his family about the need for safety precautions in the home.

PATIENT TEACHING
Inform the patient about safety measures and seizure precautions. Discuss the importance of following the prescribed medication regimen and the need for drug level monitoring, as indicated. Refer him to social service or community resources, if appropriate.

N

Neck pain

Neck pain may originate from any neck structure, ranging from the meninges and cervical vertebrae to its blood vessels, muscles, and lymphatic tissue. This symptom can also be referred from other areas of the body. Its location, onset, and pattern help determine its origin and underlying causes. Neck pain usually results from trauma and degenerative, congenital, inflammatory, metabolic, and neoplastic disorders.

Act now *If the patient's neck pain is due to trauma, first ensure proper cervical spine immobilization, preferably with a long backboard* and a Philadelphia collar. (See Applying a Philadelphia collar.) *Then take the patient's vital signs, and perform a quick neurologic examination. If he shows signs of respiratory distress, give oxygen. Intubation or tracheostomy and mechanical ventilation may be necessary. Ask the patient (or a family member, if the patient can't answer) how the injury occurred. Then examine the neck for abrasions, swelling, lacerations, erythema, and ecchymoses.*

ASSESSMENT
History
If the patient hasn't sustained trauma, inquire about the severity and onset of his neck pain. Where specifically in the neck does he feel pain? Does anything relieve or

APPLYING A PHILADELPHIA COLLAR

A lightweight molded polyethylene collar designed to hold the neck straight with the chin slightly elevated and tucked in, the Philadelphia cervical collar immobilizes the cervical spine, decreases muscle spasms, and relieves some pain. It also prevents further injury and promotes healing. To apply the collar, fit it snugly around the patient's neck and attach the Velcro fasteners or buckles at the back. Be sure to check the patient's airway and his neurovascular status to ensure that the collar isn't too tight. Make sure that the collar isn't placed too high in front, which can hyperextend the neck. In a patient with a neck sprain, hyperextension may cause the ligaments to heal in a shortened position; in a patient with a cervical spine fracture, it could cause serious neurologic damage.

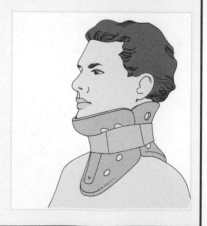

NECK PAIN:
CAUSES AND ASSOCIATED FINDINGS

MAJOR ASSOCIATED SIGNS AND SYMPTOMS

COMMON CAUSES	Arm pain	Back pain	Brudzinski's sign	Decreased level of consciousness	Decreased range of motion	Deformity	Dysphagia	Dyspnea	Ecchymoses	Fatigue	Fever	Headache	Hemoptysis	Hoarseness
Ankylosing spondylitis	●	●			●					●	●			
Cervical extension injury	●	●										●		
Cervical fibrositis														
Cervical spine fracture					●	●						●		
Cervical spine infection (acute)					●	●	●				●			
Cervical spine tumor					●									
Cervical spondylosis	●				●									
Cervical stenosis	●				●									
Esophageal trauma							●						●	
Herniated cervical disk	●	●			●						●			
Hodgkin's lymphoma										●				
Laryngeal cancer							●	●			●		●	●
Lymphadenitis											●			
Meningitis			●	●								●		
Neck sprain					●				●					
Osteoporosis		●				●								
Paget's disease						●						●		
Rheumatoid arthritis					●	●				●				
Spinous process fracture					●	●								
Subarachnoid hemorrhage			●	●								●		
Thyroid trauma							●	●						
Torticollis														
Tracheal trauma							●	●					●	●

Kernig's sign	Lymphadenopathy	Malaise	Muscle spasms	Nuchal rigidity	Paralysis	Paresthesia	Swelling	Tenderness	Weakness
		•		•					
			•	•			•		
								•	
					•				
			•			•		•	•
					•	•			•
						•			•
					•	•			
							•		
							•		•
	•	•					•		•
	•								
	•	•						•	
•				•					
			•				•		
								•	
					•	•			•
	•	•					•	•	•
							•	•	
•				•					
							•		
				•	•				

worsen the pain? Is there a particular event that precipitates the pain? Also, ask about the development of other symptoms such as headaches. Next, focus on the patient's current and past illnesses and injuries, diet, drug history, and family health history.

Physical examination

Thoroughly inspect the patient's neck, shoulders, and cervical spine for swelling, masses, erythema, and ecchymoses. Assess active range of motion (ROM) in his neck by having him perform flexion, extension, rotation, and lateral side bending. Note the degree of pain produced by these movements. Examine his posture, and test and compare bilateral muscle strength. Check the sensation in his arms, and assess his hand grasp and arm reflexes. Attempt to elicit Brudzinski's and Kernig's signs if there isn't a history of neck trauma, and palpate the cervical lymph nodes for enlargement. (See *Neck pain: Causes and associated findings.*)

Pediatric pointers

The most common causes of neck pain in children are meningitis and trauma. Congenital torticollis can, rarely, cause neck pain.

MEDICAL CAUSES

● *Ankylosing spondylitis.* Intermittent, moderate to severe neck pain and stiffness with severely restricted ROM is characteristic of ankylosing spondylitis. Intermittent low back pain and stiffness and arm pain are generally worse in the morning or after periods of inactivity and are usually relieved after exercise. Related findings also include low-grade fever, limited chest expansion, malaise, anorexia, fatigue and, occasionally, iritis.
● *Cervical extension injury.* Anterior or posterior neck pain may develop within hours or days after a whiplash injury. Anterior pain usually diminishes within several days, but posterior pain persists and may even intensify. Associated findings include tenderness, swelling and nuchal rigidity, arm or back pain, occipital headache, muscle spasms, blurred vision, and unilateral miosis on the affected side.
● *Cervical fibrositis.* Cervical fibrositis may produce anterior neck pain that radiates to one or both shoulders. Pain is intermittent and variable, commonly changing with weather patterns. Other findings are nonspe-

cific but usually include point tenderness over involved muscles.

- **Cervical spine fracture.** A fracture at C1 to C4 can cause sudden death; survivors may experience severe neck pain that restricts all movement, intense occipital headache, quadriplegia, deformity, and respiratory paralysis.
- **Cervical spine infection (acute).** Cervical spine infection can cause neck pain that restricts motion. Other findings include fever, possible deformity, muscle spasms, local tenderness, dysphagia, paresthesia, and muscle weakness.
- **Cervical spine tumor.** Metastatic tumors typically produce persistent neck pain that increases with movement and isn't relieved by rest; primary tumors cause mild to severe pain along a specific nerve root. Other findings depend on the lesions and may include paresthesia, arm and leg weakness that progresses to atrophy and paralysis, and bladder and bowel incontinence.
- **Cervical spondylosis.** Cervical spondylosis is a degenerative process that produces posterior neck pain that restricts movement and is aggravated by it. Pain may radiate down either arm and may accompany paresthesia, weakness, and stiffness.
- **Cervical stenosis.** Cervical stenosis is a progressive disorder, commonly asymptomatic, that may cause nonspecific neck and arm pain, paresthesia, muscle weakness or paralysis, and decreased ROM.
- **Esophageal trauma.** An esophageal mucosal tear or a pulsion diverticulum may produce mild neck pain, chest pain, edema, hemoptysis, and dysphagia.
- **Herniated cervical disk.** Herniated cervical disk characteristically causes variable neck pain that restricts movement and is aggravated by it. It also causes referred pain along a specific dermatome, paresthesia and other sensory disturbances, and arm weakness.
- **Hodgkin's lymphoma.** Hodgkin's lymphoma may eventually result in generalized pain that may affect the neck. Lymphadenopathy, the classic sign, may accompany paresthesia, muscle weakness, fever, fatigue, weight loss, malaise, and hepatomegaly.
- **Laryngeal cancer.** Neck pain that radiates to the ear develops late in laryngeal cancer. The patient may also develop dysphagia, dyspnea, hemoptysis, stridor, hoarseness, and cervical lymphadenopathy.
- **Lymphadenitis.** With lymphadenitis, enlarged and inflamed cervical lymph nodes

cause acute pain and tenderness. Fever, chills, and malaise may also occur.

- **Meningitis.** Neck pain may accompany characteristic nuchal rigidity of meningitis. Related findings include fever, headache, photophobia, positive Brudzinski's and Kernig's signs, and a decreased level of consciousness (LOC).
- **Neck sprain.** Minor sprains typically produce pain, slight swelling, stiffness, and restricted ROM. Ligament rupture causes pain, marked swelling, ecchymosis, muscle spasms, and nuchal rigidity with head tilt.
- **Osteoporosis.** Neck pain is rare with osteoporosis, which usually affects the thoracic or lumbar vertebrae. Cervical vertebrae involvement produces tenderness and deformity.
- **Paget's disease.** Paget's disease is a slowly developing disease that's commonly asymptomatic in its early stages. As it progresses, cervical vertebrae deformity may produce severe, persistent neck pain, along with paresthesia and arm weakness or paralysis.
- **Rheumatoid arthritis (RA).** Although RA typically affects peripheral joints, it can also involve the cervical vertebrae. Acute inflammation may cause moderate to severe pain that radiates along a specific nerve root accompanied by increased warmth, swelling, and tenderness in involved joints. Stiffness may restrict the patient's ROM. He may also experience paresthesia and muscle weakness, low-grade fever, anorexia, malaise, fatigue and, possibly, neck deformity. Some pain and stiffness remain after the acute phase.
- **Spinous process fracture.** Fracture near the cervicothoracic junction produces acute pain radiating to the shoulders. Associated findings include swelling, exquisite tenderness, restricted ROM, muscle spasms, and deformity.
- **Subarachnoid hemorrhage.** In subarachnoid hemorrhage, Kernig's and Brudzinski's signs are present. The patient may also develop a headache, possibly describing it as "the worst headache of my life."

Alert *Subarachnoid hemorrhage is a life-threatening condition. In addition to Kernig's and Brudzinski's signs and a headache, it may also cause moderate to severe neck pain and rigidity and a decreased LOC.*

- **Thyroid trauma.** Besides mild to moderate neck pain, thyroid trauma may cause local swelling and ecchymosis. If a hematoma forms, it can cause dyspnea.

- *Torticollis.* With torticollis, severe neck pain accompanies recurrent unilateral stiffness and muscle spasms that produce a characteristic head tilt.
- *Tracheal trauma.* Fracture of the tracheal cartilage, a life-threatening condition, produces moderate to severe neck pain and respiratory difficulty. Torn tracheal mucosa produces mild to moderate pain and may result in airway occlusion, hemoptysis, hoarseness, and dysphagia.

NURSING CONSIDERATIONS
Promote the patient's comfort by giving an anti-inflammatory and an analgesic, as needed. Prepare him for diagnostic tests, such as X-rays, computed tomography scan, blood tests, and cerebrospinal fluid analysis.

PATIENT TEACHING
Inform the patient about the need for activity restrictions. Teach him how to apply the cervical collar, if needed. Reinforce the importance of performing exercises, as indicated.

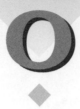

Ocular deviation

Ocular deviation refers to abnormal eye movement that may be conjugate (both eyes move together) or disconjugate (one eye moves separately from the other). This common sign may result from ocular, neurologic, endocrine, and systemic disorders that interfere with the muscles, nerves, or brain centers governing eye movement. Occasionally, it signals a life-threatening disorder such as a ruptured cerebral aneurysm. (See *Ocular deviation: Characteristics and causes in cranial nerve damage.*)

Normally, eye movement is directly controlled by the extraocular muscles innervated by the oculomotor, trochlear, and abducens nerves (cranial nerves III, IV, and VI). Together, these muscles and nerves direct a visual stimulus to corresponding parts of the retina. Disconjugate ocular deviation may result from unequal muscle tone (nonparalytic strabismus) or from muscle paralysis associated with cranial nerve damage (paralytic strabismus). Conjugate ocular deviation may result from disorders that affect the centers in the cerebral cortex and brain stem responsible for conjugate eye movement. Typically, such disorders cause gaze palsy—difficulty moving the eyes in one or more directions.

Act now   *If the patient displays ocular deviation, take his vital signs immediately and assess him for an altered level of consciousness (LOC), pupil changes, motor or sensory dysfunction, and severe headache. If possible, ask the patient's family about behavioral changes. Is there a history of recent head trauma? Respiratory support may be necessary. Also, prepare the patient for emergency neurologic tests such as a computed tomography (CT) scan.*

ASSESSMENT
History

If the patient isn't in distress, ask how long he has had the ocular deviation. Is it accompanied by double vision, eye pain, or headache? Also, ask if he's noticed associated motor or sensory changes or fever.

Determine whether the patient's history includes hypertension, diabetes, allergies, and thyroid, neurologic, or muscular disorders. Then obtain a thorough ocular history. Has the patient ever had extraocular muscle imbalance, eye or head trauma, or eye surgery?

Physical examination

During the physical examination, observe the patient for partial or complete ptosis. Does he spontaneously tilt his head or turn his face to compensate for ocular deviation? Check for eye redness or periorbital edema. Assess visual acuity, and then evaluate extraocular muscle function by testing the six cardinal fields of gaze. Test for near vision with a handheld eye chart held approximately 14″ (35.5 cm) in front of the patient's face.

Pediatric pointers

The most common cause of ocular deviation in children is nonparalytic strabismus. Normally, children achieve binocular vision by age 3 to 4 months. Although severe strabismus is readily apparent, mild strabismus

OCULAR DEVIATION: CHARACTERISTICS AND CAUSES IN CRANIAL NERVE DAMAGE

CHARACTERISTICS	CRANIAL NERVE (CN) AND EXTRAOCULAR MUSCLES INVOLVED	PROBABLE CAUSES
Inability to move the eye upward, downward, inward, and outward; drooping eyelid; and, except in diabetes, a dilated pupil in the affected eye	Oculomotor nerve (CN III); medial rectus, superior rectus, inferior rectus, and inferior oblique muscles	Cerebral aneurysm, diabetes, temporal lobe herniation from increased intracranial pressure, brain tumor
Loss of downward and outward movement in the affected eye	Trochlear nerve (CN IV); superior oblique muscle	Head trauma
Loss of outward movement in the affected eye	Abducens nerve (CN VI); lateral rectus muscle	Brain tumor

must be confirmed by tests for misalignment, such as the corneal light reflex test and the cover test. Testing is crucial—early corrective measures help preserve binocular vision and cosmetic appearance. Also, mild strabismus may indicate retinoblastoma, a tumor that may be asymptomatic before age 2 except for a characteristic whitish reflex in the pupil.

MEDICAL CAUSES

- *Brain tumor.* The nature of ocular deviation depends on the site and extent of the tumor. Associated signs and symptoms include headaches that are most severe in the morning, behavioral changes, memory loss, dizziness, confusion, vision loss, motor and sensory dysfunction, aphasia and, possibly, signs of hormonal imbalance. The patient's LOC may slowly deteriorate from lethargy to coma. Late signs include papilledema, vomiting, increased systolic blood pressure, widening pulse pressure, and decorticate posture.
- *Cavernous sinus thrombosis.* In cavernous sinus thrombosis, ocular deviation may be accompanied by diplopia, photophobia, exophthalmos, orbital and eyelid edema, corneal haziness, diminished or absent pupillary reflexes, and impaired visual acuity. Other features include high fever, headache, malaise, nausea and vomiting, seizures, and tachycardia. Retinal hemorrhage and papilledema are late signs.

- *Cerebral aneurysm.* When an aneurysm near the internal carotid artery compresses the oculomotor nerve, it may produce features that resemble third cranial nerve palsy. Typically, ocular deviation and diplopia are the presenting signs. Other cardinal findings include ptosis, a dilated pupil on the affected side, and a severe, unilateral headache, usually in the frontal area. Rupture of the aneurysm abruptly intensifies the pain, which may be accompanied by nausea and vomiting. Bleeding from the site causes meningeal irritation, resulting in nuchal rigidity, back and leg pain, fever, irritability, occasional seizures, and blurred vision. Other signs and symptoms associated with intracranial bleeding include hemiparesis, dysphagia, and visual defects.
- *Diabetes mellitus.* A leading cause of isolated third cranial nerve palsy, especially in the middle-age patient with long-standing mild diabetes, diabetes mellitus may cause ocular deviation and ptosis. Typically, the patient also complains of a sudden onset of diplopia and pain.
- *Encephalitis.* Encephalitis may cause ocular deviation and diplopia. Typically, it begins abruptly with fever, headache, and vomiting, followed by signs of meningeal irritation (for example, nuchal rigidity) and of neuronal damage (for example, seizures, aphasia, ataxia, hemiparesis, cranial nerve palsies, and photophobia). The patient's

PROTECTIVE EYE COVERING

Provide a protective cover for the eye until it can be examined by an ophthalmologist. To do this, make padding by wrapping gauze loosely around your hand several times to form a "donut" with a central opening diameter large enough to avoid pressure on the globe. Secure with an over and under wrap of gauze to form a firm edge.

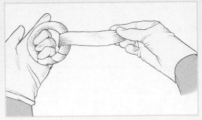

Apply the donut over the orbit of the eye, avoiding contact with the globe.

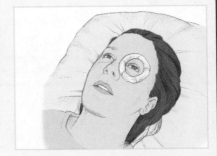

Lay an eye shield (or styrofoam cup) on top of the donut.

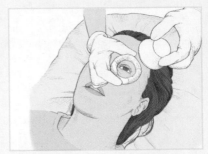

Apply an eye patch to the unaffected eye to prevent consensual movement of and further trauma to the affected eye. Secure the eye patch and eye shield by wrapping 4" gauze around the head several times.

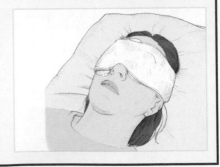

LOC may rapidly deteriorate from lethargy to coma.

- *Head trauma.* The nature of ocular deviation depends on the site and extent of head trauma. The patient may have visible soft-tissue injury, bony deformity, facial edema, and clear or bloody otorrhea or rhinorrhea. Besides these obvious signs of trauma, he may also develop blurred vision, diplopia, nystagmus, behavioral changes, headache, motor and sensory dysfunction, and a decreased LOC that may progress to coma. Signs of increased intracranial pressure—such as bradycardia, increased systolic pressure, and widening pulse pressure—may also occur.

- *Multiple sclerosis (MS).* Ocular deviation may be an early sign of MS. Accompanying it are diplopia, blurred vision, and sensory dysfunction such as paresthesia. Other signs and symptoms include nystagmus, constipation, muscle weakness, paralysis, spasticity, hyperreflexia, intention tremor, gait ataxia, dysphagia, dysarthria, impotence, and emotional instability. In addition, the patient may experience urinary frequency, urgency, and incontinence.

- *Myasthenia gravis.* Ocular deviation may accompany the more common presenting signs of diplopia and ptosis. Myasthenia gravis may affect only the eye muscles, or it may progress to other muscle groups, causing altered facial expression, difficulty chewing, dysphagia, weakened voice, and impaired fine hand movements. Signs of respiratory distress reflect weakness of the diaphragm and other respiratory muscles.

- *Ophthalmoplegic migraine.* Most common in young adults, ophthalmoplegic migraine produces ocular deviation and diplopia that persist for days after the pain subsides. Associated signs and symptoms include unilateral headache, possibly with ptosis on the same side; temporary hemiplegia; and sensory deficits. Irritability, depression, or slight confusion may also occur.

- *Orbital blowout fracture.* In orbital blowout fracture, the inferior rectus muscle may become entrapped, resulting in limited extraocular movement and ocular deviation. Typically, the patient's upward gaze is absent; other directions of gaze may be affected if edema is dramatic. The globe may also be displaced downward and inward. Associated signs and symptoms include pain, diplopia, nausea, periorbital edema, and ecchymosis.

- *Orbital cellulitis.* Orbital cellulitis may cause a sudden onset of ocular deviation and diplopia. Other signs and symptoms include unilateral eyelid edema and erythema, hyperemia, chemosis, and extreme orbital pain. Purulent discharge makes eyelashes matted and sticky. Proptosis is a late sign.

- *Orbital tumor.* Ocular deviation occurs as the tumor gradually enlarges. Associated findings include proptosis, diplopia and, possibly, blurred vision.

- *Stroke.* Stroke is a life-threatening disorder that may cause ocular deviation, depending on the site and extent of the stroke. Accompanying features are also variable and include an altered LOC, contralateral hemiplegia and sensory loss, dysarthria, dysphagia, homonymous hemianopsia, blurred vision, and diplopia. In addition, the patient may develop urine retention or incontinence or both, constipation, behavioral changes, headache, vomiting, and seizures.

- *Thyrotoxicosis.* The patient with thyrotoxicosis may also experience exophthalmos—proptotic or protruding eyes—which, in turn, causes limited extraocular movement and ocular deviation. Usually, the patient's upward gaze weakens first, followed by diplopia. Other features are lid retraction, a wide-eyed staring gaze, excessive tearing, edematous eyelids and, sometimes, an inability to close the eyes. Cardinal features of thyrotoxicosis include tachycardia, palpitations, weight loss despite increased appetite, diarrhea, tremors, an enlarged thyroid, dyspnea, nervousness, diaphoresis, heat intolerance, and an atrial or ventricular gallop.

NURSING CONSIDERATIONS

Continue to monitor the patient's vital signs and neurologic status if you suspect an acute neurologic disorder. Take seizure precautions, if necessary. Also, prepare the patient for diagnostic tests, such as blood studies, orbital and skull X-rays, and a CT scan. If the source of the condition is related to trauma, the eye may require a protective covering until treatment is initiated. (See *Protective eye covering.*)

PATIENT TEACHING

Inform the patient and his family about the disorder and its treatment. Explain changes in LOC that should be reported. Provide information related to maintaining a safe environment. Teach techniques to reduce environmental and situational stress. Discuss the importance of follow-up care with a specialist.

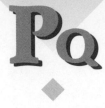

Pallor

Pallor is abnormal paleness or loss of skin color, which may develop suddenly or gradually. Although generalized pallor affects the entire body, it's most apparent on the face, conjunctiva, oral mucosa, and nail beds. Localized pallor commonly affects a single limb.

Skin color and the thickness and vascularity of underlying subcutaneous tissue affect the detection of pallor. Subtle lightening of skin color may be difficult to detect in dark-skinned persons — for example, the conjunctiva and oral mucosa may occasionally be the only areas in which pallor is evident.

Pallor may result from decreased peripheral oxyhemoglobin or decreased total oxyhemoglobin. The former reflects diminished peripheral blood flow associated with peripheral vasoconstriction or arterial occlusion or with low cardiac output. (Transient peripheral vasoconstriction may occur with exposure to cold, causing nonpathologic pallor.) The latter usually results from anemia, the chief cause of pallor. (See *How pallor develops.*)

Act now *If generalized pallor suddenly develops, quickly look for signs of shock, such as tachycardia, hypotension, oliguria, and a decreased level of consciousness (LOC). Prepare to rapidly infuse fluids or blood. Keep emergency resuscitation equipment nearby.*

ASSESSMENT
History
If the patient's condition permits, take a complete history. Does he have a history of anemia or a chronic disorder that might lead to pallor, such as renal failure, heart failure, or diabetes? Ask about his diet, noting his intake of green vegetables.

Explore the pallor more fully. When did the patient first notice it? Is the pallor constant or intermittent? Does it occur when he's exposed to the cold or when he experiences emotional stress? Investigate associated signs and symptoms, such as dizziness, fainting, orthostasis, weakness and fatigue on exertion, dyspnea, chest pain, palpitations, or loss of libido. Ask the female patient about menstrual irregularities. If the pallor is confined to one or both legs, ask the patient if walking is painful. Do his legs feel cold or numb? If the pallor is confined to his fingers, ask about tingling and numbness.

Physical examination
Start the physical examination by taking the patient's vital signs. Be sure to check for orthostatic hypotension. Auscultate the heart for gallops and murmurs and the lungs for crackles. Check the patient's skin temperature — cold extremities commonly occur with vasoconstriction or arterial occlusion. Also, note skin ulceration. Examine the abdomen for splenomegaly. Finally, palpate peripheral pulses. An absent pulse in a pale extremity may indicate arterial occlusion, whereas a weak pulse may indicate low cardiac output.

HOW PALLOR DEVELOPS

Pallor may result from decreased peripheral oxyhemoglobin or decreased total oxyhemoglobin. This chart illustrates the progression to pallor.

```
Low cardiac output ─────┐
                        ↓
Arterial occlusion ──→ Decreased peripheral ──→ Decreased
                       perfusion                 oxyhemoglobin to
                        ↑                         tissues
Peripheral ─────────────┘                            ↓
vasoconstriction                                   Pallor
                                                     ↑
Anemia ──────────────→ Decreased serum ──→ Decreased oxygen-
                       hemoglobin           carrying capacity of
                                            blood
```

Pediatric pointers

In children, pallor can stem from a congenital heart defect or chronic lung disease.

MEDICAL CAUSES

● *Anemia.* Typically, pallor develops gradually with anemia. The patient's skin may also appear sallow or grayish. Other effects include fatigue, dyspnea, tachycardia, bounding pulse, atrial gallop, systolic bruit over the carotid arteries and, possibly, crackles and bleeding tendencies.

● *Arterial occlusion (acute).* Pallor develops abruptly in the extremity with the occlusion, which usually results from an embolus. A line of demarcation develops, separating the cool, pale, cyanotic, and mottled skin below the occlusion from the normal skin above it. Accompanying the pallor may be severe pain, intense intermittent claudication, paresthesia, and paresis in the affected extremity. Absent pulses and increased capillary refill time below the occlusion are also characteristic.

● *Arterial occlusive disease (chronic).* With chronic arterial occlusive disease, pallor is specific to an extremity—usually one leg, but occasionally, both legs or an arm. It develops gradually from obstructive arteriosclerosis or a thrombus and is aggravated by elevating the extremity. Associated findings include intermittent claudication, weakness, cool skin, diminished pulses in the extremity and, possibly, ulceration and gangrene.

● *Cardiac arrhythmias.* Serious reductions in cardiac output caused by complete heart block and attacks of tachyarrhythmia may lead to pallor. Other features include an irregular, rapid, or slow pulse as well as dizziness, weakness and fatigue, hypotension, confusion, palpitations, diaphoresis, oliguria and, possibly, loss of consciousness.

● *Frostbite.* Pallor is localized to the frostbitten area, such as the feet, hands, or ears. Typically, the area feels cold, waxy and, perhaps, hard in deep frostbite. The skin doesn't blanch and sensation may be absent. As the area thaws, the skin turns purplish blue. Blistering and gangrene may then follow if the frostbite is severe.

● *Orthostatic hypotension.* With orthostatic hypertension, pallor occurs abruptly on rising from a recumbent position to a sitting or standing position. A precipitous drop in blood pressure, an increase in heart rate, and dizziness are also characteristic. At times, the patient loses consciousness for several minutes.

- **Raynaud's disease.** Pallor of the fingers upon exposure to cold or stress is a hallmark of Raynaud's disease. Typically, the fingers abruptly turn pale and then cyanotic; with rewarming, they become red and paresthetic. With chronic disease, ulceration may occur.
- **Shock.** Two forms of shock initially cause an acute onset of pallor and cool, clammy skin. With hypovolemic shock, other early signs and symptoms include restlessness, thirst, slight tachycardia, and tachypnea. As shock progresses, the skin becomes increasingly clammy, the pulse becomes more rapid and thready, and hypotension develops with narrowing pulse pressure. Other signs and symptoms include oliguria, subnormal body temperature, and a decreased LOC. With cardiogenic shock, the signs and symptoms are similar, but usually more profound.
- **Vasopressor syncope.** The sudden onset of pallor immediately precedes or accompanies loss of consciousness during syncopal attacks. These common fainting spells may be triggered by emotional stress or pain and usually last only a few seconds or minutes. Before loss of consciousness, the patient may exhibit diaphoresis, nausea, yawning, hyperpnea, weakness, confusion, tachycardia, and dim vision. He then develops bradycardia, hypotension, a few clonic jerks, and dilated pupils with loss of consciousness.

NURSING CONSIDERATIONS

If the patient has chronic generalized pallor, prepare him for blood studies and, possibly, bone marrow biopsy. If he has localized pallor, he may require arteriography or other diagnostic studies to accurately determine the cause.

When pallor results from low cardiac output, administer blood and fluids. The patient may also require a diuretic, a cardiotonic, and an antiarrhythmic. Frequently monitor his vital signs, intake and output, electrocardiogram results, and hemodynamic status.

PATIENT TEACHING

If the patient's pallor is related to anemia, explain the importance of an iron-rich diet and rest. If he has pallor due to frostbite or Raynaud's disease, inform him about cold protection measures. If pallor is related to orthostatic hypotension, explain the need to stand up slowly and to sit down when dizziness occurs.

Palpitations

Defined as a conscious awareness of one's heartbeat, palpitations are usually felt over the precordium or in the throat or neck. The patient may describe them as pounding, jumping, turning, fluttering, or flopping or as missing or skipping beats. Palpitations may be regular or irregular, fast or slow, and paroxysmal or sustained.

Although usually insignificant, palpitations may result from a cardiac or metabolic disorder and from the effects of certain drugs. Nonpathologic palpitations may occur with a newly implanted prosthetic valve because the valve's clicking sound heightens the patient's awareness of his heartbeat. Transient palpitations may accompany emotional stress, such as fright, anger, or anxiety, or physical stress, such as exercise and fever. They can also accompany the use of stimulants, such as tobacco and caffeine.

To help characterize palpitations, ask the patient to simulate their rhythm by tapping his finger on a hard surface. An irregular "skipped beat" rhythm points to premature ventricular contractions, whereas an episodic racing rhythm that ends abruptly suggests paroxysmal atrial tachycardia.

Act now *If the patient complains of palpitations, ask him about dizziness and shortness of breath. Then inspect for pale, cool, clammy skin. Take the patient's vital signs, noting hypotension and an irregular or abnormal pulse. If these signs are present, suspect cardiac arrhythmia. Prepare to begin cardiac monitoring and, if necessary, to assist with synchronized cardioversion or defibrillation. Start an I.V. line to administer an antiarrhythmic, if needed.*

ASSESSMENT
History

If the patient isn't in distress, perform a complete cardiac history and physical examination. Ask if he has a cardiovascular or pulmonary disorder, which may produce arrhythmias. Does he have a history of hypertension or hypoglycemia? Be sure to obtain a drug history. Has he recently started cardiac glycoside therapy? Also, ask about caffeine, tobacco, amphetamine, and alcohol consumption.

Physical examination

Perform a complete cardiac and pulmonary assessment. Then explore associated symptoms, such as weakness, fatigue, and angina. Finally, auscultate for gallops, murmurs, and abnormal breath sounds. Cardiac monitoring may be indicated when a cardiac arrhythmia is suspected. (See *Palpitations: Causes and associated findings,* pages 226 and 227.)

Pediatric pointers

Palpitations in children commonly result from fever and congenital heart defects, such as patent ductus arteriosus and septal defects. Because many children can't describe this complaint, focus your attention on objective measurements, such as cardiac monitoring, physical examination, and laboratory tests.

MEDICAL CAUSES

- *Anemia.* Palpitations may occur with anemia, especially on exertion. Pallor, fatigue, and dyspnea are also common. Associated signs include a systolic ejection murmur, bounding pulse, tachycardia, crackles, an atrial gallop, and a systolic bruit over the carotid arteries.
- *Anxiety attack (acute).* Anxiety is the most common cause of palpitations. With this disorder, palpitations may be accompanied by diaphoresis, facial flushing, trembling, and an impending sense of doom. Almost invariably, the patient hyperventilates, which may lead to dizziness, weakness, and syncope. Other typical findings include tachycardia, precordial pain, shortness of breath, restlessness, and insomnia.
- *Cardiac arrhythmias.* Paroxysmal or sustained palpitations may be accompanied by dizziness, weakness, and fatigue. The patient may also experience an irregular, rapid, or slow pulse rate as well as decreased blood pressure, confusion, pallor, oliguria, and diaphoresis.
- *Hypertension.* With hypertension, the patient may be asymptomatic or may complain of sustained palpitations alone or with headache, dizziness, tinnitus, and fatigue. His blood pressure typically exceeds 140/90 mm Hg.
- *Hypocalcemia.* Typically, hypocalcemia produces palpitations, weakness, and fatigue. It progresses from paresthesia to muscle tension and carpopedal spasms. The patient may also exhibit muscle twitching, hyperactive deep tendon reflexes, chorea, and positive Chvostek's and Trousseau's signs.
- *Hypoglycemia.* When the blood glucose level drops significantly, the sympathetic nervous system triggers adrenaline production. This may cause sustained palpitations, which may be accompanied by fatigue, irritability, hunger, cold sweats, tremors, tachycardia, anxiety, and headache. Eventually, the patient may develop central nervous system reactions. These include blurred or double vision, muscle weakness, hemiplegia, and an altered LOC.
- *Mitral prolapse.* A valvular disorder, mitral prolapse may cause paroxysmal palpitations accompanied by sharp, stabbing, or aching precordial pain. The hallmark of this disorder, however, is a midsystolic click followed by an apical systolic murmur. Associated signs and symptoms may include dyspnea, dizziness, severe fatigue, migraine headache, anxiety, paroxysmal tachycardia, crackles, and peripheral edema.
- *Mitral stenosis.* Early features of mitral stenosis—a valvular disorder—typically include sustained palpitations accompanied by exertional dyspnea, fatigue, paroxysmal nocturnal dyspnea, and atrial fibrillations. Auscultation also reveals a loud S_1 or opening snap and a rumbling diastolic murmur at the apex. Patients may also experience related signs and symptoms, such as an atrial gallop and, with advanced mitral stenosis, orthopnea, dyspnea at rest, peripheral edema, jugular vein distention, ascites, and hepatomegaly.
- *Pheochromocytoma.* Pheochromocytoma, a rare adrenal medulla tumor causes episodic hypermetabolism, commonly associated with paroxysmal palpitations. The cardinal sign is dramatically elevated blood pressure, which may be sustained or paroxysmal. Associated signs and symptoms include tachycardia, headache, chest or abdominal pain, diaphoresis, warm and pale or flushed skin, paresthesia, tremors, insomnia, nausea and vomiting, and anxiety.
- *Sick sinus syndrome.* A patient with sick sinus syndrome may experience palpitations as well as bradycardia, tachycardia, chest pain, syncope, and heart failure.
- *Thyrotoxicosis.* A characteristic symptom of thyrotoxicosis, sustained palpitations may be accompanied by tachycardia, dyspnea, weight loss despite increased appetite, diarrhea, tremors, nervousness, diaphoresis, heat

PALPITATIONS:
CAUSES AND ASSOCIATED FINDINGS

MAJOR ASSOCIATED SIGNS AND SYMPTOMS

COMMON CAUSES	Bradycardia	Confusion	Crackles	Decreased blood pressure	Decreased LOC	Diaphoresis	Dizziness	Dyspnea	Facial flushing	Fatigue	Headache	Increased blood pressure	Insomnia	Murmur
Anemia			●	●				●		●				●
Acute anxiety						●	●	●	●				●	
Cardiac arrhythmias							●			●				
Hypertension							●			●	●	●		
Hypocalcemia				●						●				
Hypoglycemia		●				●	●			●	●			
Mitral prolapse				●			●	●		●				●
Mitral stenosis							●			●				●
Pheochromocytoma						●					●	●	●	
Sick sinus syndrome	●													
Thyrotoxicosis							●	●						
Wolff-Parkinson-White syndrome														

intolerance and, possibly, exophthalmos and an enlarged thyroid. The patient may also experience an atrial or ventricular gallop.

● *Wolff-Parkinson-White (WPW) syndrome.* Seen in children and adolescents, WPW syndrome results in recurrent palpitations and frequent episodes of paroxysmal tachycardia.

OTHER CAUSES

● *Drugs.* Cardiac glycosides and other drugs that precipitate cardiac arrhythmias or increase cardiac output can cause palpitations. Ganglionic blockers, beta-adrenergic blockers, calcium channel blockers, atropine, minoxidil, and sympathomimetics, such as cocaine, can also cause palpitations.

● *Exercise.* Palpitations can occur normally with exercise. Patients with coronary heart disease, hypertension, mitral valve prolapse, and cardiomegaly may experience palpitations with exercise.

● *Herbal remedies.* Ginseng and other herbal remedies may cause adverse reactions that include palpitations and an irregular heartbeat.

NURSING CONSIDERATIONS

Prepare the patient for diagnostic tests, such as an electrocardiogram and Holter monitoring. Provide supplemental oxygen, as indicated. Assess the patient for electrolyte imbalances as a potential cause for the condi-

Muscle twitching	Nausea	Pallor	Peripheral edema	Precordial pain	Syncope	Tachycardia	Tremors	Weakness
		•				•		
					•	•	•	•
								•
•								•
						•	•	
			•	•		•		
			•					
	•					•	•	•
					•	•	•	
							•	•
						•		

Paralysis, the total loss of voluntary motor function, results from severe cortical or pyramidal tract damage. It can occur with a cerebrovascular disorder, degenerative neuromuscular disease, trauma, tumor, or central nervous system infection.

Alert *Acute paralysis may be an early indicator of a life-threatening disorder such as Guillain-Barré syndrome.*

Paralysis can be local or widespread, symmetrical or asymmetrical, transient or permanent, and spastic or flaccid. It's commonly classified according to location and severity as paraplegia (sometimes transient paralysis of the legs), quadriplegia (permanent paralysis of the arms, legs, and body below the level of the spinal lesion), or hemiplegia (unilateral paralysis of varying severity and permanence). Incomplete paralysis with profound weakness (paresis) may precede total paralysis in some patients.

Act now *If paralysis has developed suddenly, suspect trauma or an acute vascular insult. After ensuring that the patient's spine is properly immobilized, quickly determine his level of consciousness (LOC) and take his vital signs. Elevated systolic blood pressure, widening pulse pressure, and bradycardia may signal increasing intracranial pressure (ICP). If possible, elevate the patient's head 30 degrees to decrease ICP.*

Evaluate the patient's respiratory status, and be prepared to administer oxygen, insert an artificial airway, or provide intubation and mechanical ventilation as needed. To help determine the nature of the patient's injury, ask him for an account of the precipitating events. If he can't respond, try to find an eyewitness.

tion. To alleviate the anxiety that may arise with palpitations, provide a quiet, comfortable environment.

PATIENT TEACHING

If the patient's palpitations are related to anxiety, provide information about anxiety and stress management. Refer him to community support services for stress management and therapy. Reinforce the need to avoid caffeine and provide information on alcohol and smoking cessation programs, as appropriate.

ASSESSMENT
History

If the patient is in no immediate danger, perform a complete neurologic assessment. Start with the history, relying on family members for information if necessary. Ask about the onset, duration, intensity, and progression of paralysis and about the events preceding its development. Focus medical history questions on the incidence of degenerative neurologic or neuromuscular disease, recent infectious illness, sexually transmitted disease, cancer, or injury. Explore related signs and symptoms, noting fever, headache, vision disturbances, dysphagia, nausea and vomiting, bowel or bladder dysfunction, muscle pain or weakness, and fatigue.

Physical examination

Perform a complete neurologic examination, testing cranial nerve, motor, and sensory function and deep tendon reflexes (DTRs). Assess strength in all major muscle groups, and note muscle atrophy. (See *Testing muscle strength,* pages 230 and 231.) Document all findings to serve as a baseline.

Pediatric pointers

Although children may develop paralysis from an obvious cause — such as trauma, an infection, or a tumor — it may also arise from a hereditary or congenital disorder, such as Werdnig-Hoffmann disease, spina bifida, or cerebral palsy.

MEDICAL CAUSES

● *Amyotrophic lateral sclerosis (ALS).* ALS, an invariably fatal disorder, produces spastic or flaccid paralysis in the body's major muscle groups, eventually progressing to total paralysis. Earlier findings include progressive muscle weakness, fasciculations, and muscle atrophy, usually beginning in the arms and hands. Cramping and hyperreflexia are also common. Involvement of respiratory muscles and the brain stem produces dyspnea and respiratory distress. Progressive cranial nerve paralysis causes dysarthria, dysphagia, drooling, choking, and difficulty chewing.
● *Bell's palsy.* Transient, unilateral facial muscle paralysis occurs in Bell's palsy, a disease of cranial nerve VII. (See *Recognizing unilateral Bell's palsy.*) The affected muscles sag, and eyelid closure may be impossible. Other signs include increased tearing, drooling, diminished or absent corneal reflex, and possible difficulty with hearing or pain in the ear.
● *Botulism.* Botulism, a bacterial toxin infection, can cause rapidly descending muscle weakness that progresses to paralysis within 2 to 4 days after eating contaminated food. Respiratory muscle paralysis leads to dyspnea and respiratory arrest. Nausea, vomiting, diarrhea, blurred or double vision, bilateral mydriasis, dysarthria, and dysphagia are some early findings.

● *Brain abscess.* Advanced abscess in the frontal or temporal lobe can cause hemiplegia accompanied by other late findings, such as ocular disturbances, unequal pupils, a decreased LOC, ataxia, tremors, and signs of infection.
● *Brain tumor.* A tumor affecting the motor cortex of the frontal lobe may cause contralateral hemiparesis that progresses to hemiplegia. The onset is gradual, but paralysis is permanent without treatment. In early stages, frontal headache and behavioral changes may be the only indicators. Eventually, seizures, aphasia, and signs of increased ICP (decreased LOC and vomiting) develop.
● *Conversion disorder.* Hysterical paralysis, a classic symptom of conversion disorder, is characterized by the loss of voluntary movement with no obvious physical cause. It can affect any muscle group, appears and disappears unpredictably, and may occur with histrionic behavior (manipulative, dramatic, vain, irrational) or a strange indifference.
● *Encephalitis.* Variable paralysis develops in the late stages of encephalitis. Earlier signs and symptoms include rapidly decreasing LOC (possibly coma), fever, headache, photophobia, vomiting, signs of meningeal irritation (nuchal rigidity, positive Kernig's and Brudzinski's signs), aphasia, ataxia, nystagmus, ocular palsies, myoclonus, and seizures.
● *Guillain-Barré syndrome.* Guillain-Barré syndrome is characterized by a rapidly developing, but reversible, ascending paralysis. It commonly begins as leg muscle weakness and progresses symmetrically, sometimes affecting even the cranial nerves, producing dysphagia, nasal speech, and dysarthria. Other effects include transient paresthesia, orthostatic hypotension, tachycardia, diaphoresis, and bowel and bladder incontinence.

Alert *Respiratory muscle paralysis may be life-threatening.*
● *Head trauma.* Cerebral injury can cause paralysis due to cerebral edema and increased ICP. The onset is usually sudden. Location and extent vary, depending on the injury. Associated findings also vary, but include a decreased LOC, headache, blurred or double vision, nausea and vomiting, and focal neurologic disturbances. Sensory disturbances, such as paresthesia and loss of sensation, may also occur.

- *Migraine headache.* Hemiparesis, scotomas, paresthesia, confusion, dizziness, photophobia, nausea and vomiting, or other transient symptoms may precede the onset of a throbbing unilateral headache and may persist after it subsides.
- *Multiple sclerosis (MS).* With MS, paralysis commonly waxes and wanes until the later stages, when it may become permanent. Its extent can range from monoplegia to quadriplegia. In most patients, vision and sensory disturbances (paresthesia) are the earliest symptoms. Later findings are widely variable and may include muscle weakness and spasticity, nystagmus, hyperreflexia, intention tremor, gait ataxia, dysphagia, dysarthria, impotence, and constipation. Urinary frequency, urgency, and incontinence may also occur.
- *Myasthenia gravis.* With myasthenia gravis, a neuromuscular disease, profound muscle weakness and abnormal fatigability may produce paralysis of certain muscle groups. Paralysis is usually transient in early stages, but becomes more persistent as the disease progresses. Associated findings depend on the areas of neuromuscular involvement; they include weak eye closure, ptosis, diplopia, lack of facial mobility, dysphagia, nasal speech, and frequent nasal regurgitation of fluids. Neck muscle weakness may cause the patient's jaw to drop and his head to bob. Respiratory muscle involvement can lead to respiratory distress — dyspnea, shallow respirations, and cyanosis.
- *Neurosyphilis.* Irreversible hemiplegia may occur in the late stages of neurosyphilis. Dementia, cranial nerve palsies, tremors, and abnormal reflexes are other late findings.
- *Parkinson's disease.* Tremors, bradykinesia, and lead-pipe or cogwheel rigidity are the classic signs of Parkinson's disease. Extreme rigidity can progress to paralysis, particularly in the extremities. In most cases, paralysis resolves with prompt treatment of the disease.
- *Peripheral nerve trauma.* Severe injury to a peripheral nerve or group of nerves results in the loss of motor and sensory function in the innervated area. Muscles become flaccid and atrophied, and reflexes are lost. If transection isn't complete, paralysis may be temporary.
- *Peripheral neuropathy.* Typically, peripheral neuropathy produces muscle weakness

(Text continues on page 232.)

RECOGNIZING UNILATERAL BELL'S PALSY

Bell's palsy usually causes a unilateral facial paralysis. This produces a distorted appearance with an inability to wrinkle the forehead, close the eyelid, smile, show the teeth, or puff out the cheek.

Distorted appearance

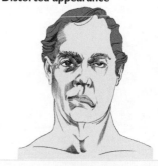

Wrinkling the forehead

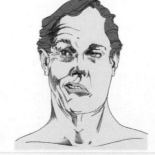

Smiling

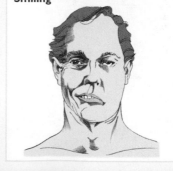

TESTING MUSCLE STRENGTH

Obtain an overall picture of the patient's motor function by testing strength in 10 selected muscle groups. Ask the patient to attempt normal range-of-motion movements against your resistance. If the muscle group is weak, vary the amount of resistance as necessary to permit accurate assessment. If necessary, position the patient so his limbs don't have to resist gravity, and repeat the test.

ARM MUSCLES

Biceps. With your hand on the patient's hand, have him flex his forearm against your resistance. Watch for biceps contraction.

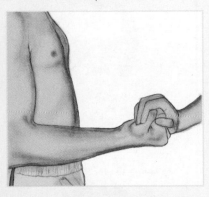

Deltoid. With the patient's arm fully extended, place one hand over his deltoid muscle and the other on his wrist. Ask him to abduct his arm to a horizontal position against your resistance; as he does so, palpate for deltoid contraction.

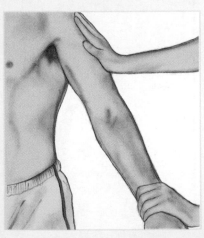

Triceps. Have the patient abduct and hold his arm midway between flexion and extension. Hold and support his arm at the wrist, and ask him to extend it against your resistance. Watch for triceps contraction.

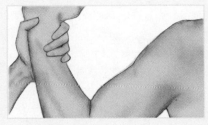

Dorsal interossei. Have the patient extend and spread his fingers, and tell him to try to resist your attempt to squeeze them together.

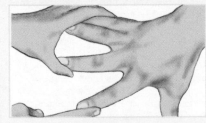

Forearm and hand (grip). Have the patient grasp your middle and index fingers and squeeze as hard as he can. To prevent pain or injury to the examiner, the examiner should cross his fingers.

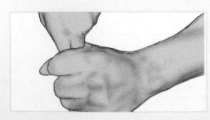

Rate muscle strength on a scale from 0 to 5:

0 = Total paralysis
1 = Visible or palpable contraction, but no movement
2 = Full muscle movement with force of gravity eliminated
3 = Full muscle movement against gravity, but no movement against resistance
4 = Full muscle movement against gravity; partial movement against resistance
5 = Full muscle movement against gravity and resistance—normal strength.

LEG MUSCLES

Anterior tibial. With the patient's leg extended, place your hand on his foot and ask him to dorsiflex his ankle against your resistance. Palpate for anterior tibial contraction.

Extensor hallucis longus. With your finger on the patient's great toe, have him dorsiflex the toe against your resistance. Palpate for extensor hallucis contraction.

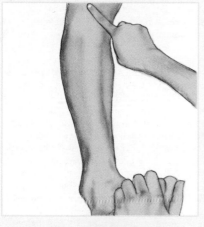

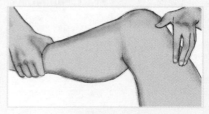

Quadriceps. Have the patient bend his knee slightly while you support his lower leg. Then ask him to extend the knee against your resistance; as he's doing so, palpate for quadriceps contraction.

Psoas. While you support his leg, have the patient raise his knee and then flex his hip against your resistance. Watch for psoas contraction.

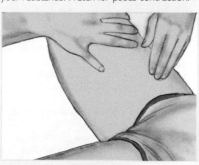

Gastrocnemius. With the patient on his side, support his foot and ask him to plantarflex his ankle against your resistance. Palpate for gastrocnemius contraction.

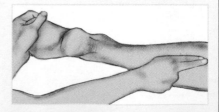

and sensory disturbances in the extremities that may lead to flaccid paralysis and atrophy. Related effects include paresthesia, loss of vibration sensation, hypoactive or absent DTRs, neuralgia, and skin changes such as anhidrosis.

- **Poliomyelitis.** Poliomyelitis can produce insidious, permanent flaccid paralysis, muscle wasting, and hyporeflexia. Sensory function remains intact, but the patient loses voluntary muscle control. Signs and symptoms before paralysis also include muscle weakness, headache, fever, nuchal rigidity, and nausea and vomiting.
- **Rabies.** Rabies, an acute disorder, produces progressive flaccid paralysis, vascular collapse, coma, and death within 2 weeks of contact with an infected animal. Prodromal signs and symptoms — paresthesia and itching at the bite site accompanied by fever, headache, hyperesthesia, photophobia, tachycardia, malaise, alternating rage and calm, hydrophobia, shallow respirations, and excessive salivation, lacrimation, and perspiration — develop almost immediately. Within 2 to 10 days, a phase of excitement begins, marked by agitation, cranial nerve dysfunction (pupillary changes, hoarseness, facial weakness, ocular palsies), tachycardia or bradycardia, cyclic respirations, high fever, urine retention, and drooling.
- **Seizure disorders.** Seizures, particularly focal seizures, can cause transient local paralysis (Todd's paralysis). Any part of the body may be affected, although paralysis tends to occur contralateral to the side of the irritable focus.
- **Spinal cord injury.** Complete spinal cord transection results in permanent spastic paralysis below the level of injury. Reflexes may return after spinal shock resolves. Partial transection causes variable paralysis and paresthesia, depending on the location and extent of injury.
- **Spinal cord tumors.** Paresis, pain, paresthesia, and variable sensory loss may occur along the nerve distribution pathway served by the affected cord segment. Eventually, these symptoms may progress to spastic paralysis with hyperactive DTRs (unless the tumor is in the cauda equina, which produces hyporeflexia) and, perhaps, bladder and bowel incontinence. Paralysis is permanent without treatment.
- **Stroke.** A stroke involving the motor cortex can produce contralateral paresis or paral-

ysis. The onset may be sudden or gradual, and paralysis may be transient or permanent. Associated signs and symptoms vary widely and may include headache, vomiting, seizures, decreased LOC and mental acuity, dysarthria, dysphagia, ataxia, contralateral paresthesia or sensory loss, apraxia, agnosia, aphasia, vision disturbances, emotional lability, and bowel and bladder dysfunction.
- **Subarachnoid hemorrhage.** A potentially life-threatening disorder, subarachnoid hemorrhage can produce sudden paralysis. The condition may be temporary, resolving with decreasing edema, or permanent, if tissue destruction has occurred. Other acute effects are severe headache, mydriasis, photophobia, aphasia, a sharply decreased LOC, nuchal rigidity, vomiting, and seizures.
- **Syringomyelia.** Syringomyelia, a degenerative spinal cord disease, produces segmental paresis, leading to flaccid paralysis of the hands and arms. Reflexes are absent, and loss of pain and temperature sensation is distributed over the neck, shoulders, and arms in a capelike pattern.
- **Thoracic aortic aneurysm.** Occlusion of spinal arteries by a ruptured thoracic aortic aneurysm may cause the sudden onset of transient bilateral paralysis. Severe chest pain radiating to the neck, shoulders, back, and abdomen and a sensation of tearing in the thorax are prominent symptoms. Related findings include syncope, pallor, diaphoresis, dyspnea, tachycardia, cyanosis, diastolic heart murmur, and abrupt loss of radial and femoral pulses or wide variations in pulses and blood pressure between the arms and legs. Paradoxically, however, the patient appears to be in shock, and his systolic blood pressure is either normal or elevated.
- **Transient ischemic attack (TIA).** Episodic TIAs may cause transient unilateral paresis or paralysis accompanied by paresthesia, blurred or double vision, dizziness, aphasia, dysarthria, a decreased LOC, and other site-dependent effects.
- **West Nile encephalitis.** A brain infection, West Nile encephalitis is caused by West Nile virus, a mosquito-borne flavivirus endemic to Africa, the Middle East, western Asia, and the United States. Mild infections are common and include fever, headache, and body aches, which are sometimes accompanied by a skin rash and swollen lymph glands. More severe infections are marked by headache, high fever, neck stiff-

ness, stupor, disorientation, coma, tremors, occasional convulsions, paralysis and, rarely, death.

OTHER CAUSES

● *Drugs.* Therapeutic use of neuromuscular blockers, such as pancuronium or curare, produces paralysis.
● *Electroconvulsive therapy (ECT).* ECT can produce acute, but transient, paralysis.

NURSING CONSIDERATIONS

Because a paralyzed patient is particularly susceptible to complications of prolonged immobility, provide frequent position changes, meticulous skin care, and frequent chest physiotherapy. He may benefit from passive range-of-motion exercises to maintain muscle tone, application of splints to prevent contractures, and the use of footboards or other devices to prevent footdrop. If his cranial nerves are affected, the patient will have difficulty chewing and swallowing. Provide a liquid or soft diet, and keep suction equipment on hand in case aspiration occurs. Feeding tubes or total parenteral nutrition may be necessary with severe paralysis. Paralysis and accompanying vision disturbances may make ambulation hazardous; provide a call light and show the patient how to call for help. As appropriate, arrange for physical, speech, or occupational therapy.

PATIENT TEACHING

Provide information and referrals to home care and other support services, which may include social services, occupational therapy, speech therapy, physical therapy, and wound care. Assess the home environment and provide information to the family about safety measures and physical alterations that may be required to allow wheelchair access and maneuverability. Provide teaching on equipment that may be needed and used at home.

Pleural friction rub

Commonly resulting from a pulmonary disorder or trauma, a pleural friction rub is a loud, coarse, grating, creaking, or squeaking sound that may be auscultated over one or both lungs during late inspiration or early expiration. It's heard best over the low axilla or the anterior, lateral, or posterior bases of the lung fields with the patient upright. Sometimes intermittent, it may resemble crackles or a pericardial friction rub. (See *Comparing auscultation findings,* pages 234 and 235.)

A pleural friction rub indicates inflammation of the visceral and parietal pleural lining, which causes congestion and edema. The resultant fibrinous exudate covers both pleural surfaces, displacing the fluid that's normally between them and causing the surfaces to rub together.

Act now *If you detect a pleural friction rub, quickly look for signs of respiratory distress: shallow or decreased respirations, dyspnea, increased accessory muscle use, intercostal or suprasternal retractions, cyanosis, nasal flaring, and crowing, wheezing, or stridor. Check for hypotension, tachycardia, and a decreased level of consciousness.*

If you detect signs of distress, open and maintain an airway. Endotracheal intubation and supplemental oxygen may be necessary. Insert a large-bore I.V. line to deliver drugs and fluids. Elevate the patient's head 30 degrees. Monitor the patient's cardiac status constantly, and check his vital signs frequently.

ASSESSMENT
History

If the patient isn't in severe distress, explore related symptoms. Ask whether he has had chest pain; if so, ask him to describe its location and severity. How long does his chest pain last? Does the pain radiate to his shoulder, neck, or upper abdomen? Does it worsen with breathing, movement, coughing, or sneezing? Does it abate if he splints his chest, holds his breath, or exerts pressure or lies on the affected side? Is he experiencing nausea or vomiting, shortness of breath with exertion, or fever?

Ask the patient about a history of rheumatoid arthritis, a respiratory or cardiovascular disorder, recent trauma, asbestos exposure, or radiation therapy. If he smokes, obtain a history in pack-years.

Physical examination

Characterize the pleural friction rub by auscultating the lungs with the patient sitting upright and breathing deeply and slowly through his mouth. Is the friction rub unilateral or bilateral? Also, listen for absent or diminished breath sounds, noting their loca-

(Text continues on page 236.)

COMPARING AUSCULTATION FINDINGS

During auscultation, you may detect a pleural friction rub, a pericardial friction rub, or crackles — three abnormal sounds that are commonly confused. Use this chart to help clarify auscultation findings.

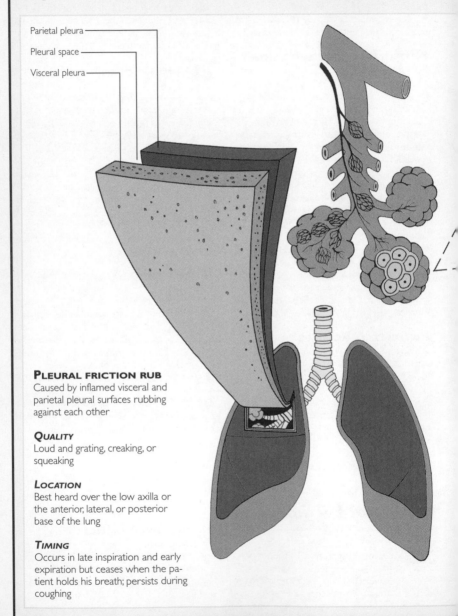

Parietal pleura

Pleural space

Visceral pleura

PLEURAL FRICTION RUB
Caused by inflamed visceral and parietal pleural surfaces rubbing against each other

QUALITY
Loud and grating, creaking, or squeaking

LOCATION
Best heard over the low axilla or the anterior, lateral, or posterior base of the lung

TIMING
Occurs in late inspiration and early expiration but ceases when the patient holds his breath; persists during coughing

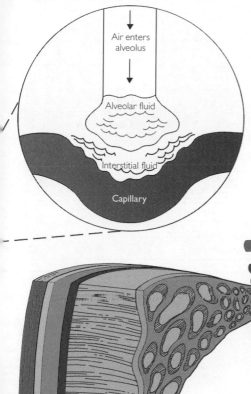

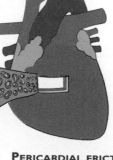

CRACKLES
Caused by air suddenly entering fluid-filled airways

QUALITY
Nonmusical clicking or rattling

LOCATION
Best heard at less distended and more dependent areas of the lungs, usually at the bases

TIMING
Occurs chiefly during inspiration

Air enters alveolus

Alveolar fluid

Interstitial fluid

Capillary

PERICARDIAL FRICTION RUB
Caused by inflamed layers of the peri-cardium rubbing against each other

QUALITY
Hard and grating, scratching, or crunching

LOCATION
Best heard along the lower left sternal border

TIMING
Occurs in relation to heartbeat; most noticeable during deep inspiration and continues even when the patient holds his breath

Endocardium

Myocardium

Visceral pericardium

Pericardial space

Parietal pericardium

Fibrous pericardium

PLEURAL FRICTION RUB:
CAUSES AND ASSOCIATED FINDINGS

MAJOR ASSOCIATED SIGNS AND SYMPTOMS

COMMON CAUSES	Altered respirations	Arthralgias	Chest pain	Cough	Crackles	Cyanosis	Decreased breath sounds	Diaphoresis	Dyspnea	Fatigue	Fever	Headache	Hemoptysis
Asbestosis			●	●	●				●				
Lung cancer			●	●					●	●	●		●
Pleurisy			●		●	●	●		●	●	●		
Pneumonia, bacterial	●		●	●	●	●			●		●	●	
Pulmonary embolism			●	●	●	●	●	●	●		●		●
Rheumatoid arthritis		●								●	●		
Systemic lupus erythematosus	●	●			●				●		●	●	
Tuberculosis, pulmonary				●	●				●	●	●		●

tion and timing in the respiratory cycle. Do abnormal breath sounds clear with coughing? Observe the patient for clubbing and pedal edema, which may indicate a chronic disorder. Then palpate for decreased chest motion, and percuss for flatness or dullness. (See *Pleural friction rub: Causes and associated findings*.)

Pediatric pointers
Auscultate for a pleural friction rub in a child who has grunting respirations, reports chest pain, or protects his chest by holding it or lying on one side. A pleural friction rub in a child is usually an early sign of pleurisy.

Geriatric pointers
In elderly patients, the intensity of pleuritic chest pain may mimic that of cardiac chest pain.

MEDICAL CAUSES
● *Asbestosis.* Besides a pleural friction rub, asbestosis may cause exertional dyspnea, cough, chest pain, and crackles. Clubbing is a late sign.

● *Lung cancer.* A pleural friction rub may be heard in the affected area of the lung. Other effects include cough (with possible hemoptysis), dyspnea, chest pain, weight loss, anorexia, fatigue, clubbing, fever, and wheezing.

● *Pleurisy.* A pleural friction rub occurs early in pleurisy. However, the cardinal symptom is sudden, intense chest pain that's usually unilateral and located in the lower and lateral parts of the chest. Deep breathing, coughing, or thoracic movement aggravates the pain. Decreased breath sounds and inspiratory crackles may be heard over the painful area. Other findings include dyspnea, tachypnea, tachycardia, cyanosis, fever, and fatigue.

● *Pneumonia (bacterial).* A pleural friction rub occurs with bacterial pneumonia, which usually starts with a dry, painful, hacking cough that rapidly becomes productive. Related effects develop suddenly and may in-

	Jugular vein distension	Muscle weakness	Restlessness	Syncope	Tachycardia	Tachypnea	Weight loss	Wheezing
							•	•
					•	•		
					•	•		
	•		•	•	•			•
		•					•	
							•	
							•	

clude shaking chills, high fever, headache, dyspnea, pleuritic chest pain, tachypnea, tachycardia, grunting respirations, nasal flaring, dullness to percussion, and cyanosis. Auscultation reveals decreased breath sounds and fine crackles.

- *Pulmonary embolism.* An embolism can cause a pleural friction rub over the affected area of the lung. Usually, the first symptom is sudden dyspnea, which may be accompanied by angina or unilateral pleuritic chest pain. Other clinical features include a nonproductive cough or a cough that produces blood-tinged sputum, tachycardia, tachypnea, low-grade fever, restlessness, and diaphoresis. Less-common findings include massive hemoptysis, chest splinting, leg edema and, with a large embolus, cyanosis, syncope, and jugular vein distention. Crackles, diffuse wheezing, decreased breath sounds, and signs of circulatory collapse may also occur.
- *Rheumatoid arthritis (RA).* RA occasionally causes a unilateral pleural friction rub, but

more typical early findings include fatigue, persistent low-grade fever, weight loss, and vague arthralgia and myalgia. Later findings include warm, swollen, painful joints as well as joint stiffness after inactivity, subcutaneous nodules on the elbows, joint deformity, and muscle weakness and atrophy.

- *Systemic lupus erythematosus.* Pulmonary involvement can cause a pleural friction rub, hemoptysis, dyspnea, pleuritic chest pain, and crackles. More characteristic effects include a butterfly rash, nondeforming joint pain and stiffness, and photosensitivity. Fever, anorexia, weight loss, and lymphadenopathy may also occur.
- *Tuberculosis (pulmonary).* With pulmonary tuberculosis, a pleural friction rub may occur over the affected part of the lung. Early signs and symptoms include chronic cough, weight loss, night sweats, low-grade fever, malaise, dyspnea, anorexia, and easy fatigability. Progression of the disorder usually produces pleuritic pain, fine crackles over the upper lobes, and a productive cough with blood-streaked sputum.

OTHER CAUSES

- *Medical treatments.* Thoracic surgery and radiation therapy can cause a pleural friction rub.

NURSING CONSIDERATIONS

Continue to monitor the patient's respiratory status and vital signs. If the patient's persistent dry, hacking cough tires him, administer an antitussive. (Avoid giving an opioid, which can further depress respirations.) Administer oxygen and an antibiotic. Prepare the patient for diagnostic tests such as chest X-rays.

PATIENT TEACHING

Because pleuritic pain commonly accompanies a pleural friction rub, teach the patient splinting maneuvers to increase his comfort. Also, apply a heating pad over the affected area and administer an analgesic for pain relief. Although coughing may be painful, instruct the patient not to suppress it because coughing and deep breathing help prevent respiratory complications. Inform him that the pain associated with a pleural friction rub may persist even after the cause has been resolved.

Pulse pressure, widened

Pulse pressure is the difference between systolic and diastolic blood pressures. Normally, systolic pressure is about 40 mm Hg higher than diastolic pressure. Widened pulse pressure—a difference of more than 50 mm Hg—commonly occurs as a physiologic response to fever, hot weather, exercise, anxiety, anemia, or pregnancy. However, it can also result from certain neurologic disorders—especially life-threatening increased intracranial pressure (ICP)—or from cardiovascular disorders that cause blood backflow into the heart with each contraction such as aortic insufficiency. Widened pulse pressure can easily be identified by monitoring arterial blood pressure and is commonly detected during routine sphygmomanometric recordings.

Act now *If the patient's level of consciousness (LOC) is decreased and you suspect that his widened pulse pressure results from increased ICP, check his vital signs. Maintain a patent airway, and prepare to hyperventilate the patient with a handheld resuscitation bag to help reduce partial pressure of carbon dioxide levels and, thus, ICP. Perform a thorough neurologic examination to serve as a baseline for assessing subsequent changes. Use the Glasgow Coma Scale to evaluate the patient's LOC. (See* Glasgow Coma Scale, *page 196.) Also, check cranial nerve (CN) function—especially in CNs III, IV, and VI—and assess pupillary reactions, reflexes, and muscle tone. (See* Exit points for the cranial nerves.) *The patient may require an ICP monitor. If you don't suspect increased ICP, ask about associated symptoms, such as chest pain, shortness of breath, weakness, fatigue, or syncope. Check for edema and auscultate for murmurs.*

ASSESSMENT
History
Obtain the patient's history, including a family medical history. Obtain a drug history. Has he experienced chest pain, shortness of breath, weakness, fatigue, or syncope? Ask the patient whether he recently had a fever. Ask about prolonged exposure to hot weather, excessive exercise, anxiety, or anemia.

Physical examination
Assess the patient for signs and symptoms of heart failure, such as crackles, dyspnea, and jugular vein distention. Check for changes in skin temperature and color and strength of peripheral pulses. Evaluate the patient's LOC. Auscultate the heart for the presence of a murmur, and check for peripheral edema.

Pediatric pointers
Increased ICP causes widened pulse pressure in a child. Patent ductus arteriosus (PDA) can also cause it, but this sign may not be evident at birth. The older child with PDA experiences exertional dyspnea, with pulse pressure that widens even further on exertion.

Geriatric pointers
Widened pulse pressure has been identified as a more powerful predictor of cardiovascular events in elderly patients than either increased systolic or diastolic blood pressure.

MEDICAL CAUSES
● *Aortic insufficiency.* With acute aortic insufficiency, pulse pressure widens progressively as the valve deteriorates, and a bounding pulse and an atrial or a ventricular gallop develop. These signs may be accompanied by chest pain, palpitations, pallor, pulsus bisferiens, and strong, abrupt carotid pulsations. Other signs of heart failure, such as crackles, dyspnea, and jugular vein distention, may also be present. Auscultation may reveal several murmurs, such as an early diastolic murmur (common) and an apical diastolic rumble (Austin Flint murmur).
● *Arteriosclerosis.* With arteriosclerosis, reduced arterial compliance causes progressive widening pulse pressure, which becomes permanent without treatment of the underlying disorder. This sign is preceded by moderate hypertension and is accompanied by signs of vascular insufficiency, such as claudication, angina, and speech and vision disturbances.
● *Febrile disorders.* Fever can cause widened pulse pressure. Accompanying symptoms vary depending on the specific disorder.
● *Increased ICP.* Widening pulse pressure is an intermediate to late sign of increased ICP. Although a decreased LOC is the earliest and most sensitive indicator of this life-threatening condition, the onset and progression of widening pulse pressure also parallel rising

EXIT POINTS FOR THE CRANIAL NERVES

As this illustration shows, 10 of the 12 pairs of cranial nerves (CNs) exit from the brain stem. The remaining two pairs—the olfactory and optic nerves—exit from the forebrain.

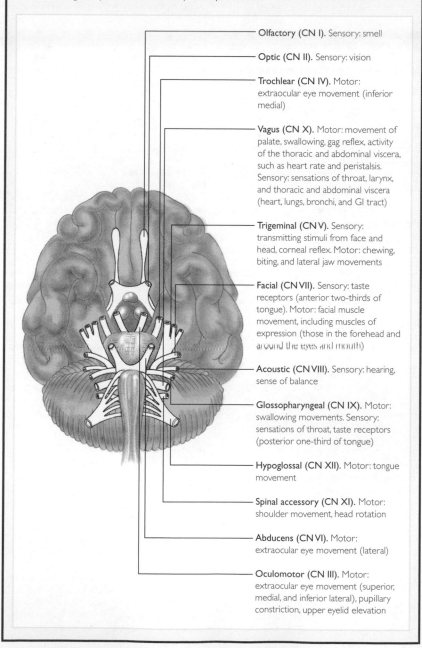

Olfactory (CN I). Sensory: smell

Optic (CN II). Sensory: vision

Trochlear (CN IV). Motor: extraocular eye movement (inferior medial)

Vagus (CN X). Motor: movement of palate, swallowing, gag reflex, activity of the thoracic and abdominal viscera, such as heart rate and peristalsis. Sensory: sensations of throat, larynx, and thoracic and abdominal viscera (heart, lungs, bronchi, and GI tract)

Trigeminal (CN V). Sensory: transmitting stimuli from face and head, corneal reflex. Motor: chewing, biting, and lateral jaw movements

Facial (CN VII). Sensory: taste receptors (anterior two-thirds of tongue). Motor: facial muscle movement, including muscles of expression (those in the forehead and around the eyes and mouth)

Acoustic (CN VIII). Sensory: hearing, sense of balance

Glossopharyngeal (CN IX). Motor: swallowing movements. Sensory: sensations of throat, taste receptors (posterior one-third of tongue)

Hypoglossal (CN XII). Motor: tongue movement

Spinal accessory (CN XI). Motor: shoulder movement, head rotation

Abducens (CN VI). Motor: extraocular eye movement (lateral)

Oculomotor (CN III). Motor: extraocular eye movement (superior, medial, and inferior lateral), pupillary constriction, upper eyelid elevation

ICP. (Even a gap of only 50 mm Hg can signal a rapid deterioration in the patient's condition.) Assessment reveals Cushing's triad: bradycardia, hypertension, and respiratory pattern changes. Other findings include headache, vomiting, and impaired or unequal motor movement. The patient may also exhibit vision disturbances, such as blurring or photophobia, and pupillary changes.

NURSING CONSIDERATIONS

If the patient displays increased ICP, continually reevaluate his neurologic status and compare your findings carefully with those of previous evaluations. Stay alert for restlessness, confusion, unresponsiveness, or a decreased LOC. Keep in mind, however, that increasing ICP is commonly signaled by subtle changes in the patient's condition, rather than the abrupt development of any one sign or symptom.

PATIENT TEACHING

Explain needed dietary modifications such as restricted sodium and saturated fats. Stress the importance of planning rest periods. If the patient has a decreased LOC, discuss specific safety measures. If the condition is related to increased body temperature, discuss fever management, proper cooling measures if exposed to excessive heat for long periods, and proper fluid consumption with the patient.

Pulse rhythm abnormality

An abnormal pulse rhythm is an irregular expansion and contraction of the peripheral arterial walls. It may be persistent or sporadic and rhythmic or arrhythmic. Detected by palpating the radial or carotid pulse, an abnormal rhythm is typically reported first by the patient, who complains of feeling palpitations. This important finding reflects an underlying cardiac arrhythmia, which may range from benign to life-threatening. Arrhythmias are commonly associated with cardiovascular, renal, respiratory, metabolic, and neurologic disorders as well as the effects of drugs, diagnostic tests, and treatments. (See *Abnormal pulse rhythm: A clue to cardiac arrhythmias,* pages 242 to 245.)

Act now   If the patient has an abnormal pulse rhythm, quickly assess for signs of reduced cardiac output, such as a decreased level of consciousness (LOC), hypotension, or dizziness. Promptly obtain an electrocardiogram (ECG) and possibly a chest X-ray, and begin cardiac monitoring. Insert an I.V. line for administration of emergency cardiac drugs, and give oxygen by nasal cannula or mask. Closely monitor the patient's vital signs, pulse quality, and cardiac rhythm because accompanying bradycardia or tachycardia may result in poor tolerance of the abnormal rhythm and cause further deterioration of cardiac output. Keep emergency intubation, cardioversion, and suction equipment handy.

ASSESSMENT
History

If the patient's condition permits, ask if he's experiencing pain. If so, ask about its onset and location. Does the pain radiate? Ask about a history of heart disease and treatments for arrhythmias. Obtain a drug history and check compliance. Also, ask about caffeine or alcohol intake. Digoxin toxicity, cessation of an antiarrhythmic, and the use of a sympathomimetic (such as epinephrine), quinidine, caffeine, cocaine, methamphetamine, or alcohol may cause arrhythmias.

Physical examination

Check the patient's apical and peripheral arterial pulses. An apical rate exceeding a peripheral arterial rate indicates a pulse deficit, which may also cause associated signs and symptoms of low cardiac output. Evaluate heart sounds: A long pause between S_1 (*lub*) and S_2 (*dub*) may indicate a conduction defect. A faint or absent S_1 and an easily audible S_2 may indicate atrial fibrillation or flutter. You may hear the two heart sounds close together on certain beats — possibly indicating premature atrial contractions — or other variations in heart rate or rhythm. Take the patient's apical and radial pulses while you listen for heart sounds. With some arrhythmias, such as premature ventricular contractions, you may hear the beat with your stethoscope but not feel it over the radial artery. This indicates an ineffective contraction that failed to produce a peripheral pulse. Next, count the apical pulse for 60 seconds, noting the frequency of skipped peripheral beats. Report your findings to the physician.

Pediatric pointers

Arrhythmias also produce pulse rhythm abnormalities in children.

MEDICAL CAUSES

● *Arrhythmias.* An abnormal pulse rhythm may be the only sign of a cardiac arrhythmia. The patient may complain of palpitations, a fluttering heartbeat, or weak and skipped beats. Pulses may be weak and rapid or slow. Depending on the specific arrhythmia, dull chest pain or discomfort and hypotension may occur. Associated findings, if any, reflect decreased cardiac output. Neurologic findings, for example, include confusion, dizziness, light-headedness, a decreased LOC and, sometimes, seizures. Other findings include decreased urine output, dyspnea, tachypnea, pallor, and diaphoresis.

NURSING CONSIDERATIONS

Be prepared to administer sedation if the patient requires cardioversion therapy. Check his vital signs frequently to detect bradycardia, tachycardia, hypertension or hypotension, tachypnea, and dyspnea. Also, monitor intake, output, and daily weight.

Collect blood samples for serum electrolyte, cardiac enzyme, and drug level studies. Prepare the patient for a chest X-ray and a 12-lead ECG. If possible, obtain a previous ECG with which to compare current findings. Prepare the patient for 24-hour Holter monitoring.

Assist the patient with ambulation, as necessary. To prevent falls and injury, raise the side rails of his bed and don't leave him unattended while he's sitting or walking.

If indicated, prepare the patient for transfer to a cardiac or intensive care unit.

PATIENT TEACHING

Instruct the patient to keep a diary of activities and symptoms that develop to correlate with the incidence of arrhythmias. Educate him about the importance of avoiding tobacco and caffeine, both of which increase arrhythmia. Provide information on smoking cessation programs. Discuss strategies to improve medication compliance.

Teach the patient how to take his pulse rate and advise him to notify his physician if he detects an abnormality. Explain the signs and symptoms he should report to his physician immediately as well as those necessitating immediate emergency care.

Pulsus paradoxus

[Paradoxical pulse]

Pulsus paradoxus is an exaggerated decline in blood pressure during inspiration. Normally, systolic pressure falls less than 10 mm Hg during inspiration. In pulsus paradoxus, it falls more than 10 mm Hg. (See *Comparing arterial pressure waves,* pages 246 and 247.) When systolic pressure falls more than 20 mm Hg, the peripheral pulses may be barely palpable or may disappear during inspiration.

Pulsus paradoxus is thought to result from an exaggerated inspirational increase in negative intrathoracic pressure. Normally, systolic pressure drops during inspiration because of blood pooling in the pulmonary system. This, in turn, reduces left ventricular filling and stroke volume and transmits negative intrathoracic pressure to the aorta. Conditions associated with large intrapleural pressure swings, such as asthma, or those that reduce left-sided heart filling, such as pericardial tamponade, produce pulsus paradoxus.

To accurately detect and measure pulsus paradoxus, use a sphygmomanometer or an intra-arterial monitoring device. Inflate the blood pressure cuff 10 to 20 mm Hg beyond the peak systolic pressure. Then deflate the cuff at a rate of 2 mm Hg/second until you hear the first Korotkoff sound during expiration. Note the systolic pressure. As you continue to slowly deflate the cuff, observe the patient's respiratory pattern. If pulsus paradoxus is present, Korotkoff sounds will disappear with inspiration and return with expiration. Continue to deflate the cuff until you hear Korotkoff sounds during inspiration and expiration and, again, note the systolic pressure. Subtract this reading from the first one to determine the degree of pulsus paradoxus. A difference of more than 10 mm Hg is abnormal.

You can also detect pulsus paradoxus by palpating the radial pulse over several cycles of slow inspiration and expiration. Marked pulse diminution during inspiration indicates pulsus paradoxus. When you check for pulsus paradoxus, remember that irregular heart rhythms and tachycardia cause variations in

(Text continues on page 244.)

ABNORMAL PULSE RHYTHM: A CLUE TO CARDIAC ARRHYTHMIAS

An abnormal pulse rhythm may be your only clue that the patient has a cardiac arrhythmia, but this sign won't help you pinpoint the specific type of arrhythmia. For that, you need a cardiac monitor or an electrocardiogram (ECG) machine. These devices record the electrical current generated by the heart's conduction system and display the information on an oscilloscope

ARRHYTHMIA

Sinus arrhythmia

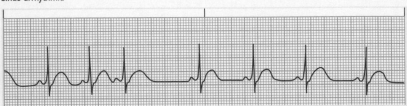

Premature atrial contractions (PACs)

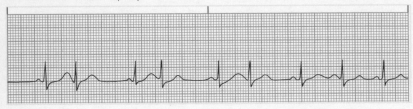

Paroxysmal atrial tachycardia

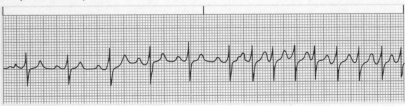

Atrial fibrillation

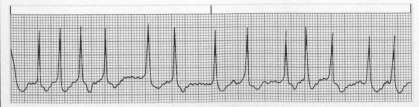

screen or a strip-chart recorder. ECG machines and cardiac monitors can identify conduction defects and electrolyte imbalances as well as rhythm disturbances.

The ECG strips below show some common cardiac arrhythmias that can cause abnormal pulse rhythms.

PULSE RHYTHM AND RATE	CLINICAL IMPLICATIONS
Irregular rhythm; fast, slow, or normal rate	◆ Reflex vagal tone inhibition (heart rate increases with inspiration and decreases with expiration) is related to the normal respiratory cycle. ◆ Sinus arrhythmia may result from drugs such as in digoxin toxicity. ◆ It occurs most commonly in children and in young adults.
Irregular rhythm during PACs; fast, slow, or normal rate	◆ Occasional PAC may be normal. ◆ Isolated PACs indicate atrial irritation—for example, from anxiety or excessive caffeine intake. Increasing PACs may herald other atrial arrhythmias. ◆ PACs may result from heart failure, chronic obstructive pulmonary disease (COPD), or the use of cardiac glycosides, aminophylline, or an adrenergic agent.
Regular rhythm with abrupt onset and termination of arrhythmia; heart rate exceeding 140 beats/minute	◆ Paroxysmal atrial tachycardia may occur in otherwise normal, healthy persons experiencing physical or psychological stress, hypoxia, or digoxin toxicity; with the use of marijuana; or with excessive consumption of caffeine or other stimulants. ◆ It may precipitate angina or heart failure.
Irregular rhythm; atrial rate exceeding 400 beats/minute; ventricular rate varies	◆ Atrial fibrillation may result from heart failure, COPD, hypertension, sepsis, pulmonary embolus, mitral valve disease, digoxin toxicity (rarely), atrial irritation, postcoronary bypass, or valve replacement surgery. ◆ Because atria don't contract, preload isn't consistent, so cardiac output changes with each beat; emboli may also result.

(continued)

Arrhythmia

Premature junctional contractions (PJCs)

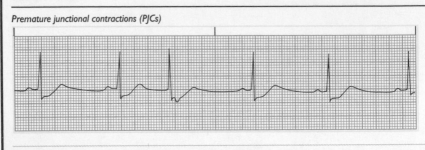

Second-degree atrioventricular (AV) heart block, Type I (Wenckebach)

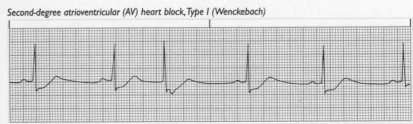

Second-degree AV heart block, Type II

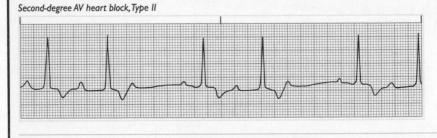

Premature ventricular contractions (PVCs) (multifocal)

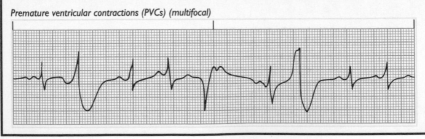

pulse amplitude and must be ruled out before true pulsus paradoxus can be identified.

Act now Pulsus paradoxus may signal cardiac tamponade — a life-threatening complication of pericardial effusion that occurs when sufficient blood or fluid accumulates to compress the heart. When you detect pulsus paradoxus, quickly take the patient's other vital signs. Check for addi-

PULSE RHYTHM AND RATE	CLINICAL IMPLICATIONS
Irregular rhythm during PJCs; fast, slow, or normal rate	◆ PJCs may result from myocardial infarction (MI) or ischemia, excessive caffeine intake and, most commonly, with digoxin toxicity (from enhanced automaticity).
Irregular ventricular rhythm; fast, slow, or normal rate	◆ Type I heart block is commonly transient, but it may progress to complete heart block. ◆ It may result from an inferior wall MI, digoxin or quinidine toxicity, vagal stimulation, electrolyte imbalance, or arteriosclerotic heart disease.
Irregular ventricular rhythm; slow or normal rate	◆ Type II heart block may progress to complete heart block. ◆ It may result from a degenerative disease of the conduction system, ischemia of the AV node in an anterior MI, anteroseptal infarction, electrolyte imbalance, or digoxin or quinidine toxicity.
Usually irregular rhythm with a long pause after the premature beat; fast, slow, or normal rate	◆ PVCs arise from different ventricular sites or from the same site with changing patterns of conduction. ◆ These contractions may result from caffeine or alcohol consumption, stress, myocardial ischemia or infarction, myocardial irritation by pacemaker electrodes, hypocalcemia, hypercalcemia, digoxin toxicity, or exercise.

tional signs and symptoms of cardiac tamponade, such as dyspnea, tachypnea, diaphoresis, jugular vein distention, tachycardia, narrowed pulse pressure, and hypotension. Emergency pericardiocente- *sis to aspirate blood or fluid from the pericardial sac may be necessary. Then evaluate the effectiveness of pericardiocentesis by measuring the degree of*

COMPARING ARTERIAL PRESSURE WAVES

The waveforms shown here help differentiate a normal arterial pulse from pulsus alternans, pulsus bisferiens, and pulsus paradoxus.

Normal arterial pulse

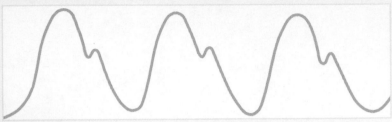

Pulsus alternans

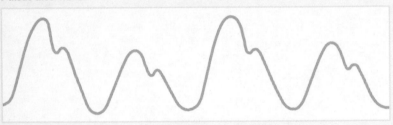

Pulsus bisferiens

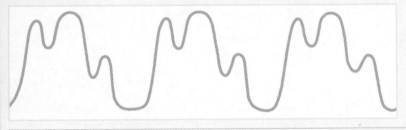

Pulsus paradoxus

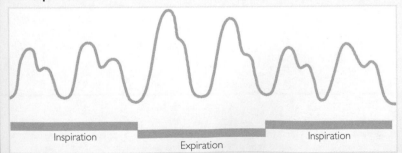

The percussion wave in a *normal arterial pulse* reflects ejection of blood into the aorta (early systole). The tidal wave is the peak of the pulse wave (later systole), and the dicrotic notch marks the beginning of diastole.

Pulsus alternans is a beat-to-beat alternation in pulse size and intensity. Although the rhythm of pulsus alternans is regular, the volume varies. If you take the blood pressure of a patient with this abnormality, you'll first hear a loud Korotkoff sound and then a soft sound. The two sounds will alternate continually. Pulsus alternans commonly accompanies states of poor contractility that occur with left-sided heart failure.

Pulsus bisferiens is a double-beating pulse with two systolic peaks. The first beat reflects pulse pressure and the second reverberation from the periphery. Pulsus bisferiens commonly occurs with aortic insufficiency (aortic stenosis, aortic regurgitation), hypertrophic cardiomyopathy or high cardiac output states.

Pulsus paradoxus is an exaggerated decline in blood pressure during inspiration, resulting from an increase in negative intrathoracic pressure. Pulsus paradoxus that exceeds 10 mm Hg is considered abnormal and may result from cardiac tamponade, constrictive pericarditis, or severe lung disease.

pulsus paradoxus; it should decrease after aspiration.

ASSESSMENT
History
If you've ruled out cardiac tamponade, obtain the patient's history. Does he have a history of chronic cardiac or pulmonary disease? Ask about the development of associated signs and symptoms, such as cough or chest pain.

Physical examination
Auscultate for abnormal breath sounds and assess the patient's respiratory status, oxygenation, and effort. Assess the patient's vital signs and cardiovascular system, and monitor his cardiac rhythm.

Pediatric pointers
Pulsus paradoxus commonly occurs in children who have chronic pulmonary disease. It typically arises during an acute asthma attack. Children with pericarditis may also develop pulsus paradoxus due to cardiac tamponade, although this disorder more commonly affects adults. Pulsus paradoxus above 20 mm Hg is a reliable indicator of cardiac tamponade in children; a change of 10 to 20 mm Hg is equivocal.

MEDICAL CAUSES
● *Cardiac tamponade.* Pulsus paradoxus commonly occurs with cardiac tamponade, but it may be difficult to detect if intrapericardial pressure rises abruptly and profound hypotension occurs. With severe tamponade, assessment also reveals these classic findings: hypotension, diminished or muffled heart sounds, and jugular vein distention. Related findings include chest pain, pericardial friction rub, narrowed pulse pressure, anxiety, restlessness, clammy skin, and hepatomegaly. Characteristic respiratory signs and symptoms include dyspnea, tachypnea, and cyanosis; the patient typically sits up and leans forward to facilitate breathing.

If cardiac tamponade develops gradually, pulsus paradoxus may be accompanied by weakness, anorexia, and weight loss. The patient may also report chest pain, but he won't have muffled heart sounds or severe hypotension.
● *Chronic obstructive pulmonary disease (COPD).* The wide fluctuations in intrathoracic pressure that characterize COPD pro-

duce pulsus paradoxus and possibly tachycardia. Other findings vary but may include dyspnea, tachypnea, wheezing, productive or nonproductive cough, accessory muscle use, barrel chest, and clubbing. The patient may show labored, pursed-lip breathing after exertion or even at rest. He typically sits up and leans forward to facilitate breathing. Auscultation reveals decreased breath sounds, rhonchi, and crackles. Weight loss, cyanosis, and edema may occur.

● *Pericarditis (chronic constrictive).* Pulsus paradoxus can occur in up to 50% of patients with chronic constrictive pericarditis. Other findings include pericardial friction rub, chest pain, exertional dyspnea, orthopnea, hepatomegaly, and ascites. Patients also exhibit peripheral edema and Kussmaul's sign—jugular vein distention that becomes more prominent on inspiration.

● *Pulmonary embolism (massive).* Decreased left ventricular filling and stroke volume in massive pulmonary embolism produce pulsus paradoxus as well as syncope and severe apprehension, dyspnea, tachypnea, and pleuritic chest pain. The patient appears cyanotic, with jugular vein distention. He may succumb to circulatory collapse, with hypotension and a weak, rapid pulse. Pulmonary infarction may produce hemoptysis along with decreased breath sounds and a pleural friction rub over the affected area.

● *Right ventricular infarction.* Infarction may produce pulsus paradoxus and elevated jugular venous or central venous pressure. Other findings are similar to those of myocardial infarction.

NURSING CONSIDERATIONS

Prepare the patient for an echocardiogram to visualize cardiac motion and help determine the causative disorder. If a pulmonary embolus is suspected, prepare the patient for a ventilation/perfusion scan. A helical CT scan of the chest or pulmonary arteriogram may also be indicated. Also, monitor his vital signs and frequently check the degree of paradox. An increase in the degree of paradox may indicate recurring or worsening cardiac tamponade or impending respiratory arrest in severe COPD. Vigorous respiratory treatment, such as chest physiotherapy, may avert the need for endotracheal intubation.

PATIENT TEACHING

Provide information about the disorder and symptoms to immediately report to the physician. Teach the patient techniques to conserve energy and decrease oxygen demands on the body. Provide information on diagnostic tests and treatment for pulsus paradoxus, including probable oxygen therapy.

Pupillary changes

Pupillary changes include nonreactive pupils or pupils that are sluggish. Nonreactive (fixed) pupils fail to constrict in response to light or to dilate when the light is removed. The development of a unilateral or bilateral nonreactive response indicates an important change in the patient's condition and may signal a life-threatening emergency and possibly brain death. It also occurs with the use of certain optic drugs.

A sluggish pupillary reaction is an abnormally slow pupillary response to light. It can occur in one pupil or both, unlike the normal reaction, which is always bilateral. A sluggish reaction accompanies degenerative disease of the central nervous system and diabetic neuropathy. It can occur normally in the elderly, whose pupils become smaller and less responsive with age.

Act now *If the patient is unconscious and develops unilateral or bilateral nonreactive pupils, quickly take his vital signs. Stay alert for decerebrate or decorticate posture, bradycardia, elevated systolic blood pressure, widened pulse pressure, and the development of other untoward changes in the patient's condition. Remember, a unilateral dilated, nonreactive pupil may be an early sign of uncal brain herniation. Emergency surgery to decrease intracranial pressure (ICP) may be necessary. If the patient isn't already being treated for increased ICP, insert an I.V. line to administer a diuretic, an osmotic, or a corticosteroid. You may also need to start the patient on controlled hyperventilation.*

ASSESSMENT
History

If the patient is conscious, obtain a brief history. Does he use eyedrops? If so, what type and when did he last instill them? Also ask if he's experiencing pain and, if so, try to determine its location, intensity, and duration.

Physical examination

Check the patient's visual acuity in both eyes. Then test the pupillary reaction to accommodation: Normally, both pupils constrict equally as the patient shifts his glance from a distant to a near object.

Next, hold a penlight at the side of each eye and examine the cornea and iris for abnormalities. Measure intraocular pressure (IOP) with a tonometer, or estimate IOP by placing your second and third fingers over the patient's closed eyelid. If the eyeball feels rock-hard, suspect elevated IOP. Ophthalmoscopic and slit-lamp examinations of the eye will need to be performed. If the patient has experienced ocular trauma, don't manipulate the affected eye. After the examination, be sure to cover the affected eye with a protective metal shield, but don't let the shield rest on the globe.

To assess pupillary reaction to light, first test the patient's direct light reflex. Darken the room, and cover one of the patient's eyes while you hold open the opposite eyelid. Using a bright penlight, bring the light toward the patient from the side and shine it directly into his opened eye. If normal, the pupil will promptly constrict. Next, test the consensual light reflex. Hold both of the patient's eyelids open, and shine the light into one eye while watching the pupil of the opposite eye. If normal, both pupils will promptly constrict. Repeat both procedures to test light reflexes in the opposite eye. A sluggish reaction in one or both pupils indicates dysfunction of cranial nerves (CNs) II and III, which mediate the pupillary light reflex. (See *Innervation of direct and consensual light reflexes,* page 250.)

Pediatric pointers

Children have nonreactive and sluggish pupils for the same reasons as adults. The most common cause is oculomotor nerve palsy from increased ICP.

MEDICAL CAUSES

- *Adie's syndrome.* Adie's syndrome produces an abrupt onset of unilateral mydriasis along with a sluggish or nonreactive pupillary response. It may also produce blurred vision and cramplike eye pain. Eventually, both eyes may be affected. Musculoskeletal assessment reveals hypoactive or absent deep tendon reflexes (DTRs) in the arms and legs.

- *Botulism.* Bilateral mydriasis and nonreactive pupils usually appear 12 to 36 hours after ingestion of tainted food. Other early findings include blurred vision, diplopia, ptosis, strabismus, and extraocular muscle palsies, along with anorexia, nausea, vomiting, diarrhea, and dry mouth. Vertigo, deafness, hoarseness, nasal voice, dysarthria, and dysphagia follow. Progressive muscle weakness and absent DTRs usually evolve over 2 to 4 days, resulting in severe constipation and paralysis of respiratory muscles with respiratory distress.

- *Diabetic neuropathy.* A patient with long-standing diabetes mellitus may have a sluggish pupillary response. Additional findings include orthostatic hypotension, syncope, dysphagia, episodic constipation or diarrhea, painless bladder distention with overflow incontinence, retrograde ejaculation, and impotence.

- *Encephalitis.* As encephalitis progresses, initially sluggish pupils become dilated and nonreactive. Decreased accommodation and other symptoms of cranial nerve palsies, such as dysphagia, develop. Within 48 hours after onset, encephalitis causes a decreased level of consciousness, high fever, headache, vomiting, and nuchal rigidity. Aphasia, ataxia, nystagmus, hemiparesis, and photophobia may occur with seizures.

- *Familial amyloid polyneuropathy.* Familial amyloid polyneuropathy produces sluggish or nonreactive pupils and miosis. Corneal opacities may affect visual acuity. The patient may also experience anhidrosis, orthostatic hypotension, alternating diarrhea and constipation, and impotence. Initially, he'll experience paresthesia and possibly pain in the feet and lower legs; later, absent DTRs and thinning legs will develop.

- *Glaucoma (acute angle-closure).* An ophthalmic emergency, examination reveals a moderately dilated, nonreactive pupil in the affected eye. Conjunctival injection, corneal clouding, and decreased visual acuity also occur. The patient experiences a sudden onset of blurred vision, followed by excruciating pain in and around the affected eye. He commonly reports seeing halos around white lights at night. Severely elevated IOP commonly induces nausea and vomiting.

- *Herpes zoster.* The patient with herpes zoster affecting the nasociliary nerve may

INNERVATION OF DIRECT AND CONSENSUAL LIGHT REFLEXES

The pupillary light reflex consists of two reactions—direct and consensual. Normally, shining a light directly onto the retina of one eye stimulates the parasympathetic nerves to cause brisk constriction of that pupil—the *direct light reflex*. The pupil of the opposite eye also constricts—the *consensual light reflex*.

The optic nerve (cranial nerve [CN] II) mediates the afferent arc of this reflex from each eye, whereas the oculomotor nerve (CN III) mediates the efferent arc to both eyes. A nonreactive or sluggish response in one or both pupils indicates dysfunction of these cranial nerves, usually due to degenerative disease of the central nervous system.

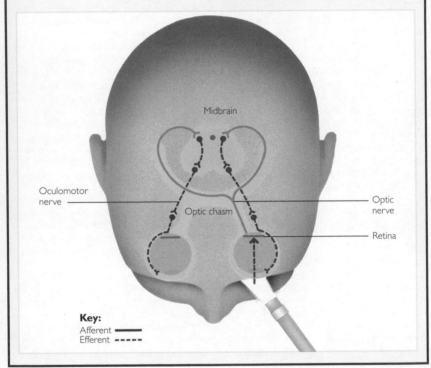

Midbrain

Oculomotor nerve

Optic chasm

Optic nerve

Retina

Key:
Afferent ——————
Efferent ----------

have a sluggish pupillary response. Examination of the conjunctiva reveals follicles. Additional ocular findings include a serous discharge, absence of tears, ptosis, and extraocular muscle palsy.

- *Iris disease (degenerative or inflammatory).* Iris disease causes pupillary nonreactivity in the affected eyes. Visual acuity may also decrease.
- *Midbrain lesions.* Although rare, midbrain lesions produce bilateral midposition nonreactive pupils. Other findings include loss of upward gaze, coma, central neurogenic hy-

perventilation, bradycardia, hemiparesis or hemiplegia, and decorticate or decerebrate posture.
- *Multiple sclerosis (MS).* MS may produce small, irregularly shaped pupils that react better to accommodation than to light. Additional ocular findings may include ptosis, nystagmus, diplopia, and blurred vision. In most cases, vision problems and sensory impairment, such as paresthesia, are the earliest indications along with weakness, numbness, tingling, and unsteadiness. Features that may occur later include intention tremor, spastici-

ty, hyperreflexia, and gait ataxia as well as muscle weakness and paralysis, dysphagia and dysarthria, constipation, and urinary urgency, frequency, and incontinence. The patient may also develop impotence and emotional instability.

● *Ocular trauma.* Severe damage to the iris or optic nerve may produce a nonreactive, dilated pupil in the affected eye (traumatic iridoplegia). This sign is usually transitory but can be permanent. Slit-lamp examination commonly reveals a V-shaped notch in the pupillary rim, indicating a tear in the iris sphincter muscle. The patient usually experiences eye pain and may also develop eye edema and ecchymoses.

● *Oculomotor nerve palsy.* The first signs of this oculomotor ophthalmoplegia commonly include a dilated, nonreactive pupil and loss of the accommodation reaction. These findings may occur in one eye or both, depending on whether the palsy is unilateral or bilateral. Among the causes of total third cranial nerve palsy is life-threatening brain herniation. Central herniation causes bilateral midposition nonreactive pupils, whereas uncal herniation initially causes a unilateral dilated, nonreactive pupil. Other common findings include diplopia, ptosis, outward deviation of the eye, and inability to elevate or adduct the eye. Additional findings depend on the underlying cause of the palsy.

● *Tertiary syphilis.* A sluggish pupillary reaction (especially in Argyll Robertson pupils) occurs in the late stage of neurosyphilis, along with marked weakness of the extraocular muscles, visual field defects and, possibly, cataractous changes in the lens. The patient may complain of orbital rim pain that worsens at night. He may also exhibit lid edema, decreased visual acuity, and exophthalmos. Tertiary lesions appear on the skin and mucous membranes. Liver, respiratory, cardiovascular, and additional neurologic dysfunction may also occur.

● *Uveitis.* A small, nonreactive pupil that appears suddenly with severe eye pain, conjunctival injection, diminished vision, and photophobia typifies anterior uveitis. With posterior uveitis, similar features develop insidiously, along with blurred vision and a distorted pupil shape.

● *Wernicke's disease.* Initially, Wernicke's disease produces an intention tremor accompanied by a sluggish pupillary reaction. Later, pupils may become nonreactive. Additional ocular findings include diplopia, gaze paralysis, nystagmus, ptosis, decreased visual acuity, and conjunctival injection. The patient may also exhibit orthostatic hypotension, tachycardia, ataxia, apathy, and confusion.

OTHER CAUSES

● *Drugs.* Instillation of a topical mydriatic and a cycloplegic may induce a temporarily nonreactive pupil in the affected eye. Opiates, such as heroin and morphine, cause pinpoint pupils with a minimal light response that can be seen only with a magnifying glass. And atropine poisoning produces widely dilated, nonreactive pupils.

NURSING CONSIDERATIONS

If the patient is conscious, monitor his pupillary light reflex to detect changes. If he's unconscious, close his eyes to prevent corneal exposure. (Use tape to secure the eyelids, if needed.) A sluggish pupillary reaction isn't diagnostically significant, although it occurs with various disorders.

PATIENT TEACHING

Stress the importance of regular ophthalmologic examinations. Provide information and techniques to use to reduce photophobia. Teach the patient self-care techniques related to diabetes. Provide information on maintaining a safe home environment.

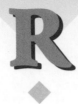

Respirations, grunting

Characterized by a deep, low-pitched grunting sound at the end of each breath, grunting respirations are a chief sign of respiratory distress in infants and children. They may be soft and heard only on auscultation, or loud and clearly audible without a stethoscope. Typically, the intensity of grunting respirations reflects the severity of respiratory distress. The grunting sound coincides with closure of the glottis, an effort to increase end-expiratory pressure in the lungs and prolong alveolar gas exchange, thereby enhancing ventilation and perfusion.

Grunting respirations indicate intrathoracic disease with lower respiratory involvement. Though most common in children, they sometimes occur in adults who are in severe respiratory distress. Whether they occur in children or in adults, grunting respirations demand immediate medical attention.

Act now *If the patient exhibits grunting respirations, quickly place him in a comfortable position and check for signs of respiratory distress:*
- *accessory muscle use*
- *cyanotic lips or nail beds*
- *decreased level of consciousness.*
- *hypotension (less than 90/60 mm Hg in adults or poor capillary refill in children)*
- *nasal flaring*
- *substernal, subcostal, or intercostal retractions, or shoulder elevations*
- *tachycardia (a minimum of 160 beats/minute in infants, 120 to 140 beats/minute in children ages 1 to 5, 120 beats/minute in children older than age 5, or 100 beats/minute in adults)*
- *tachypnea (a minimum respiratory rate of 60 breaths/minute in infants, 40 breaths/minute in children ages 1 to 5, 30 breaths/minute in children older than age 5, or 20 breaths/minute in adults)*
- *wheezing*

If you detect any of these signs, monitor oxygen saturation, and administer oxygen and prescribed medications such as a bronchodilator. Also, have emergency equipment available and prepare to intubate the patient if necessary. Obtain arterial blood gas (ABG) analysis to determine oxygenation status.

ASSESSMENT
History
After addressing the child's respiratory status, ask his parents when the grunting respirations began. Is he usually healthy with normal growth and development? If the patient is a premature infant, find out his gestational age. Ask the parents if anyone in the home has recently had an upper respiratory tract infection. Has the child had signs and symptoms of such an infection, such as a runny nose, cough, low-grade fever, or anorexia? Does he have a history of frequent colds or upper respiratory tract infections? Does he have a history of respiratory syncytial virus? Ask the parents to describe changes in the child's activity level or feeding pattern to determine if the child is lethargic or less alert than usual.

Physical examination
Begin the physical examination by inspecting the rate, depth, and ease of respirations and

any signs of respiratory distress. Auscultate the lungs, especially the lower lobes. Note diminished or abnormal sounds, such as crackles or sibilant rhonchi, which may indicate mucus or fluid buildup. Also, characterize the color, amount, and consistency of discharge or sputum. Note the characteristics of the cough, if any. Observe for abrupt behavior changes and lowered level of consciousness.

MEDICAL CAUSES

● *Asthma.* Grunting respirations and wheezing may be apparent during a severe asthma attack, usually triggered by an upper respiratory tract infection or an allergic response. As the attack progresses, dyspnea, chest tightness, and coughing occur. Patients may have a silent chest if air movement is poor. Immediate bronchodilator and corticosteroid therapy is needed.

● *Heart failure.* A late sign of left-sided heart failure, grunting respirations accompany increasing pulmonary edema. Associated features include a productive cough, crackles, jugular vein distention, and chest wall retractions. Cyanosis may also be evident, depending on the underlying congenital cardiac defect.

● *Pneumonia.* Life-threatening bacterial pneumonia is common after an upper respiratory tract infection or cold. *Pneumocystis carinii (jiroveci)* pneumonia commonly affects children infected with human immunodeficiency virus. It causes grunting respirations accompanied by high fever, tachypnea, nonproductive or scantly productive cough, anorexia, and lethargy. Auscultation reveals diminished breath sounds, scattered crackles, and sibilant rhonchi over the affected lung. As the disorder progresses, patients may also develop severe dyspnea, substernal and subcostal retractions, nasal flaring, cyanosis, and increasing lethargy. Some infants display GI signs, such as vomiting, diarrhea, and abdominal distention. Oxygen therapy is often needed.

● *Respiratory distress syndrome.* The result of lung immaturity in a premature infant (less than 37 weeks' gestation) usually of low birth weight, respiratory distress syndrome initially causes audible expiratory grunting along with intercostal, subcostal, or substernal retractions accompanied by tachycardia and tachypnea. Later, as respiratory distress tires the infant, apnea or irregular respirations replace the grunting. Severe respiratory distress is characterized by cyanosis, frothy sputum, dramatic nasal flaring, lethargy, bradycardia, and hypotension. Eventually, the infant becomes unresponsive. Auscultation reveals harsh, diminished breath sounds and crackles over the base of the lungs on deep inspiration. Oliguria and peripheral edema may also occur. This disease can occur in all age groups, as a result of aspiration, infection, embolism, shock, trauma, and other causes. Findings are similar in all ages.

NURSING CONSIDERATIONS

Closely monitor the patient's condition. Keep emergency equipment nearby in case respiratory distress worsens. Prepare to administer oxygen using an oxygen hood or tent. Continually monitor ABG levels and deliver the minimum amount of oxygen possible, to avoid causing retinopathy of prematurity from excessively high oxygen levels.

Begin inhalation therapy with a bronchodilator, and administer an I.V. antimicrobial if the patient has pneumonia (or, in some cases, status asthmaticus). Follow these measures with chest physical therapy, as necessary. (See *Positioning an infant for chest physical therapy,* pages 254 and 255.)

Prepare the patient for chest X-rays. Because sedatives are contraindicated during respiratory distress, the restless child must be restrained during testing, as necessary. To prevent exposure to radiation, wear a lead apron and cover the child's genital area with a lead shield. If a blood culture is ordered, be sure to record on the laboratory slip current antibiotic use.

Remember to explain all procedures to the patient's parents and to provide emotional support.

PATIENT TEACHING

Teach the patient's parents how to perform respiratory care and therapy in the home. Instruct them in the proper use of prescribed medications. Explain signs and symptoms that require immediate attention. If the grunting is related to asthma, teach the parents measures to assist them in managing the condition and reducing allergins in the home environment.

(Text continues on page 256.)

POSITIONING AN INFANT FOR CHEST PHYSICAL THERAPY

An infant with grunting respirations may need chest physical therapy to mobilize and drain excess lung secretions. Auscultate first to locate congested areas, and determine the best drainage position. Then review the illustrations here, which show the various drainage positions and where to place your hands for percussion. Use the fingers of one hand to perform percussion. Vibrate these fingers and move them toward the infant's head to facilitate drainage.

Hold the infant upright and about 30 degrees forward to percuss and drain the apical segments of the upper lobes.

Place the infant in a supine position to percuss and drain the anterior segments of the upper lobes.

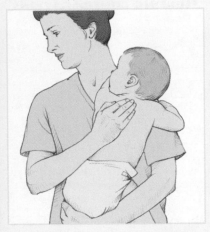

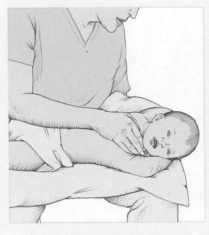

Use this position to percuss and drain the posterior segments of the upper lobes.

Hold the infant at a 45-degree angle on his side with his head down about 15 degrees to percuss and drain the right middle lobe.

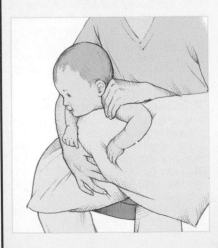

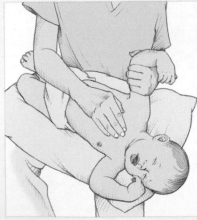

Place the infant in a supine position with his head 30 degrees lower than his feet to percuss and drain the anterior segments of the lower lobes.

Place the infant in a prone position with his head down 30 degrees to percuss and drain the posterior basal segments of the lower lobes.

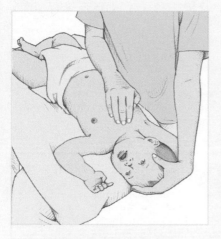

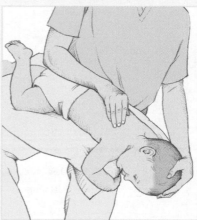

Place the infant on his side with his head down 30 degrees to percuss and drain the lateral basal segments of the lower lobes. Repeat this on the other side.

Use a prone position to percuss and drain the superior segments of the lower lobes.

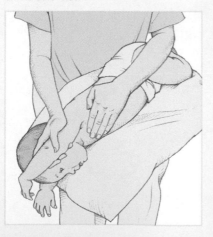

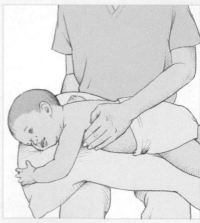

Respirations, shallow

Respirations are shallow when a diminished volume of air enters the lungs during inspiration. In an effort to obtain enough air, the patient with shallow respirations usually breathes at an accelerated rate. However, as he tires or as his muscles weaken, this compensatory increase in respirations diminishes, leading to inadequate gas exchange and such signs as dyspnea, cyanosis, confusion, agitation, loss of consciousness, and tachycardia.

Shallow respirations may develop suddenly or gradually and may last briefly or become chronic. They're a key sign of respiratory distress and neurologic deterioration. Causes include inadequate central respiratory control over breathing, neuromuscular disorders, increased resistance to airflow into the lungs, respiratory muscle fatigue or weakness, voluntary alterations in breathing, decreased activity from prolonged bed rest, pain, procedural sedation, and substance abuse.

Act now *If you observe shallow respirations, stay alert for impending respiratory failure or arrest. Is the patient severely dyspneic or agitated or frightened? Look for signs of airway obstruction. Use suction as necessary. If an adult patient is choking, use the Heimlich maneuver unless the patient becomes unresponsive. Then place the patient supine, attempt four rescue breaths and perform five abdominal thrusts to try to expel the foreign object.*

If the patient is also wheezing, check for stridor, nasal flaring, and accessory muscle use. Administer oxygen with a face mask or a handheld resuscitation bag. Attempt to calm the patient. Administer epinephrine I.V. Insert an artificial airway and prepare for endotracheal intubation and ventilatory support. Measure his tidal volume and minute volume with a Wright respirometer to determine the need for mechanical ventilation. (See Measuring lung volumes.) If the emergency is less acute,

---

MEASURING LUNG VOLUMES

Use a Wright respirometer to measure tidal volume (the amount of air inspired with each breath) and minute volume (the volume of air inspired in a minute — or tidal volume multiplied by respiratory rate). You can connect the respirometer to an intubated patient's airway via an endotracheal tube (shown here) or a tracheostomy tube. If the patient isn't intubated, connect the respirometer to a face mask, making sure that the seal over his mouth and nose is airtight.

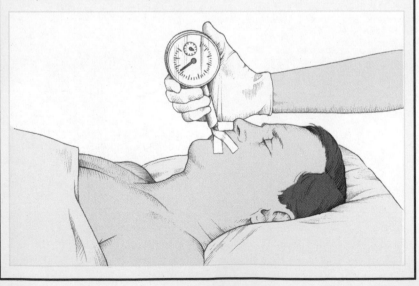

check arterial blood gas (ABG) levels, heart rate, blood pressure, and oxygen saturation. Tachycardia, increased or decreased blood pressure, poor minute volume, and deteriorating ABG levels or oxygen saturation signal the need for intubation and mechanical ventilation, whether the patient is conscious or unconscious.

ASSESSMENT
History
If the patient isn't in severe respiratory distress, begin with the history. Ask about chronic illness and surgery or trauma. Has he had a tetanus booster in the past 10 years? Does he have asthma, allergies, or a history of heart failure or vascular disease? Does he have a chronic respiratory disorder or respiratory tract infection, tuberculosis, or a neurologic or neuromuscular disease? Does he smoke or has he smoked in the past? Obtain a drug history as well, and explore the possibility of drug abuse.

Ask about the patient's shallow respirations. When did they begin? How long do they last? What makes them subside? What aggravates them? Ask about changes in appetite, weight, activity level, and behavior.

Physical examination
Begin the physical examination by assessing the patient's level of consciousness (LOC) and his orientation to time, person, and place. Observe spontaneous movements, and test muscle strength and deep tendon reflexes (DTRs). Next, inspect the chest for deformities or abnormal movements such as intercostal retractions. Inspect the extremities for cyanosis and digital clubbing.

Now, palpate for expansion and diaphragmatic tactile fremitus, and percuss for hyperresonance or dullness. Auscultate for diminished, absent, or adventitious breath sounds and for abnormal or distant heart sounds. Do you note peripheral edema? Finally, examine the abdomen for distention, tenderness, or masses. (See *Shallow respirations: Causes and associated findings,* pages 258 to 261.)

Pediatric pointers
In children, shallow respirations commonly indicate a life-threatening condition. Airway obstruction can occur rapidly because of narrow passageways; if it does, administer back blows or chest thrusts but not abdominal thrusts, which can damage internal organs.

Causes of shallow respirations in infants and children include idiopathic (infant) respiratory distress syndrome, acute epiglottiditis, diphtheria, aspiration of a foreign body, croup, acute bronchiolitis, cystic fibrosis, and bacterial pneumonia.

Observe the child to detect apnea. As needed, use humidification and suction, and administer supplemental oxygen. Give parenteral fluids to ensure adequate hydration. Chest physiotherapy may be required.

Geriatric pointers
Stiffness or deformity of the chest wall associated with aging may cause shallow respirations.

MEDICAL CAUSES
- *Acute respiratory distress syndrome (ARDS).* Initially, life-threatening ARDS produces rapid, shallow respirations and dyspnea, at times after the patient appears stable. Hypoxemia leads to intercostal and suprasternal retractions, diaphoresis, and fluid accumulation, causing rhonchi and crackles. As hypoxemia worsens, the patient exhibits more difficulty breathing, restlessness, apprehension, a decreased LOC, cyanosis and, possibly, tachycardia.
- *Amyotrophic lateral sclerosis (ALS).* Respiratory muscle weakness in ALS causes progressive shallow respirations. Exertion may result in increased weakness and respiratory distress. ALS initially produces upper extremity muscle weakness and wasting, which in several years affect the trunk, neck, tongue, and muscles of the larynx, pharynx, and lower extremities. Associated signs and symptoms include muscle cramps and atrophy, hyperreflexia, slight spasticity of the legs, coarse fasciculations of the affected muscle, impaired speech, and difficulty chewing and swallowing.
- *Asthma.* With asthma, bronchospasm and hyperinflation of the lungs cause rapid, shallow respirations. In adults, mild persistent signs and symptoms may worsen during severe attacks. Related respiratory effects include expiratory wheezing, rhonchi, dry cough, dyspnea, prolonged expirations, intercostal and supraclavicular retractions on inspiration, nasal flaring, and accessory muscle use. Chest tightness, tachycardia, diaphoresis, and flushing or cyanosis may occur.

(Text continues on page 260.)

SHALLOW RESPIRATIONS: CAUSES AND ASSOCIATED SYMPTOMS

MAJOR ASSOCIATED SIGNS AND SYMPTOMS

COMMON CAUSES	Accessory muscle use	Anxiety	Asymmetrical chest expansion	Chest pain	Chest tightness	Costal retractions	Cough	Crackles	Cyanosis	Decreased breath sounds	Decreased LOC	Diaphoresis	Diplopia	Dysarthnia	Dysphagia	Dyspnea	Fatigue	Fever
Acute respiratory distress syndrome		●				●		●	●		●	●				●		
Amyotrophic lateral sclerosis														●	●			
Asthma	●				●	●	●					●				●		
Atelectasis		●				●	●		●	●		●				●		
Botulism													●	●	●			
Bronchiectasis							●	●								●	●	●
Chronic bronchitis							●		●	●						●		
Coma											●							
Emphysema	●						●		●	●						●		
Flail chest			●					●										
Fractured ribs																		
Guillain-Barré syndrome														●	●			
Kyphoscoliosis																●	●	
Muscular dystrophy																		
Myasthenia gravis									●				●		●	●	●	
Obesity									●							●		
Parkinson's disease														●	●		●	
Pleural effusion				●		●				●						●		
Pneumonia				●			●	●	●	●		●				●	●	●

	Flushing	Gait disturbance	Headache	Hemoptysis	Hyperreflexia	Jaw pain & stiffness	Low blood pressure	Muscle weakness	Mydriasis	Nasal flaring	Nausea & vomiting	Pain	Paralysis	Peripheral edema	Pleural friction rub	Prolonged expiration	Restlessness	Rhonchi	Stridor	Tachycardia	Tachypnea	Weakness	Weight loss	Wheezing
																	●	●		●				
					●			●														●		
	●									●						●				●				●
																				●	●			
								●	●		●		●											
				●														●					●	●
			●	●										●										●
								●					●											
								●								●					●			
							●					●								●				
												●												
								●					●											
												●												
								●																
								●																
															●									
		●																					●	
										●										●	●		●	
			●									●							●	●				

(continued)

MAJOR ASSOCIATED SIGNS AND SYMPTOMS

COMMON CAUSES	Accessory muscle use	Anxiety	Asymmetrical chest expansion	Chest pain	Chest tightness	Costal retractions	Cough	Crackles	Cyanosis	Decreased breath sounds	Decreased LOC	Diaphoresis	Diplopia	Dysarthria	Dysphagia	Dyspnea	Fatigue	Fever
Pneumothorax	●	●		●			●		●	●						●		
Pulmonary edema		●					●	●	●			●				●		
Pulmonary embolism				●			●	●	●							●		●
Spinal cord injury																		
Tetanus												●		●	●			
Upper airway obstruction							●		●	●						●		

● **Atelectasis.** Decreased lung expansion or pleuritic pain causes a sudden onset of rapid, shallow respirations. Other signs and symptoms include dry cough, dyspnea, tachycardia, anxiety, cyanosis, tachypnea, hypoxia, and diaphoresis. Examination reveals dullness on percussion, decreased breath sounds and vocal fremitus, inspiratory lag, and substernal or intercostal retractions.

● **Botulism.** With botulism, progressive muscle weakness and paralysis initially cause shallow respirations. Within 4 days, the patient develops respiratory distress from respiratory muscle paralysis. Early signs and symptoms include bilateral mydriasis and nonreactive pupils, anorexia, nausea, vomiting, diarrhea, dry mouth, blurred vision, diplopia, ptosis, strabismus, and extraocular muscle palsies. Other signs quickly follow, including vertigo, deafness, hoarseness, constipation, nasal voice, dysarthria, and dysphagia.

● **Bronchiectasis.** Increased secretions obstruct airflow in the lungs, leading to shallow respirations and a productive cough with copious, foul-smelling, mucopurulent sputum (a classic finding). Other findings include hemoptysis, wheezing, rhonchi, coarse crackles during inspiration, and late-stage clubbing. The patient may complain of weight loss, fatigue, exertional weakness and dyspnea, fever, malaise, and halitosis.

● **Chronic bronchitis.** Airway obstruction causes chronic shallow respirations. Chronic bronchitis may begin with a nonproductive, hacking cough that later becomes productive. It may also cause diminished breath sounds, wheezing, intermittent dyspnea, hemoptysis, morning headache, cyanosis, pedal edema, weight gain, and distant heart sounds.

● **Coma.** Rapid, shallow respirations result from neurologic dysfunction or restricted chest movement.

● **Emphysema.** Increased breathing effort causes muscle fatigue, leading to chronic shallow respirations. The patient may also display dyspnea, anorexia, malaise, tachy-

Flushing	Gait disturbance	Headache	Hemoptysis	Hyperreflexia	Jaw pain & stiffness	Low blood pressure	Muscle weakness	Mydriasis	Nasal flaring	Nausea & vomiting	Pain	Paralysis	Peripheral edema	Pleural friction rub	Prolonged expiration	Restlessness	Rhonchi	Stridor	Tachycardia	Tachypnea	Weakness	Weight loss	Wheezing
																●			●	●			
						●											●		●	●			●
																	●		●	●			●
						●						●											
				●	●														●				
																			●	●			●

pnea, diminished breath sounds, cyanosis, pursed-lip breathing, accessory muscle use, barrel chest, chronic productive cough, and clubbing (a late sign).
- *Flail chest.* With flail chest, decreased air movement results in rapid, shallow respirations, paradoxical chest wall motion from rib instability, tachycardia, hypotension, ecchymoses, cyanosis, and pain over the affected area.
- *Fractured ribs.* Pain on inspiration and possibly expiration may cause shallow respirations.
- *Guillain-Barré syndrome.* Progressive ascending paralysis causes a rapid or progressive onset of shallow respirations. Muscle weakness begins in the lower limbs and extends finally to the face. Associated findings include paresthesia, dysarthria, diminished or absent corneal reflex, nasal speech, dysphagia, ipsilateral loss of facial muscle control, and flaccid paralysis.

Alert *In Guillain-Barré syndrome, monitor respirations carefully because the patient may need to be intubated if he goes into respiratory failure.*
- *Kyphoscoliosis.* Skeletal cage distortion can eventually cause rapid, shallow respirations from reduced lung capacity. It also causes back pain, fatigue, tracheal deviation, and dyspnea.
- *Muscular dystrophy.* With progressive thoracic deformity and muscle weakness, shallow respirations may occur along with waddling gait, contractures, scoliosis, lordosis, and muscle atrophy or hypertrophy.
- *Myasthenia gravis.* The progression of myasthenia gravis causes respiratory muscle weakness marked by shallow respirations, dyspnea, and cyanosis. Other effects include fatigue, weak eye closure, ptosis, diplopia, and difficulty chewing and swallowing.
- *Obesity.* Morbid obesity may cause shallow respirations due to the work of breathing associated with movement of the chest wall. Heart and breath sounds may be distant.

Alert *Morbid obesity may contribute to hypoventilation syndrome with decreased LOC, dyspnea, peripheral edema, and hypoxia requiring assisted ventilation.*

● *Parkinson's disease.* Fatigue and weakness lead to progressive shallow respirations. Typically, Parkinson's disease slowly progresses to increased rigidity (lead-pipe or cogwheel), masklike facies, stooped posture, shuffling gait, dysphagia, drooling, dysarthria, and pill-rolling tremor.

● *Pleural effusion.* With pleural effusion, restricted lung expansion causes shallow respirations, beginning suddenly or gradually. Other findings include nonproductive cough, weight loss, dyspnea, and pleuritic chest pain. Examination reveals pleural friction rub, tachycardia, tachypnea, decreased chest motion, flatness on percussion, egophony, decreased or absent breath sounds, and decreased tactile fremitus.

● *Pneumonia.* Pulmonary consolidation results in rapid, shallow respirations. The patient may experience dyspnea; fever; shaking chills; pleuritic chest pain; cough with dark, thick, or bloody sputum; tachycardia; decreased breath sounds; crackles; and rhonchi. He may also develop myalgia, fatigue, anorexia, headache, abdominal pain, cyanosis, and diaphoresis.

● *Pneumothorax.* Pneumothorax causes a sudden onset of shallow respirations and dyspnea. Related effects include sudden sharp, severe chest pain (commonly unilateral) worsening with movement, which may be accompanied by tachycardia, tachypnea, nonproductive cough, cyanosis, accessory muscle use, asymmetrical chest expansion, anxiety, restlessness, hyperresonance or tympany on the affected side, subcutaneous crepitation, decreased vocal fremitus, and diminished or absent breath sounds on the affected side.

● *Pulmonary edema.* Pulmonary vascular congestion causes rapid, shallow respirations. Early signs and symptoms include exertional dyspnea, orthopnea, paroxysmal nocturnal dyspnea, nonproductive cough, tachycardia, tachypnea, dependent crackles, and a ventricular gallop. Severe pulmonary edema produces more rapid, labored respirations and a productive cough with frothy, bloody sputum. Other signs and symptoms of severe pulmonary edema include widespread crackles, wheezing and rhonchi, worsening tachycardia, arrhythmias, cya-

nosis, hypotension, thready pulse, anxiety, and cold, clammy skin.

● *Pulmonary embolism.* Pulmonary embolism causes sudden, rapid, shallow respirations and severe dyspnea with angina or pleuritic chest pain. Other clinical features include tachycardia, tachypnea, a nonproductive cough or a productive cough with blood-tinged sputum, low-grade fever, restlessness, diaphoresis, pleural friction rub, crackles, diffuse wheezing, dullness on percussion, decreased breath sounds, and signs of circulatory collapse. Less common findings are massive hemoptysis, chest splinting, leg edema, and (with a large embolism) cyanosis, syncope, and jugular vein distention.

● *Spinal cord injury.* Diaphragmatic breathing and shallow respirations may occur in injury to the C5 to C8 area. Other findings include quadriplegia with flaccidity followed by spastic paralysis, areflexia, hypotension, sensory loss below the level of the injury, and bowel and bladder incontinence.

● *Tetanus.* With tetanus, a now rare disorder, spasm of the intercostal muscles and diaphragm causes shallow respirations. Late findings typically include jaw pain and stiffening, difficulty opening the mouth, tachycardia, fever, profuse diaphoresis, hyperactive DTRs, dysphagia, and opisthotonos.

● *Upper airway obstruction.* Partial airway obstruction causes acute shallow respirations with sudden gagging and dry, paroxysmal coughing accompanied by hoarseness, stridor, and tachycardia. Other findings include dyspnea, decreased breath sounds, wheezing, and cyanosis.

OTHER CAUSES

● *Drugs.* Opioids, sedatives and hypnotics, tranquilizers, neuromuscular blockers, magnesium sulfate, and anesthetics can produce slow, shallow respirations.

● *Surgery.* After abdominal or thoracic surgery, pain associated with chest splinting and decreased chest wall motion may cause shallow respirations.

NURSING CONSIDERATIONS

Prepare the patient for such diagnostic tests as ABG analysis, pulmonary function tests, chest X-rays, or bronchoscopy.

Position the patient as nearly upright as possible to ease his breathing. (Help a postoperative patient splint his incision while coughing.) If he's taking a drug that depresses respirations, follow all precautions, and monitor him closely. Ensure adequate hydration, and use humidification as needed to thin secretions and to relieve inflamed, dry, or irritated airway mucosa. Administer humidified oxygen, a bronchodilator, a mucolytic, an expectorant, or an antibiotic as ordered.

Turn the patient frequently. He may require chest physiotherapy, incentive spirometry, or intermittent positive-pressure breathing. Monitor the patient for increasing lethargy, which may indicate rising carbon dioxide levels. Have emergency equipment at the patient's bedside.

PATIENT TEACHING

Have the patient cough and deep-breathe every hour to clear secretions and to counteract possible hypoventilation. Provide information and teaching related to respiratory therapy and equipment that may be needed upon discharge. Provide emotional support to the patient and his family.

Respirations, stertorous

Characterized by a harsh, rattling, or snoring sound, stertorous respirations usually result from the vibration of relaxed oropharyngeal structures during sleep or coma, causing partial airway obstruction. Less commonly, these respirations result from retained mucus in the upper airway.

This common sign occurs in about 10% of normal individuals, especially middle-age, obese men. It may be aggravated by the use of alcohol or a sedative before bed, which increases oropharyngeal flaccidity, and by sleeping in the supine position, which allows the relaxed tongue to slip back into the airway. The major pathologic causes of stertorous respirations are obstructive sleep apnea and life-threatening upper airway obstruction associated with an oropharyngeal tumor or with uvular or palatal edema. This obstruction may also occur during the postictal phase of a generalized seizure when mucus secretions or a relaxed tongue blocks the airway or during postsurgery or conscious sedation.

Occasionally, stertorous respirations are mistaken for stridor, which is another sign of upper airway obstruction. However, stridor indicates laryngeal or tracheal obstruction, whereas stertorous respirations signal higher airway obstruction.

Act now *If you detect stertorous respirations, check the patient's mouth and throat for edema, redness, masses, or foreign objects. If edema is marked, quickly take his vital signs, including oxygen saturation. Observe the patient for signs and symptoms of respiratory distress, such as dyspnea, tachypnea, accessory muscle use, intercostal muscle retractions, and cyanosis. Elevate the head of the bed 30 degrees to help ease breathing and reduce edema. Then administer supplemental oxygen by nasal cannula or face mask, and prepare to intubate the patient, perform a tracheostomy, or provide mechanical ventilation. Insert an I.V. line for fluid and drug access, and begin cardiac monitoring.*

ASSESSMENT
History

Ask the patient about signs of sleep deprivation, such as personality changes, headaches, daytime somnolence, or decreased mental acuity. When possible, ask a family member whether the patient snores. If so, does his snoring awaken others? Does the snoring improve if he sleeps with the window open? Does the patient talk in his sleep or sleepwalk?

Physical examination

Perform a complete respiratory assessment. Examine the head, nose, and throat. If you detect stertorous respirations while the patient is sleeping, observe his breathing pattern for 3 to 4 minutes. Do noisy respirations cease when he turns on his side and recur when he assumes a supine position? Watch carefully for periods of apnea and note their length. Monitor the patient's level of oxygenation.

Pediatric pointers

In children, the most common cause of stertorous respirations is nasal or pharyngeal obstruction secondary to tonsillar or adenoid hypertrophy or the presence of a foreign body.

Geriatric pointers

Encourage the patient to seek treatment for sleep apnea.

MEDICAL CAUSES

● *Airway obstruction.* Regardless of its cause, partial airway obstruction may lead to stertorous respirations accompanied by wheezing, dyspnea, tachypnea and, later, intercostal retractions and nasal flaring. If the obstruction becomes complete, the patient abruptly loses his ability to talk and displays diaphoresis, tachycardia, and inspiratory chest movement but absent breath sounds. Severe hypoxemia rapidly ensues, resulting in cyanosis, loss of consciousness, and cardiopulmonary collapse.

● *Obstructive sleep apnea.* Loud and disruptive snoring is a major characteristic of obstructive sleep apnea, which commonly affects the obese. Typically, snoring alternates with periods of sleep apnea, which usually end with loud gasping sounds. Alternating tachycardia and bradycardia may occur.

Episodes of snoring and apnea recur in a cyclic pattern throughout the night. Sleep disturbances, such as somnambulism and talking during sleep, may also occur. Some patients display hypertension and ankle edema. Most awaken in the morning with a generalized headache, feeling tired and unrefreshed. The most common complaint is excessive daytime sleepiness. Lack of sleep may cause depression, hostility, and decreased mental acuity.

OTHER CAUSES

● *Endotracheal intubation, suction, or surgery.* These procedures may cause significant palatal or uvular edema, resulting in stertorous respirations.

NURSING CONSIDERATIONS

Continue to monitor the patient's respiratory status carefully. Administer a corticosteroid or an antibiotic and cool, humidified oxygen to reduce palatal and uvular inflammation and edema.

Laryngoscopy and bronchoscopy, to rule out airway obstruction, or formal sleep studies may be necessary.

PATIENT TEACHING

If excessive weight is related to the condition, discuss the importance and methods of weight loss. Explain the assembly and use of a continuous or bilevel positive airway pressure device for a patient with sleep apnea. Teach the patient to elevate his head while sleeping. Provide information and recommend a smoking cessation program if the patient smokes.

Retractions, costal and sternal

A cardinal sign of respiratory distress in infants and in children, retractions are visible indentations of the soft tissue covering the chest wall. They may be suprasternal (directly above the sternum and clavicles), intercostal (between the ribs), subcostal (below the lower costal margin of the rib cage), or substernal (just below the xiphoid process). Retractions may be mild or severe, producing barely visible to deep indentations.

Normally, infants and young children use abdominal muscles for breathing, unlike older children and adults, who use the diaphragm. When breathing requires extra effort, accessory muscles assist respiration, especially inspiration. Retractions typically accompany accessory muscle use.

Alert *A severely agitated child or a child crying in pain may also have sternal retractions.*

Act now *If you detect retractions in a child, check quickly for other signs of respiratory distress, such as cyanosis, tachypnea, tachycardia, and decreased oxygen saturation. Also, prepare the child for suctioning, insertion of an artificial airway, and oxygen administration.*

Observe the depth and location of retractions. Also note the rate, depth, and quality of respirations. Look for accessory muscle use, nasal flaring during inspiration, or grunting during expiration. If the child has a cough, record the color, consistency, and odor of sputum. Note whether the child appears restless or lethargic. Finally, auscultate the child's lungs to detect abnormal breath sounds. (See *Observing retractions.*)

ASSESSMENT
History

After the child's condition has been stabilized, obtain his medical history from his parents. Was he born prematurely? What was his birth weight? Was the delivery complicated? Ask about recent signs of an upper respiratory tract infection, such as runny nose, cough, and low-grade fever. How of-

Observing Retractions

When you observe retractions in infants and children, remember to note their exact location—an important clue to the cause and severity of respiratory distress. For example, subcostal and substernal retractions usually result from lower respiratory tract disorders; suprasternal retractions occur in upper respiratory tract disorders.

Mild intercostal retractions alone may be normal. However, intercostal retractions accompanied by subcostal and substernal retractions may indicate moderate respiratory distress. Deep suprasternal retractions typically indicate severe distress.

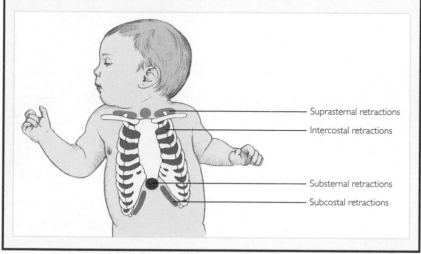

Suprasternal retractions
Intercostal retractions
Substernal retractions
Subcostal retractions

ten has the child had respiratory problems during the past year? Has he been in contact with anyone who has had a cold, the flu, or other respiratory ailments? Did he ever have respiratory syncytial virus? Did he aspirate food, liquid, or a foreign body? Inquire about a personal or family history of allergies or asthma.

Physical examination

If the child isn't in distress, complete a cardiopulmonary assessment. Take the child's vital signs, including his temperature. Monitor the child's level of oxygenation and breath sounds.

Pediatric pointers

When examining a child for retractions, remember that crying may accentuate the contractions.

Geriatric pointers

Although retractions may occur at any age, they're more difficult to visualize in an older patient who's obese or who has chronic chest wall stiffness or deformity.

MEDICAL CAUSES

- *Asthma attack.* Intercostal and suprasternal retractions may accompany an asthma attack. They're preceded by dyspnea, wheezing, a hacking cough, and pallor. Related features include cyanosis or flushing, crackles, rhonchi, diaphoresis, tachycardia, tachypnea, a frightened, anxious expression and, in patients with severe distress, nasal flaring.
- *Bronchiolitis.* Most common in children younger than age 2 years, bronchiolitis is an acute lower respiratory tract infection that may cause intercostal and subcostal retractions, nasal flaring, tachypnea, dyspnea, cough, restlessness, and slight fever. Periodic apnea may occur in infants younger than age 6 months.
- *Croup (spasmodic).* Croup causes attacks of a barking cough, stridor, inspiratory crackles, expiratory wheezing, hoarseness, dyspnea, and restlessness. As distress worsens,

the child may display suprasternal, substernal, and intercostal retractions accompanied by nasal flaring, tachycardia, cyanosis, and an anxious, frantic expression. Croup attacks usually subside within a few hours but tend to recur and may require intubation.

- *Epiglottiditis.* A life-threatening bacterial infection, epiglottiditis may precipitate severe respiratory distress with suprasternal, substernal, and intercostal retractions as well as stridor, nasal flaring, cyanosis, and tachycardia. Early features include the sudden onset of a barking cough and high fever, sore throat, hoarseness, dysphagia, drooling, dyspnea, and restlessness. The child becomes panicky as edema makes breathing difficult. Total airway occlusion may occur in 2 to 5 hours.
- *Heart failure.* Usually linked to a congenital heart defect in children, heart failure may cause intercostal and substernal retractions along with nasal flaring, progressive tachypnea and, in severe respiratory distress, grunting respirations, edema, and cyanosis. Other findings include productive cough, crackles, jugular vein distention, tachycardia, right upper quadrant pain, anorexia, and fatigue.
- *Laryngotracheobronchitis (acute).* A viral infection, substernal and intercostal retractions typically follow low to moderate fever, runny nose, poor appetite, barking cough, hoarseness, and inspiratory stridor. Associated signs and symptoms include shallow, rapid respirations as well as tachycardia, restlessness, irritability, and pale, cyanotic skin.
- *Pneumonia (bacterial).* Bacterial pneumonia begins with signs and symptoms of acute infection, such as high fever and lethargy, which are followed by subcostal and intercostal retractions, nasal flaring, dyspnea, tachypnea, grunting respirations, cyanosis, and a productive cough. Auscultation may reveal diminished breath sounds, scattered crackles, and sibilant rhonchi over the affected lung. GI effects may include vomiting, diarrhea, and abdominal distention.
- *Respiratory distress syndrome.* Substernal and subcostal retractions are an early sign of respiratory distress syndrome — a life-threatening condition that affects premature neonates shortly after birth. Associated early signs include tachypnea, tachycardia, and expiratory grunting. As respiratory distress worsens, intercostal and suprasternal retractions typically occur, and apnea or irregular respirations replace grunting. Other effects include nasal flaring, cyanosis, lethargy, and eventual unresponsiveness as well as bradycardia and hypotension. Auscultation may detect crackles over the lung bases on deep inspiration and harsh, diminished breath sounds. Oliguria and peripheral edema may occur.

NURSING CONSIDERATIONS

Monitor the child's vital signs. Keep suction equipment and an appropriate-sized airway at the bedside. If the infant weighs less than 15 lb (6.8 kg), place him in an oxygen hood. If he weighs more, place him in a cool mist tent instead. Perform chest physical therapy with postural drainage to help mobilize and drain excess lung secretions. (See *Positioning an infant for chest physical therapy,* pages 254 and 255.) A bronchodilator or, occasionally, a steroid may also be used.

Prepare the child for chest X-rays, cultures, pulmonary function tests, and arterial blood gas analysis. Explain the procedures to his parents as well, and have them calm and comfort the child.

PATIENT TEACHING

Instruct the patient or a family member on proper administration of medication at home. Provide instructions for providing a humidified environment. Stress the importance of maintaining adequate hydration. Provide information on the use of respiratory equipment and techniques to administer respiratory therapies at home.

Scrotal swelling

Scrotal swelling occurs when a condition affecting the testicles, epididymis, or scrotal skin produces edema or a mass; the penis may be involved. Scrotal swelling can affect males of any age. It can be unilateral or bilateral and painful or painless.

The sudden onset of painful scrotal swelling suggests torsion of a testicle or testicular appendages, especially in a prepubescent male. This emergency requires immediate surgery to untwist and stabilize the spermatic cord or to remove the appendage.

Act now *If severe pain accompanies scrotal swelling, ask when the swelling began. Using a Doppler stethoscope, evaluate blood flow to the testicle. If it's decreased or absent, suspect testicular torsion and prepare the patient for surgery. Withhold food and fluids, insert an I.V. line, and apply an ice pack to the scrotum to reduce pain and swelling. An attempt may be made to untwist the cord manually, but even if this is successful, the patient may still require surgery for stabilization.*

ASSESSMENT
History
If the patient isn't in distress, obtain his medical history. Ask about injury to the scrotum, urethral discharge, cloudy urine, increased urinary frequency, and dysuria. Is he sexually active? When was his last sexual contact? Does he have a history of sexually transmitted disease? Find out about recent illnesses, particularly mumps. Does the patient have a history of prostate surgery or prolonged catheterization? Is the swelling affected by changing his body position or level of activity?

Physical examination
Take the patient's vital signs, especially noting fever, and palpate his abdomen for tenderness. Then examine the entire genital area. Assess the scrotum with the patient in supine and standing positions. Note its size and color. Is the swelling unilateral or bilateral? Do you see signs of trauma or bruising? Are there rashes or lesions present? Gently palpate the scrotum for a cyst or lump. Note especially tenderness or increased firmness. Check the testicles' position in the scrotum. Finally, transilluminate the scrotum to distinguish a fluid-filled cyst from a solid mass. (A solid mass can't be transilluminated.)

Pediatric pointers
A thorough physical assessment is especially important for children with scrotal swelling, who may be unable to provide history data. In children up to age 1, a hernia or hydrocele of the spermatic cord may stem from abnormal fetal development. In infants, scrotal swelling may stem from ammonia-related dermatitis if diapers aren't changed often enough. In prepubescent males, it usually results from torsion of the spermatic cord.

Other disorders that can produce scrotal swelling in children include epididymitis (rare before age 10), traumatic orchitis from contact sports, and mumps, which usually occurs after puberty.

MEDICAL CAUSES

- *Elephantiasis of the scrotum.* With elephantiasis of the scrotum (common in some tropical countries), infection by a filaria worm obstructs lymphatic drainage, causing chronic gross scrotal edema and pain. Associated findings include other areas of pitting and, eventually, brawny edema (especially the legs), thickened subcutaneous tissue, hyperkeratosis, and skin fissures.
- *Epididymal cysts.* Located in the head of the epididymis, these cysts produce painless scrotal swelling.
- *Epididymal tuberculosis.* Epididymal tuberculosis produces an enlarged scrotal mass separated from the testicle. Other findings include palpable beading along the vas deferens, induration of the prostate or seminal vesicles, and pus or tubercle bacilli in urine.
- *Epididymitis.* Key features of inflammation are pain, extreme tenderness, and swelling in the groin and scrotum. The patient waddles to avoid pressure on the groin and scrotum during walking. He may have high fever, malaise, urethral discharge and cloudy urine, and lower abdominal pain on the affected side. His scrotal skin may be hot, red, dry, flaky, and thin.
- *Gumma.* Gumma is a rare, painless nodule — usually associated with benign tertiary syphilis — that can affect any bone or organ. If it affects the testicle, it causes edema.
- *Hernia.* Herniation of bowel into the scrotum can cause swelling and a soft or unusually firm scrotum. Occasionally, bowel sounds can be auscultated in the scrotum.
- *Hydrocele.* Fluid accumulation produces gradual scrotal swelling that's usually painless. The scrotum may be soft and cystic or firm and tense. Palpation reveals a round, nontender scrotal mass.
- *Idiopathic scrotal edema.* Swelling occurs quickly with idiopathic scrotal edema and usually disappears within 24 hours. The affected testicle is pink.
- *Orchitis (acute).* Mumps, syphilis, or tuberculosis may precipitate acute orchitis, which causes sudden painful swelling of one or, at times, both testicles. Related findings include a hot, reddened scrotum accompanied by fever of up to 104° F (40° C), chills, lower abdominal pain, nausea, vomiting, and extreme weakness. Urinary signs are usually absent.
- *Scrotal burns.* Burns cause swelling within 24 hours of injury. Depending on the burn's severity, associated findings may include severe pain, erythema, chafing, tissue sloughing, and maceration with a weeping exudate.
- *Scrotal trauma.* Blunt trauma causes scrotal swelling with bruising and severe pain. The scrotum may appear dark or bluish.
- *Spermatocele.* This usually painless cystic mass lies above and behind the testicle and contains opaque fluid and sperm. Its onset may be acute or gradual. Less than 1 cm in diameter, it's movable and may be transilluminated.
- *Testicular torsion.* Most common between ages 12 and 25 years, testicular torsion — a urologic emergency — causes scrotal swelling with sudden, severe pain and, possibly, elevation of the affected testicle within the scrotum. It may also cause nausea and vomiting.
- *Testicular tumor.* Typically painless, smooth, and firm, a testicular tumor produces swelling and a sensation of excessive weight in the scrotum.
- *Torsion of a hydatid of Morgagni.* Torsion of a hydatid of Morgagni — a small, pea-sized cyst — severs its blood supply, causing hard, painful swelling on the testicle's upper pole.

OTHER CAUSES

- *Surgery.* An effusion of blood from surgery can produce a hematocele, leading to scrotal swelling.

NURSING CONSIDERATIONS

Keep the patient on bed rest and administer an antibiotic. Provide adequate fluids, fiber, and stool softeners. Place a rolled towel between the patient's legs and under the scrotum to help reduce severe swelling. Or, if the patient has mild or moderate swelling, advise him to wear a loose-fitting athletic supporter lined with a soft cotton dressing. For several days, administer an analgesic to relieve his pain. Encourage sitz baths, and apply heat or ice packs to decrease inflammation.

Prepare the patient for needle aspiration of fluid-filled cysts and other diagnostic tests, such as lung tomography and computed tomography scan of the abdomen, to rule out malignant tumors.

PATIENT TEACHING

Encourage the patient to perform regular testicular self-examinations. Explain the importance of wearing a scrotal support for comfort and to decrease edema.

Seizures, generalized tonic-clonic

Like other types of seizures, generalized tonic-clonic seizures are caused by the paroxysmal, uncontrolled discharge of central nervous system (CNS) neurons, leading to neurologic dysfunction. Unlike most other types of seizures, however, this cerebral hyperactivity isn't confined to the original focus or to a localized area but extends to the entire brain.

A generalized tonic-clonic seizure may begin with or without an aura. As seizure activity spreads to the subcortical structures, the patient loses consciousness, falls to the ground, and may utter a loud cry that's precipitated by air rushing from the lungs through the vocal cords. His body stiffens (tonic phase), and then undergoes rapid, synchronous muscle jerking and hyperventilation (clonic phase). Tongue biting, incontinence, diaphoresis, profuse salivation, and signs of respiratory distress may also occur. The seizure usually stops after 2 to 5 minutes. The patient then regains consciousness but displays confusion. He may complain of headache, fatigue, muscle soreness, and arm and leg weakness and may sleep for hours.

Alert *If the seizure persists for longer than 5 minutes, emergency treatment is required.*

Generalized tonic-clonic seizures usually occur singly. The patient may be asleep or awake and active. (See *What happens during a generalized tonic-clonic seizure,* page 270.) Possible complications include respiratory arrest due to airway obstruction from secretions, status epilepticus (occurring in 5% to 8% of patients), head or spinal injuries and bruises, Todd's paralysis and, rarely, cardiac arrest. Life-threatening status epilepticus is marked by prolonged seizure activity or by rapidly recurring seizures with no intervening periods of recovery. It's most commonly triggered by abrupt discontinuation of anticonvulsant therapy.

Generalized seizures may be caused by a brain tumor, a vascular disorder, head trauma, an infection, a metabolic defect, drug or alcohol withdrawal syndrome, exposure to toxins, or a genetic defect. Generalized seizures may also result from a focal seizure. With recurring seizures, or epilepsy, the cause may be unknown.

Act now *If you witness the beginning of the seizure, first check the patient's airway, breathing, and circulation, and make sure that the cause isn't asystole or a blocked airway. Stay with the patient and ensure a patent airway. Focus your care on observing the seizure and protecting the patient. Place a towel under his head to prevent injury, loosen his clothing, and move sharp or hard objects out of his way. Never try to restrain the patient or force a hard object into his mouth; you might chip his teeth or fracture his jaw.*

If possible, turn the patient to one side during the seizure to allow secretions to drain and to prevent aspiration. Otherwise, do this at the end of the clonic phase when respirations return. (If they fail to return, check for airway obstruction and suction the patient if necessary. Cardiopulmonary resuscitation, intubation, and mechanical ventilation may be needed.)

Protect the patient after the seizure by providing a safe area in which he can rest. As he awakens, reassure and reorient him. Check his vital signs and neurologic status. Be sure to carefully record these data and your observations during the seizure.

If the seizure lasts longer than 4 minutes or if a second seizure occurs before full recovery from the first, suspect status epilepticus. Establish an airway, start an I.V. line, give supplemental oxygen, and begin cardiac monitoring. Draw blood for appropriate studies. Turn the patient on his side, with his head in a semi-dependent position, to drain secretions and prevent aspiration. Periodically turn him to the opposite side, check his arterial blood gas levels for hypoxemia, and administer oxygen by mask, increasing the flow rate if necessary. To halt the seizure, administer diazepam or lorazepam by slow I.V. push, repeated two or three times at 10- to 20-minute intervals. If the patient isn't known to have epilepsy, an I.V. bolus of dextrose 50% with thiamine may be ordered. Dextrose may stop the seizures if he has hypoglycemia. If his thiamine level is low, give thiamine to guard against further damage.

If the patient is intubated, expect to insert a nasogastric (NG) tube to prevent vomiting and aspiration. Be aware that the NG tube can trigger the gag reflex and cause vomiting in the patient who hasn't already been intubated. Be sure to record your observations and the intervals between seizures.

What happens during a generalized tonic-clonic seizure

Before the seizure

Prodromal signs and symptoms, such as myoclonic jerks, throbbing headache, and mood changes, may occur over several hours or days. The patient may have premonitions of the seizure. For example, he may report an *aura*, such as seeing a flashing light or smelling a characteristic odor.

During the seizure

If a generalized seizure begins with an aura, this indicates that irritability in a specific area of the brain quickly became widespread. Common auras include palpitations, epigastric distress rapidly rising to the throat, head or eye turning, and sensory hallucinations.

Next, *loss of consciousness* occurs as a sudden discharge of intense electrical activity overwhelms the brain's subcortical center. The patient falls and experiences brief, bilateral myoclonic contractures. Air forced through spasmodic vocal cords may produce a birdlike, piercing cry.

During the *tonic phase,* skeletal muscles contract for 10 to 20 seconds. The patient's eyelids are drawn up, his arms are flexed, and his legs are extended. His mouth opens wide and then snaps shut; he may bite his tongue. His respirations cease because of respiratory muscle spasm, and initial pallor of the skin and mucous membranes (the result of impaired venous return) changes to cyanosis secondary to apnea. The patient arches his back and slowly lowers his arms (as shown below).

Other effects include dilated, nonreactive pupils as well as greatly increased heart rate and blood pressure, increased salivation and tracheobronchial secretions, and profuse diaphoresis.

During the *clonic phase,* which lasts about 60 seconds, mild trembling progresses to violent contractures or jerks. Other motor activity includes facial grimaces (with possible tongue biting) and violent expiration of bloody, foamy saliva from clonic contractures of thoracic cage muscles. Clonic jerks slowly decrease in intensity and frequency. The patient is still apneic.

After the seizure

The patient's movements gradually cease, and he becomes unresponsive to external stimuli. Other postseizure features include stertorous respirations from increased tracheobronchial secretions, equal or unequal pupils (that become reactive), and urinary incontinence due to brief muscle relaxation. After about 5 minutes, the patient's level of consciousness increases, and he appears confused and disoriented. His muscle tone, heart rate, and blood pressure return to normal, but he is extremely sleepy.

The patient will generally fall asleep right after recovery from the seizure activity. After several hours' sleep, the patient awakens exhausted and may have a headache, sore muscles, and amnesia about the seizure.

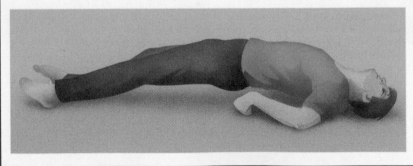

Assessment
History

Obtain the patient's medical history. Has he had generalized or focal seizures before? If so, how frequently? Do other family members have seizures? Is the patient receiving drug therapy? Is he compliant? Ask about sleep deprivation and emotional or physical stress at the time the seizure occurred. Ask about the use of alcohol or illicit drugs.

If you didn't witness the seizure, obtain a description from the patient's family. Ask when it started and how long it lasted. Did the patient report unusual sensations before the seizure began? Did the seizure start in one area of the body and spread, or did it affect the entire body immediately? Did the patient fall on a hard surface? Did his eyes or head turn? Did he turn blue? Did he lose bladder control? Did he have other seizures before recovering? Does he complain of headache and muscle soreness?

Physical examination

If the patient may have sustained a head injury, perform a complete neurologic examination, observing closely for loss of consciousness, unequal or nonreactive pupils, and focal neurologic signs. Assess his vital signs. Is he increasingly difficult to arouse when you check on him at 20-minute intervals? Examine his arms, legs, and face (including tongue) for injury, residual paralysis, or limb weakness.

Pediatric pointers

Generalized seizures are common in children. In fact, between 75% and 90% of epileptic patients experience their first seizure before age 20. Many children ages 3 months to 3 years experience generalized seizures associated with fever; some of these children later develop seizures without fever. Generalized seizures may also stem from inborn errors of metabolism, perinatal injury, brain infection, Reye's syndrome, Sturge-Weber syndrome, arteriovenous malformation, lead poisoning, hypoglycemia, and idiopathic causes. The pertussis component of the DPT vaccine may cause seizures; however, this is rare.

Alert A subtle manifestation of seizure onset in a neonate is eye deviation and lip smacking.

MEDICAL CAUSES

- *Alcohol withdrawal syndrome.* Seizures as well as status epilepticus may develop 7 to 48 hours after abrupt cessation of alcohol consumption by the individual with alcohol dependency. Restlessness, hallucinations, profuse diaphoresis, and tachycardia may also occur.

- *Brain abscess.* Generalized seizures may occur in the acute stage of abscess formation or after the abscess disappears. Decreased level of consciousness (LOC) varies from drowsiness to deep stupor according to the size and location of the abscess. Early signs and symptoms reflect increased intracranial pressure (ICP) and include constant headache, nausea, vomiting, and focal seizures. Typical later features include ocular disturbances, such as nystagmus, impaired vision, and unequal pupils. Other findings vary with the abscess site, but may include aphasia, hemiparesis, abnormal behavior, and personality changes.

- *Brain tumor.* Generalized seizures may occur, depending on the tumor's location and type. Other findings include a slowly decreasing LOC, morning headache, dizziness, confusion, focal seizures, vision loss, motor and sensory disturbances, aphasia, and ataxia. Later findings include papilledema, vomiting, increased systolic blood pressure, widening pulse pressure and, eventually, decorticate posture.

- *Cerebral aneurysm.* Occasionally, generalized seizures may occur with an aneurysm rupture. Premonitory signs and symptoms may last several days, but the onset is typically abrupt with severe headache, nausea, vomiting, and a decreased LOC. Related signs and symptoms vary according to the site and amount of bleeding, but may include nuchal rigidity, irritability, hemiparesis, hemisensory defects, dysphagia, photophobia, diplopia, ptosis, and unilateral pupil dilation.

- *Chronic renal failure.* End-stage renal failure produces the rapid onset of twitching, trembling, myoclonic jerks, and generalized seizures. Related signs and symptoms include anuria or oliguria, fatigue, malaise, irritability, decreased mental acuity, muscle cramps, peripheral neuropathies, anorexia, and constipation or diarrhea. Integumentary effects include skin color changes (yellow, brown, or bronze), pruritus, and uremic frost. Other effects include ammonia breath odor, nausea and vomiting, ecchymoses, petechiae, GI bleeding, mouth and gum ulcers, hypertension, and Kussmaul's respirations.

- *Eclampsia.* Generalized seizures are a hallmark of eclampsia. Related findings include severe frontal headache, nausea and vomiting, vision disturbances, increased blood pressure, fever of up to 104° (40° C), peripheral edema, and sudden weight gain. The patient may also exhibit oliguria, irritability, hyperactive deep tendon reflexes (DTRs), and a decreased LOC.

● *Encephalitis.* Seizures are an early sign of encephalitis, indicating a poor prognosis; they may also occur after recovery as a result of residual damage. Other findings include fever, headache, photophobia, nuchal rigidity, neck pain, vomiting, aphasia, ataxia, hemiparesis, nystagmus, irritability, cranial nerve palsies (causing facial weakness, ptosis, and dysphagia), and myoclonic jerks.

● *Epilepsy (idiopathic).* In most cases, the cause of recurrent seizures is unknown.

● *Head trauma.* In severe cases, generalized seizures may occur at the time of injury. (Months later, focal seizures may occur.) Severe head trauma may also cause a decreased LOC, leading to coma. Other signs and symptoms may include soft-tissue injury of the face, head, or neck as well as facial edema and clear or bloody drainage from the mouth, nose, or ears. The patient may also exhibit Battle's sign, lack of response to oculocephalic and oculovestibular stimulation, and bony deformity of the face, head, or neck. Motor and sensory deficits may occur along with altered respirations. Examination may reveal signs of increasing ICP, such as decreased response to painful stimuli, nonreactive pupils, bradycardia, increased systolic pressure, and widening pulse pressure. If the patient is conscious, he may exhibit visual deficits, behavioral changes, and headache.

● *Hepatic encephalopathy.* Generalized seizures may occur late in hepatic encephalopathy. Associated late-stage findings in the comatose patient include fetor hepaticus, asterixis, hyperactive DTRs, and a positive Babinski's sign.

● *Hypertensive encephalopathy.* A life-threatening disorder, hypertensive encephalopathy may cause seizures along with severely increased blood pressure, a decreased LOC, intense headache, vomiting, transient blindness, paralysis and, eventually, Cheyne-Stokes respirations.

● *Hypoglycemia.* Generalized seizures usually occur with severe hypoglycemia, accompanied by blurred or double vision, motor weakness, hemiplegia, trembling, excessive diaphoresis, tachycardia, myoclonic twitching, and a decreased LOC.

● *Hyponatremia.* Seizures develop when serum sodium levels fall below 125 mEq/L,

especially if the decrease is rapid. Hyponatremia also causes orthostatic hypotension, headache, muscle twitching and weakness, fatigue, oliguria or anuria, cold and clammy skin, decreased skin turgor, irritability, lethargy, confusion, and stupor or coma. Excessive thirst, tachycardia, nausea, vomiting, and abdominal cramps may also occur. Severe hyponatremia may cause cyanosis and vasomotor collapse, with a thready pulse.

● *Hypoparathyroidism.* Worsening tetany causes generalized seizures. Chronic hypoparathyroidism produces neuromuscular irritability and hyperactive DTRs.

● *Hypoxic encephalopathy.* Besides generalized seizures, hypoxic encephalopathy may produce myoclonic jerks and coma. Later, if the patient has recovered, dementia, visual agnosia, choreoathetosis, and ataxia may occur.

● *Multiple sclerosis (MS).* MS rarely produces generalized seizures. Characteristic findings include vision deficits, paresthesia, constipation, muscle weakness, paralysis, spasticity, hyperreflexia, intention tremor, ataxic gait, dysphagia, dysarthria, impotence, and emotional lability. Urinary frequency, urgency, and incontinence may also occur.

● *Neurofibromatosis.* Multiple brain lesions from neurofibromatosis cause focal and generalized seizures. Inspection reveals café-au-lait spots, multiple skin tumors, scoliosis, and kyphoscoliosis. Related findings include dizziness, ataxia, monocular blindness, and nystagmus.

● *Porphyria (intermittent acute).* Generalized seizures are a late sign of porphyria, indicating severe CNS involvement. Acute porphyria also causes severe abdominal pain, tachycardia, psychotic behavior, muscle weakness, and sensory loss in the trunk.

● *Sarcoidosis.* Lesions may affect the brain, causing generalized and focal seizures. Associated findings include a nonproductive cough with dyspnea, substernal pain, malaise, fatigue, arthralgia, myalgia, weight loss, tachypnea, dysphagia, skin lesions, and impaired vision.

● *Stroke.* Seizures (focal more common than generalized) may occur within 6 months of an ischemic stroke. Associated signs and symptoms vary with the location and extent of brain damage. They include a decreased LOC, contralateral hemiplegia, dysarthria, dysphagia, ataxia, unilateral sensory loss, apraxia, agnosia, and aphasia. The patient may also develop visual deficits, memory loss, poor judgment, personality changes, emotional lability, urine retention or urinary incontinence, constipation, headache, and vomiting.

OTHER CAUSES

- *Arsenic poisoning.* Besides generalized seizures, arsenic poisoning may cause a garlicky breath odor, increased salivation, and generalized pruritus. GI effects include diarrhea, nausea, vomiting, and severe abdominal pain. Related effects include diffuse hyperpigmentation, paresthesia of the extremities, alopecia, irritated mucous membranes, weakness, muscle aches, peripheral neuropathy, and sharply defined edema of the eyelids, face, and ankles.
- *Barbiturate withdrawal.* In chronically intoxicated patients, barbiturate withdrawal may produce generalized seizures 2 to 4 days after the last dose. Status epilepticus is possible.
- *Diagnostic tests.* Contrast agents used in radiologic tests may cause generalized seizures.
- *Drugs.* Toxic blood levels of some drugs, such as theophylline, lidocaine, Indocin, meperidine, penicillins, and cimetidine, may cause generalized seizures. Phenothiazines, tricyclic antidepressants, amphetamines, isoniazid, and vincristine may cause seizures in patients with preexisting epilepsy.

NURSING CONSIDERATIONS

Closely monitor the patient for recurring seizure activity. Prepare him for a computed tomography scan or magnetic resonance imaging and EEG. Monitor therapeutic drug levels. Provide a safe environment and institute seizure precautions. Continue to monitor the patient's vital signs and respiratory status. Provide supplemental oxygen, as indicated.

PATIENT TEACHING

Advise the patient's family to observe and record his seizure activity to ensure proper treatment. Emphasize the importance of strict compliance with the drug regimen and warn the patient about its possible adverse effects. Stress the importance of regular follow-up appointments for blood studies. Provide information on alcohol or drug cessation programs if the seizure was related to withdrawal or abuse.

Skin, clammy

Clammy skin—moist, cool, and commonly pale—is a sympathetic response to stress, which triggers release of the hormones epinephrine and norepinephrine. These hormones cause cutaneous vasoconstriction and secretion of cold sweat from eccrine glands, particularly on the palms, forehead, and soles.

Clammy skin typically accompanies shock, acute hypoglycemia, anxiety reactions, arrhythmias, and heat exhaustion. It also occurs as a vasovagal reaction to severe pain associated with nausea, anorexia, epigastric distress, hyperpnea, tachypnea, weakness, confusion, tachycardia, and pupillary dilation or a combination of these findings. Marked bradycardia and syncope may follow.

Act now *Clammy skin commonly accompanies emergency conditions, such as shock, acute hypoglycemia, and arrhythmias. (See Clammy skin: A key finding, page 274.)*

ASSESSMENT
History

If the patient's condition permits, obtain his medical history. Does he have type 1 diabetes mellitus or a cardiac disorder? Is he taking medication? If so, determine whether he takes an antiarrhythmic. Is he experiencing pain, chest pressure, nausea, or epigastric distress? Does he feel weak? Does he have a dry mouth? Does he have diarrhea or increased urination?

Physical examination

Check the patient's vital signs. Perform a complete cardiovascular assessment, followed by a physical assessment. Check the patient's blood glucose level. Next, examine the pupils for dilation. Also, check for abdominal distention and increased muscle tension.

Pediatric pointers

Be aware that absence of clammy skin doesn't rule out shock in infants. Clammy skin doesn't occur in infants younger than 12 months because their sweat glands aren't yet fully developed.

CLAMMY SKIN: A KEY FINDING

If you detect clammy skin while assessing a patient, stay alert because this sign commonly accompanies such emergency conditions as shock, acute hypoglycemia, and arrhythmias. Knowing what to do and how to intervene is of the utmost importance. For guidance on how to react to this finding, review these typical clinical situations.

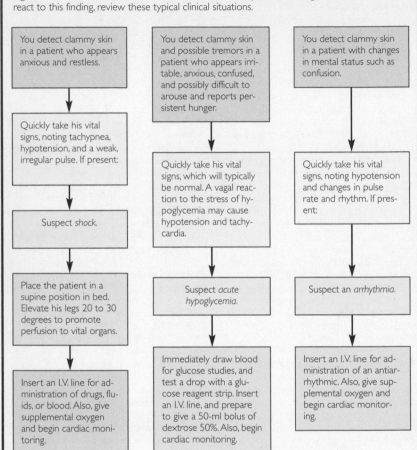

You detect clammy skin in a patient who appears anxious and restless.

↓

Quickly take his vital signs, noting tachypnea, hypotension, and a weak, irregular pulse. If present:

↓

Suspect *shock*.

↓

Place the patient in a supine position in bed. Elevate his legs 20 to 30 degrees to promote perfusion to vital organs.

↓

Insert an I.V. line for administration of drugs, fluids, or blood. Also, give supplemental oxygen and begin cardiac monitoring.

You detect clammy skin and possible tremors in a patient who appears irritable, anxious, confused, and possibly difficult to arouse and reports persistent hunger.

↓

Quickly take his vital signs, which will typically be normal. A vagal reaction to the stress of hypoglycemia may cause hypotension and tachycardia.

↓

Suspect *acute hypoglycemia*.

↓

Immediately draw blood for glucose studies, and test a drop with a glucose reagent strip. Insert an I.V. line, and prepare to give a 50-ml bolus of dextrose 50%. Also, begin cardiac monitoring.

You detect clammy skin in a patient with changes in mental status such as confusion.

↓

Quickly take his vital signs, noting hypotension and changes in pulse rate and rhythm. If present:

↓

Suspect an *arrhythmia*.

↓

Insert an I.V. line for administration of an antiarrhythmic. Also, give supplemental oxygen and begin cardiac monitoring.

Geriatric pointers

Elderly patients develop clammy skin easily because of decreased tissue perfusion. Always consider bowel ischemia in the differential diagnosis of older patients who present with cool, clammy skin — especially if abdominal pain or bloody stools occur.

MEDICAL CAUSES

● *Anxiety.* An acute anxiety attack commonly produces cold, clammy skin on the forehead, palms, and soles. Other features include pallor, dry mouth, tachycardia or bradycardia, palpitations, and hypertension or hypotension. The patient may also develop tremors, breathlessness, headache, muscle tension, nausea, vomiting, abdominal distention, diarrhea, increased urination, and sharp chest pain.

● *Arrhythmias.* Cardiac arrhythmias may produce generalized cool, clammy skin along with mental status changes, dizziness, and hypotension.

- **Cardiogenic shock.** Generalized cool, moist, pale skin accompanies confusion, restlessness, hypotension, tachycardia, tachypnea, narrowing pulse pressure, cyanosis, and oliguria.
- **Heat exhaustion.** In the acute stage of heat exhaustion, generalized cold, clammy skin accompanies an ashen appearance, headache, confusion, syncope, giddiness and, possibly, a subnormal temperature, with mild heat exhaustion. The patient may exhibit a rapid and thready pulse, nausea, vomiting, tachypnea, oliguria, thirst, muscle cramps, hypotension, blurred vision, and loss of consciousness.
- **Hypoglycemia (acute).** Generalized cool, clammy skin or diaphoresis may accompany irritability, tremors, palpitations, hunger, headache, tachycardia, and anxiety. Central nervous system disturbances include blurred vision, diplopia, confusion, motor weakness, hemiplegia, and coma. These signs and symptoms typically resolve after the patient is given glucose.
- **Hypovolemic shock.** With this common form of shock, generalized pale, cold, clammy skin accompanies subnormal body temperature, hypotension with narrowing pulse pressure, tachycardia, tachypnea, and a rapid, thready pulse. Other findings are flat neck veins, increased capillary refill time, decreased urine output, confusion, and a decreased level of consciousness.
- **Septic shock.** The cold shock stage causes generalized cold, clammy skin. Associated findings include a rapid and thready pulse, severe hypotension, persistent oliguria or anuria, and respiratory failure.

NURSING CONSIDERATIONS

Take the patient's vital signs frequently and monitor urine output. If clammy skin occurs with an anxiety reaction or pain, offer the patient emotional support, administer pain medication, and provide a quiet environment.

PATIENT TEACHING

If an underlying illness is related to the patient's clammy skin, provide information on the condition. If the condition is related to an alteration in the patient's blood glucose level, provide information on management of hypoglycemia and early signs of a falling blood glucose level. Provide information on the importance of nutrition and hydration.

Skin, mottled

Mottled skin is patchy discoloration indicating primary or secondary changes of the deep, middle, or superficial dermal blood vessels. It can result from a hematologic, immune, or connective tissue disorder. Other causes include chronic occlusive arterial disease, dysproteinemia, immobility, exposure to heat or cold, or shock. Mottled skin can be a normal reaction such as the diffuse mottling that occurs when exposure to cold causes venous stasis in cutaneous blood vessels (cutis marmorata).

Mottling that occurs with other signs and symptoms usually affects the extremities, typically indicating restricted blood flow. For example, livedo reticularis, a characteristic network pattern of reddish blue discoloration, occurs when vasospasm of the middermal blood vessels slows local blood flow in dilated superficial capillaries and small veins. Shock causes mottling from systemic vasoconstriction.

Act now *Mottled skin may indicate an emergency condition requiring rapid evaluation and intervention. If the patient is pale, cool, clammy, and mottled at the elbows and knees or all over, he may be developing hypovolemic shock. Monitor his vital signs, and note tachycardia or a weak, thready pulse. Observe the neck for flattened jugular veins, and assess the patient for anxiety. If you detect these signs and symptoms, place the patient in a supine position in bed with his legs elevated 20 to 30 degrees. Administer oxygen by nasal cannula or face mask and begin cardiac monitoring. Insert a large-bore I.V. line for rapid fluid infusion or blood product administration and prepare to insert a central line or pulmonary artery catheter. Also prepare to insert a catheter to monitor urinary output.*

Localized mottling in a pale, cool extremity that the patient describes as painful, numb, and tingling may signal acute arterial occlusion. If the patient presents with these signs and symptoms, immediately check his distal pulses. If they're absent or diminished, you'll need to insert an I.V. line in an unaffected extremity and prepare the patient for arteriography or immediate surgery.

ASSESSMENT
History

If the patient isn't in distress, obtain his medical history. Ask if the mottling began suddenly or gradually. What precipitated it? How long has he had it? Does anything relieve it? Does he have other symptoms, such as pain, numbness, or tingling in an extremity? If so, do they disappear with temperature changes?

Physical examination
Observe the patient's skin color, and palpate his arms and legs for skin texture, swelling, and temperature differences between extremities. Check capillary refill. Also, palpate for the presence (or absence) of pulses and for their quality. Note breaks in the skin, muscle appearance, and hair distribution. Assess motor and sensory function.

Pediatric pointers
A common cause of mottled skin in children is systemic vasoconstriction from shock. Other causes are the same as those for adults.

Geriatric pointers
In elderly patients, decreased tissue perfusion can easily cause mottled skin. Arterial occlusion and polycythemia vera, which are common in this age-group, may also cause mottled skin. Suspect bowel ischemia in elderly patients who present with livedo reticularis, especially if they also report abdominal pain or bloody stools.

MEDICAL CAUSES
- *Acrocyanosis.* With acrocyanosis, a rare disorder, anxiety or exposure to cold can cause vasospasm in small cutaneous arterioles. This results in persistent symmetrical blue and red mottling of the affected hands, feet, and nose.
- *Arterial occlusion (acute).* Initial signs include temperature and color changes. Pallor may change to blotchy cyanosis and livedo reticularis. Color and temperature demarcation develop at the level of the obstruction. Other effects include a sudden onset of pain in the extremity and possibly paresthesia, paresis, and a sensation of cold in the affected area. Examination reveals diminished or absent pulses, cool extremities, increased capillary refill time, pallor, and diminished reflexes.
- *Arteriosclerosis obliterans.* Atherosclerotic buildup narrows intra-arterial lumina, resulting in reduced blood flow through the affected artery. Obstructed blood flow to the ex-

tremities (most commonly the lower) produces such peripheral signs and symptoms as leg pallor, cyanosis, blotchy erythema, and livedo reticularis. Related findings include intermittent claudication (most common symptom), diminished or absent pedal pulses, and leg coolness. Other symptoms include coldness and paresthesia.
- *Buerger's disease.* A form of vasculitis, Buerger's disease produces unilateral or asymmetrical color changes and mottling, particularly livedo networking in the lower extremities. It also typically causes intermittent claudication and erythema along extremity blood vessels. During exposure to cold, the feet are cold, cyanotic, and numb; later, they're hot, red, and tingling. Other findings include impaired peripheral pulses and peripheral neuropathy. Buerger's disease is typically exacerbated by smoking.
- *Cryoglobulinemia.* A necrotizing disorder, cryoglobulinemia causes patchy livedo reticularis, petechiae, and ecchymoses. Other findings include fever, chills, urticaria, melena, skin ulcers, epistaxis, Raynaud's phenomenon, eye hemorrhage, hematuria, and gangrene.
- *Hypovolemic shock.* Vasoconstriction from shock commonly produces skin mottling, initially in the knees and elbows. As shock worsens, mottling becomes generalized. Early signs include a sudden onset of pallor, cool skin, restlessness, thirst, tachypnea, and slight tachycardia. As shock progresses, associated findings include cool, clammy skin as well as a rapid, thready pulse accompanied by hypotension, narrowed pulse pressure, decreased urine output, subnormal temperature, confusion, and a decreased level of consciousness.
- *Livedo reticularis (idiopathic or primary).* Symmetrical, diffuse mottling can involve the hands, feet, arms, legs, buttocks, and trunk. Initially, networking is intermittent and most pronounced on exposure to cold or stress; eventually, mottling persists even with warming.
- *Periarteritis nodosa.* Skin findings include asymmetrical, patchy livedo reticularis, palpable nodules along the path of medium-sized arteries, erythema, purpura, muscle wasting, ulcers, gangrene, peripheral neuropathy, fever, weight loss, and malaise.
- *Polycythemia vera.* A hematologic disorder, polycythemia vera produces livedo reticularis, hemangiomas, purpura, rubor, ulcera-

tive nodules, and scleroderma-like lesions. Other symptoms include headache, a vague feeling of fullness in the head, dizziness, vertigo, vision disturbances, dyspnea, aquagenic pruritus, and night sweats.

● *Rheumatoid arthritis (RA).* RA may cause skin mottling. Early nonspecific signs and symptoms progress to joint pain and stiffness with subcutaneous nodules, usually on the elbows.

● *Systemic lupus erythematosus (SLE).* A connective tissue disorder, SLE can cause livedo reticularis, most commonly on the outer arms. Other signs and symptoms include a butterfly rash, nondeforming joint pain and stiffness, photosensitivity, Raynaud's phenomenon, patchy alopecia, seizures, fever, anorexia, weight loss, lymphadenopathy, and emotional lability.

OTHER CAUSES

● *Immobility.* Prolonged immobility may cause bluish mottling, most noticeably in dependent extremities.

● *Thermal exposure.* Prolonged thermal exposure, such as from a heating pad or hot water bottle, may cause erythema ab igne — a localized, reticulated, brown-to-red mottling.

NURSING CONSIDERATIONS

Assess for exacerbation of the underlying condition, and refer the patient for medical treatment. Maximize circulation to the affected areas by keeping them warm and in proper alignment.

PATIENT TEACHING

If the patient has a chronic condition, such as SLE, periarteritis nodosa, or cryoglobulinemia, advise him to watch for mottled skin because it may indicate a flare-up of his disorder. Encourage the patient to avoid wearing tight clothing and to avoid overexposure to cooling or heating devices.

Splenomegaly

Because it occurs with various disorders and in up to 5% of normal adults, splenomegaly — an enlarged spleen — isn't a diagnostic sign by itself. Usually, however, it points to infection, trauma, or a hepatic, autoimmune, neoplastic, or hematologic disorder.

Because the spleen functions as the body's largest lymph node, splenomegaly can result from any process that triggers lymphadenopathy. For example, it may reflect reactive hyperplasia (a response to an infection or inflammation), proliferation or infiltration of neoplastic cells, extramedullary hemopoiesis, phagocytic cell proliferation, increased blood cell destruction, or vascular congestion associated with portal hypertension.

Splenomegaly may be detected by light palpation under the left costal margin. (See *How to palpate for splenomegaly,* page 278.) However, because this technique isn't always advisable or effective, splenomegaly may need to be confirmed by a computed tomography (CT) or radionuclide scan.

Act now *If the patient who presents with splenomegaly has a history of abdominal or thoracic trauma, don't palpate the abdomen because this may aggravate internal bleeding. Instead, examine the patient for left upper quadrant pain and signs of shock, such as tachycardia and tachypnea. If you detect these signs, suspect splenic rupture. Insert an I.V. line for emergency fluid and blood replacement, and administer oxygen. Also, catheterize the patient to evaluate urine output, and begin cardiac monitoring. Prepare the patient for possible surgery.*

ASSESSMENT
History

If you detect splenomegaly during a routine physical examination, begin by exploring associated signs and symptoms. Ask the patient if he has been unusually tired lately. Does he frequently have colds, sore throats, or other infections? Does he bruise easily? Ask about left upper quadrant pain, abdominal fullness, and early satiety.

Physical examination

Begin the physical examination by performing a complete abdominal assessment, including palpation of the spleen. Examine the patient's skin for pallor and ecchymoses, and palpate his axillae, groin, and neck for lymphadenopathy. (See *Splenomegaly: Causes and associated findings,* pages 280 and 281.)

Pediatric pointers

In addition to the causes of splenomegaly already described, children may develop sple-

How to palpate for splenomegaly

Detecting splenomegaly requires skillful and gentle palpation to avoid rupturing the enlarged spleen. Follow these steps carefully:

◆ Place the patient in the supine position, and stand at her right side. Place your left hand under the left costovertebral angle, and push lightly to move the spleen forward. Then press your right hand gently under the left front costal margin.

◆ Have the patient take a deep breath and then exhale. As she exhales, move your right hand along the tissue contours under the border of the ribs, feeling for the spleen's edge. The enlarged spleen should feel like a firm mass that bumps against your fingers. Re-

member to begin palpation low enough in the abdomen to catch the edge of a massive spleen.

◆ Grade the splenomegaly as slight (½" to 1½" [1 to 4 cm] below the costal margin), moderate (1½" to 3" [4 to 8 cm] below the costal margin), or great (greater than or equal to 3" [8 cm] below the costal margin).

◆ Reposition the patient on her right side with her hips and knees flexed slightly to move the spleen forward. Then repeat the palpation procedure.

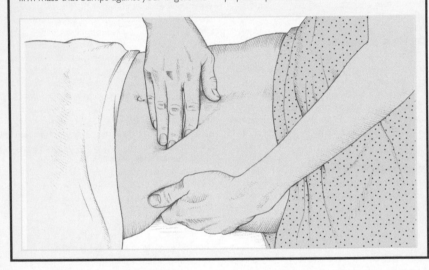

nomegaly in histiocytic disorders, congenital hemolytic anemia, Gaucher's disease, Niemann-Pick disease, hereditary spherocytosis, sickle cell disease, or beta-thalassemia (Cooley's anemia). Splenic abscess is the most common cause of splenomegaly in immunocompromised children.

MEDICAL CAUSES

● *Amyloidosis.* Marked splenomegaly may occur with amyloidosis from excessive protein deposits in the spleen. Associated signs and symptoms vary, depending on which other organs are involved. The patient may display signs of renal failure, such as oliguria and anuria, and signs of heart failure, such as dyspnea, crackles, and tachycardia. GI effects

may include constipation or diarrhea and a stiff, enlarged tongue, resulting in dysarthria.

● *Brucellosis.* With severe cases of brucellosis, splenomegaly is a major sign. Typically, this rare infection begins insidiously with fatigue, headache, backache, anorexia, arthralgia, fever, chills, sweating, and malaise. Later, it may cause hepatomegaly, lymphadenopathy, weight loss, and vertebral or peripheral nerve pain on pressure.

● *Cirrhosis.* About one-third of patients with advanced cirrhosis develop moderate to marked splenomegaly. Among other late findings are jaundice, hepatomegaly, leg edema, hematemesis, and ascites. Signs of hepatic encephalopathy — such as asterixis, fetor hepaticus, slurred speech, and a decreased level of consciousness that may progress to coma—are also common. Besides jaundice, skin effects may include severe pruritus, poor tissue turgor, spider angiomas, palmar erythema, pallor, and signs of bleeding tendencies. Endocrine effects may include menstrual irregularities or testicular atrophy, gynecomastia, and the loss of chest and axillary hair. The patient may also develop fever and right upper abdominal pain that's aggravated by sitting up or leaning forward.

- **Endocarditis (subacute infective).** Endocarditis usually causes an enlarged, but nontender, spleen. Its classic sign, however, is a suddenly changing murmur or the discovery of a new murmur in the presence of fever. Other features include anorexia, pallor, weakness, fever, night sweats, fatigue, tachycardia, weight loss, arthralgia, petechiae, hematuria and, in chronic cases, clubbing. If embolization occurs, the patient may develop chest, abdominal, or limb pain accompanied by paralysis, hematuria, and blindness. Endocarditis may produce Osler's nodes (tender, raised, subcutaneous lesions on the fingers or toes), Roth's spots (hemorrhagic areas with white centers on the retina), and Janeway lesions (purplish macules on the palms or soles).
- **Felty's syndrome.** Splenomegaly is characteristic in Felty's syndrome that occurs with chronic rheumatoid arthritis. Associated findings are joint pain and deformity, sensory or motor loss, rheumatoid nodules, palmar erythema, lymphadenopathy, and leg ulcers.
- **Hepatitis.** Splenomegaly may occur with hepatitis. More characteristic findings include hepatomegaly, vomiting, jaundice, and fatigue.
- **Histoplasmosis.** Acute disseminated histoplasmosis commonly produces splenomegaly and hepatomegaly. It may also cause lymphadenopathy, jaundice, fever, anorexia, emaciation, and signs and symptoms of anemia, such as weakness, fatigue, pallor, and malaise. Occasionally, the patient's tongue, palate, epiglottis, and larynx become ulcerated, resulting in pain, hoarseness, and dysphagia.
- **Hypersplenism (primary).** With hypersplenism, splenomegaly accompanies signs of pancytopenia—anemia, neutropenia, or thrombocytopenia. If the patient has anemia, findings may include weakness, fatigue, malaise, and pallor. If he has severe neu-

tropenia, frequent bacterial infections are likely. If he has severe thrombocytopenia, easy bruising or spontaneous, widespread hemorrhage may occur. The patient also experiences left-sided abdominal pain and a feeling of fullness after eating a small amount of food.

- **Leukemia.** Moderate to severe splenomegaly is an early sign of acute and chronic leukemia. With chronic granulocytic leukemia, splenomegaly is sometimes painful. Accompanying it may be hepatomegaly, lymphadenopathy, fatigue, malaise, pallor, fever, gum swelling, bleeding tendencies, weight loss, anorexia, and abdominal, bone, and joint pain. At times, acute leukemia also causes dyspnea, tachycardia, and palpitations. With advanced disease, the patient may display confusion, headache, vomiting, seizures, papilledema, and nuchal rigidity.
- **Lymphoma.** Moderate to massive splenomegaly is a late sign and may be accompanied by hepatomegaly, painless lymphadenopathy, scaly dermatitis with pruritus, fever, fatigue, weight loss, and malaise.
- **Malaria.** A common sign of malaria, splenomegaly is typically preceded by the malarial paroxysm of chills, followed by high fever and then diaphoresis. Related effects include headache, muscle pain, and hepatomegaly. With benign malaria, these paroxysms alternate with periods of well-being. With severe malaria, however, the patient may develop a persistent high fever, orthostatic hypotension, seizures, delirium, coma, coughing (with possible hemoptysis), vomiting, abdominal pain, diarrhea, melena, oliguria or anuria and, possibly, hemiplegia.
- **Mononucleosis (infectious).** A common sign of infectious mononucleosis, splenomegaly is most pronounced during the second and third weeks of illness. Typically, it's accompanied by a triad of signs and symptoms: sore throat, cervical lymphadenopathy, and fluctuating temperature with an evening peak of 101° to 102° F (38.3° to 38.9° C). Occasionally, hepatomegaly, jaundice, and a maculopapular rash may also occur.
- **Pancreatic cancer.** Cancer of the pancreas may cause moderate to severe splenomegaly if tumor growth compresses the splenic vein. Other characteristic findings include abdominal or back pain, anorexia, nausea and vomiting, weight loss, GI bleeding, jaundice, pruritus, skin lesions, emotional lability, weak-

SPLENOMEGALY:
CAUSES AND ASSOCIATED FINDINGS

MAJOR ASSOCIATED SIGNS AND SYMPTOMS

COMMON CAUSES	Abdominal pain	Anuria	Arthralgia	Bleeding tendencies	Decreased LOC	Diaphoresis	Diarrhea	Dysarthria	Dyspnea	Fatigue	Fever
Amyloidosis		●					●	●	●		
Brucellosis			●			●				●	●
Cirrhosis	●			●	●						●
Endocarditis, subacute infective			●							●	●
Felty's syndrome			●								
Hepatitis										●	
Histoplasmosis								●		●	
Hypersplenism, primary	●			●						●	
Leukemia	●		●						●	●	●
Lymphoma										●	●
Malaria	●	●				●	●	●		●	
Mononucleosis, infectious										●	
Pancreatic cancer	●			●						●	
Polycythemia vera	●			●					●	●	
Sarcoidosis	●			●					●	●	
Splenic rupture	●			●							
Thrombotic thrombocytopenic purpura	●		●	●						●	●

ness, and fatigue. Palpation may reveal a tender abdominal mass and hepatomegaly; auscultation reveals a bruit in the periumbilical area and left upper quadrant.

● *Polycythemia vera.* Late in polycythemia vera, the spleen may become markedly enlarged, resulting in easy satiety, abdominal fullness, and left upper quadrant or pleuritic chest pain. Signs and symptoms accompanying splenomegaly are widespread and numerous. The patient may exhibit deep, purplish red oral mucous membranes, headache, dyspnea, dizziness, vertigo, weakness, and fatigue. He may also develop finger and toe

Headache	Hepatomegaly	Impaired mentation	Jaundice	Lymphadeno-pathy	Malaise	Murmur	Oliguria	Pain	Pallor	Seizures	Skin lesions	Tachycardia	Vomiting	Weakness	Weight loss
							•					•			
•	•			•	•										•
	•	•	•						•		•				
						•		•	•		•	•		•	•
				•				•			•				
	•			•									•		
	•			•	•				•					•	
					•				•					•	
•	•	•		•	•			•			•	•	•	•	
	•				•	•					•				•
•	•					•		•					•		
	•		•	•							•				
	•		•		•			•			•			•	•
•	•	•						•			•			•	•
	•				•	•				•	•				•
											•				
•	•			•					•		•			•	

paresthesia, impaired mentation, tinnitus, blurred or double vision, scotoma, increased blood pressure, and intermittent claudication. Other signs and symptoms include pruritus, urticaria, ruddy cyanosis, epigastric distress, weight loss, hepatomegaly, and bleeding tendencies.

● *Sarcoidosis.* A granulomatous disorder, sarcoidosis may produce splenomegaly and hepatomegaly, possibly accompanied by vague abdominal discomfort. Its other signs and symptoms vary with the affected body system, but may include nonproductive cough, dyspnea, malaise, fatigue, arthralgia, myalgia, weight loss, lymphadenopathy, skin lesions, irregular pulse, impaired vision, dysphagia, and seizures.

● *Splenic rupture.* Splenomegaly may result from massive hemorrhage. The patient may also experience left upper quadrant pain, abdominal rigidity, and Kehr's sign.

● *Thrombotic thrombocytopenic purpura.* Thrombotic thrombocytopenic purpura may produce splenomegaly and hepatomegaly accompanied by fever, generalized purpura, jaundice, pallor, vaginal bleeding, and hematuria. Other effects include fatigue, weakness, headache, pallor, abdominal pain, and arthralgias. Eventually, the patient develops signs of neurologic deterioration and renal failure.

NURSING CONSIDERATIONS
Prepare the patient for diagnostic studies, such as a complete blood count, blood cultures, and radionuclide and CT scans of the spleen. Assist in managing the underlying disorder and prepare the patient for surgery, as indicated.

PATIENT TEACHING
Inform the patient about techniques to avoid infection. Emphasize the importance of complying with the drug therapy regimen and knowing its potential adverse effects. Provide postoperative teaching, if indicated.

Stridor

A loud, harsh, musical respiratory sound, stridor results from an obstruction in the trachea or larynx. Other causes include foreign-body aspiration, croup syndrome, laryngeal diphtheria, pertussis, retropharyngeal abscess, and congenital abnormalities of the larynx.

Usually heard during inspiration, this sign may also occur during expiration in severe upper airway obstruction. It may begin as low-pitched "croaking" and progress to high-pitched "crowing" as respirations become more vigorous.

Act now *If you hear stridor, quickly check the patient's vital signs, including oxygen saturation, and examine him for other signs of partial airway obstruction — choking or gagging, tachypnea, dyspnea, shallow respirations, inter-*

costal retractions, nasal flaring, tachycardia, cyanosis, and diaphoresis. (Be aware that abrupt cessation of stridor signals complete obstruction in which the patient has inspiratory chest movement but absent breath sounds. Unable to talk, he quickly becomes lethargic and loses consciousness.)

If you detect signs of airway obstruction, try to clear the airway with back blows or abdominal thrusts (Heimlich maneuver). Next, administer oxygen by nasal cannula or face mask, or prepare for emergency endotracheal (ET) intubation or tracheostomy and mechanical ventilation. (See Emergency endotracheal intubation.*) Have equipment ready to suction aspirated vomitus or blood through the ET or tracheostomy tube. Connect the patient to a cardiac monitor, and position him upright to ease his breathing.*

ASSESSMENT
History
When the patient's condition permits, obtain his medical history. First, find out when the stridor began. Has he had it before? Does he have an upper respiratory tract infection? If so, how long has he had it?

Ask about a history of allergies, tumors, and respiratory and vascular disorders. Note recent exposure to smoke or noxious fumes or gases. Next, explore associated signs and symptoms. Does stridor occur with pain or a cough?

Physical assessment
Examine the patient's mouth for excessive secretions, foreign matter, inflammation, and swelling. Assess his neck for swelling, masses, subcutaneous crepitation, and scars. Observe the patient's chest for delayed, decreased, or asymmetrical chest expansion. Auscultate for wheezes, rhonchi, crackles, rubs, and other abnormal breath sounds. Percuss for dullness, tympany, or flatness. Finally, note burns or signs of trauma, such as ecchymoses and lacerations.

Pediatric pointers
Stridor is a major sign of airway obstruction in a child. When you hear this sign, you must intervene quickly to prevent total airway obstruction. This emergency can happen more rapidly in a child because his airway is narrower than an adult's.

MEDICAL CAUSES
● *Airway trauma.* Local trauma to the upper airway commonly causes acute obstruc-

EMERGENCY ENDOTRACHEAL INTUBATION

A patient with stridor may require emergency endotracheal (ET) intubation to establish a patent airway and administer mechanical ventilation. Follow these essential steps:

- Gather the necessary equipment.
- Explain the procedure to the patient.
- Place the patient flat on his back with a small blanket or pillow under his head. This position aligns the axis of the oropharynx, posterior pharynx, and trachea.
- Check the cuff on the ET tube for leaks.
- After intubation, inflate the cuff, using the minimal leak technique.
- Check tube placement by auscultating for bilateral breath sounds or using a capnometer; observe the patient for chest expansion and feel for warm exhalations at the ET tube's opening.
- Insert an oral airway or bite block.

- Secure the ET tube and airway with tape applied to skin treated with compound benzoin tincture.
- Suction secretions from the patient's mouth and the ET tube as needed.
- Administer oxygen or initiate mechanical ventilation (or both).

After the patient has been intubated, suction secretions as needed and check cuff pressure once every shift (correcting air leaks with the minimal leak technique). Provide mouth care every 2 to 3 hours and as needed. Prepare the patient for chest X-rays to check ET tube placement, and restrain and reassure him as needed

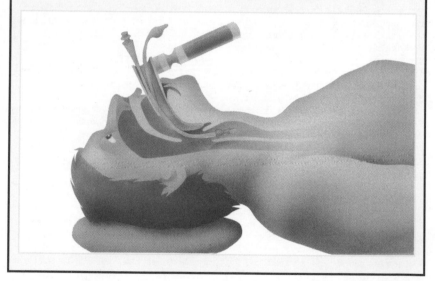

tion, resulting in the sudden onset of stridor. Accompanying this sign are dysphonia, dysphagia, hemoptysis, cyanosis, accessory muscle use, intercostal retractions, nasal flaring, tachypnea, progressive dyspnea, and shallow respirations. Palpation may reveal subcutaneous crepitation in the neck or upper chest.

- *Anaphylaxis.* With a severe allergic reaction, upper airway edema and laryngospasm cause stridor and other signs and symptoms of respiratory distress — nasal flaring, wheezing, accessory muscle use, intercostal retrac-

tions, and dyspnea. The patient may also develop nasal congestion and profuse, watery rhinorrhea. Typically, these respiratory effects are preceded by a feeling of impending doom or fear, weakness, diaphoresis, sneezing, nasal pruritus, urticaria, erythema, and angioedema. Common associated findings include chest or throat tightness, dysphagia and, possibly, signs of shock, such as hypotension, tachycardia, and cool, clammy skin.

- *Anthrax (inhalation).* Initial signs and symptoms of inhalation anthrax are flulike and include fever, chills, weakness, cough, and chest pain. The disease generally occurs in two stages with a period of recovery after the initial symptoms. The second stage develops abruptly with rapid deterioration marked by stridor, fever, dyspnea, and hypotension generally leading to death within 24 hours. Radiologic findings include mediastinitis and symmetric mediastinal widening.

● *Aspiration of a foreign body.* Sudden stridor is characteristic in this life-threatening situation. Related findings include an abrupt onset of dry, paroxysmal coughing, gagging or choking, hoarseness, tachycardia, wheezing, dyspnea, tachypnea, intercostal muscle retractions, diminished breath sounds, cyanosis, and shallow respirations. The patient typically appears anxious and distressed.

● *Epiglottiditis.* With epiglottiditis, an inflammatory condition, stridor is caused by an erythematous, edematous epiglottis that obstructs the upper airway. Stridor occurs along with fever, sore throat, and a croupy cough.

● *Hypocalcemia.* With hypocalcemia, laryngospasm can cause stridor. Other findings include paresthesia, carpopedal spasm, and positive Chvostek's and Trousseau's signs.

● *Inhalation injury.* Within 48 hours after inhalation of smoke or noxious fumes, the patient may develop laryngeal edema and bronchospasms, resulting in stridor. Associated signs and symptoms include singed nasal hairs, orofacial burns, coughing, hoarseness, sooty sputum, crackles, rhonchi, wheezes, and other signs and symptoms of respiratory distress, such as dyspnea, accessory muscle use, intercostal retractions, and nasal flaring.

● *Laryngeal tumor.* Stridor is a late sign and may be accompanied by dysphagia, dyspnea, enlarged cervical nodes, and pain that radiates to the ear. Typically, stridor is preceded by hoarseness, minor throat pain, and a mild, dry cough.

● *Laryngitis (acute).* Acute laryngitis may cause severe laryngeal edema, resulting in stridor and dyspnea. Its chief sign, however, is mild to severe hoarseness, perhaps with transient voice loss. Other findings include sore throat, dysphagia, dry cough, malaise, and fever.

● *Mediastinal tumor.* Commonly producing no symptoms at first, this type of tumor may eventually compress the trachea and bronchi, resulting in stridor. Its other effects include hoarseness, brassy cough, tracheal shift or tug, jugular vein distention, face and neck swelling, stertorous respirations, and suprasternal retractions on inspiration. The patient may also report dyspnea, dysphagia, and pain in the chest, shoulder, or arm.

● *Retrosternal thyroid.* An anatomic abnormality, retrosternal thyroid causes stridor, dysphagia, cough, hoarseness, and tracheal deviation. It can also cause signs of thyrotoxicosis.

● *Thoracic aortic aneurysm.* If this aneurysm compresses the trachea, it may cause stridor accompanied by dyspnea, wheezing, and a brassy cough. Other findings include hoarseness or complete voice loss, dysphagia, jugular vein distention, prominent chest veins, tracheal tug, paresthesia or neuralgia, and edema of the face, neck, and arms. The patient may also complain of substernal, lower back, abdominal, or shoulder pain.

OTHER CAUSES

● *Diagnostic tests.* Bronchoscopy or laryngoscopy may precipitate laryngospasm and stridor.

● *Medical treatments.* After prolonged intubation, the patient may exhibit laryngeal edema and stridor when the tube is removed. Aerosol therapy with epinephrine may reduce stridor. Reintubation may be necessary in some cases. Neck surgery, such as thyroidectomy, may cause laryngeal paralysis and stridor.

NURSING CONSIDERATIONS

Continue to monitor the patient's vital signs closely. Prepare him for diagnostic tests, such as arterial blood gas analysis and chest X-rays. Offer reassurance and calm the patient and his family. Provide ongoing assessment of the patient's respiratory status and oxygenation.

PATIENT TEACHING

Instruct the patient and his family about safety measures in the home environment if the stridor is related to aspiration of a foreign object. If the stridor is related to croup, teach the parents techniques to use to manage the condition. Teach the patient and his family about signs and symptoms that require immediate attention.

Syncope

A common neurologic sign, syncope (or fainting) refers to transient loss of consciousness associated with impaired cerebral blood supply or cerebral hypoxia. It usually occurs abruptly and lasts for seconds to minutes. An episode of syncope usually starts as a feeling of light-headedness. A patient can usually prevent an episode of syncope by lying down or sitting with his head between his knees. Typically, the patient lies motionless with his skeletal muscles relaxed but sphincter muscles controlled. However, the depth of unconsciousness varies — some patients can hear voices or see blurred outlines; others are unaware of their surroundings.

In many ways, syncope simulates death: The patient is strikingly pale with a slow, weak pulse, hypotension, and almost imperceptible breathing. If severe hypotension lasts for 20 seconds or longer, the patient may also develop convulsive, tonic-clonic movements.

Syncope may result from cardiac and cerebrovascular disorders, hypoxemia, and postural changes in the presence of autonomic dysfunction. It may also follow vigorous coughing (tussive syncope) and emotional stress, injury, shock, or pain (vasovagal syncope, or common fainting). Hysterical syncope may also follow emotional stress, but isn't accompanied by other vasodepressor effects.

Act now *If you see a patient faint, ensure a patent airway, ensure his safety, and take his vital signs. Then place the patient in a supine position, elevate his legs, and loosen any tight clothing. Stay alert for tachycardia, bradycardia, or an irregular pulse. Meanwhile, place him on a cardiac monitor to detect arrhythmias. If an arrhythmia appears, give oxygen and insert an I.V. line for drugs or fluids. Be ready to begin cardiopulmonary resuscitation. Cardioversion, defibrillation, or insertion of a temporary pacemaker may be required.*

ASSESSMENT
History
Ask the patient for information about the fainting episode. Did he feel weak, light-headed, nauseous, or sweaty just before he fainted? Did he stand quickly from a sitting or prone position? During the fainting episode, did he have muscle spasms or incontinence? How long was he unconscious? When he regained consciousness, was he alert or confused? Did he have a headache? Has he fainted before? If so, how often does it occur?

Physical examination
Perform a complete cardiac and neurologic examination. Provide continuous cardiac monitoring. Next, take the patient's vital signs and examine him for injuries that may have occurred during his fall.

Pediatric pointers
Syncope is much less common in children than in adults. It may result from a cardiac or neurologic disorder, allergies, or emotional stress.

MEDICAL CAUSES
- *Aortic arch syndrome.* With aortic arch syndrome, the patient experiences syncope and may exhibit weak or abruptly absent carotid pulses and unequal or absent radial pulses. Early signs and symptoms include night sweats, pallor, nausea, anorexia, weight loss, arthralgia, and Raynaud's phenomenon. He may also develop hypotension in the arms, paresthesia, intermittent claudication, bruits, vision disturbances, dizziness, and neck, shoulder, and chest pain.
- *Aortic stenosis.* A cardinal late sign, syncope is accompanied by exertional dyspnea and angina. Related findings include marked fatigue, orthopnea, paroxysmal nocturnal dyspnea, palpitations, and diminished carotid pulses. Typically, auscultation reveals atrial and ventricular gallops as well as a harsh, crescendo-decrescendo systolic ejection murmur that's loudest at the right sternal border of the second intercostal space.
- *Cardiac arrhythmias.* Any arrhythmia that decreases cardiac output and impairs cerebral circulation may cause syncope. Other effects — palpitations, pallor, confusion, diaphoresis, dyspnea, and hypotension — usually develop first. However, with Adams-Stokes syndrome, syncope may occur without warning. During syncope, the patient develops asystole, which may precipitate spasm and myoclonic jerks if prolonged. He also displays an ashen pallor that progresses to cyanosis, incontinence, bilateral Babinski's reflex, and fixed pupils.

- *Carotid sinus hypersensitivity.* Syncope is triggered by compression of the carotid sinus, which may be caused by turning the head to one side or by wearing a tight collar. The fainting episode is usually short.
- *Hypoxemia.* Regardless of its cause, severe hypoxemia may produce syncope. Common related effects include confusion, tachycardia, restlessness, and incoordination.
- *Orthostatic hypotension.* Syncope occurs when the patient rises quickly from a recumbent position. Look for a drop of 10 mm Hg or more in systolic or diastolic blood pressure as well as tachycardia, pallor, dizziness, blurred vision, nausea, and diaphoresis.
- *Transient ischemic attacks.* Marked by transient neurologic deficits, these attacks may produce syncope and a decreased level of consciousness. Other findings vary with the affected artery, but may include vision loss, nystagmus, aphasia, dysarthria, unilateral numbness, hemiparesis or hemiplegia, tinnitus, facial weakness, dysphagia, and a staggering or an uncoordinated gait.
- *Vagal glossopharyngeal neuralgia.* With this disorder, localized pressure may trigger pain in the base of the tongue, pharynx, larynx, tonsils, and ear, resulting in syncope that lasts for several minutes.

OTHER CAUSES
- *Drugs.* Quinidine may cause syncope — and possibly sudden death — associated with ventricular fibrillation. Prazosin may cause severe orthostatic hypotension and syncope, usually after the first dose. Occasionally, griseofulvin, levodopa, and indomethacin can produce syncope.

NURSING CONSIDERATIONS
Continue to monitor the patient's vital signs closely. Prepare the patient for an electrocardiogram, Holter monitoring, and carotid duplex, carotid Doppler, and electrophysiology studies.

PATIENT TEACHING
Advise the patient to pace his activities, to rise slowly from a recumbent position, to avoid standing still for a prolonged time, and to sit or lie down as soon as he feels faint.

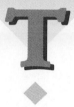

Tachycardia

Easily detected by counting the apical, carotid, or radial pulse, tachycardia is a heart rate greater than 100 beats/minute. The patient with tachycardia usually complains of palpitations or of a "racing" heart. This common sign normally occurs in response to emotional or physical stress, such as excitement, exercise, pain, anxiety, and fever. It may also result from the use of stimulants, such as caffeine and tobacco. However, tachycardia may be an early sign of a life-threatening disorder, such as cardiogenic, hypovolemic, or septic shock. It may also result from a cardiovascular, respiratory, or metabolic disorder or from the effects of certain drugs, tests, or treatments. (See *What happens in tachycardia*.)

    Act now *After detecting tachycardia, first perform electrocardiography (ECG) to examine for reduced cardiac output, which may initiate or result from tachycardia. Take the patient's other vital signs and determine his level of consciousness (LOC). If the patient has increased or decreased blood pressure and is drowsy or confused, administer oxygen and begin cardiac monitoring. Insert an I.V. line for fluid, blood product, and drug administration, and gather emergency resuscitation equipment.*

ASSESSMENT
History
If the patient's condition permits, obtain his medical history. Has he had palpitations before? If so, what treatment was he given? Explore associated symptoms: Is he dizzy or

short of breath? Is he weak or fatigued? Is he experiencing episodes of syncope or chest pain? Next, ask about a history of trauma, diabetes, or cardiac, pulmonary, or thyroid disorders. Obtain a drug history, including prescription, over-the-counter, and illegal drugs, and ask whether the patient uses alcohol.

Physical examination
Inspect the patient's skin for pallor, dehydration, or cyanosis. Assess pulses, noting peripheral edema. Assess the patient's blood

(Text continues on page 290.)

WHAT HAPPENS IN TACHYCARDIA

Tachycardia represents the heart's effort to deliver more oxygen to body tissues by increasing the rate at which blood passes through the vessels. This sign can reflect overstimulation within the sinoatrial node, the atrium, the atrioventricular node, or the ventricles.

Because heart rate affects cardiac output (cardiac output = heart rate × stroke volume), tachycardia can lower cardiac output by reducing ventricular filling time and stroke volume (the output of each ventricle at every contraction). As cardiac output plummets, arterial pressure and peripheral perfusion decrease. Tachycardia further aggravates myocardial ischemia by increasing the heart's demand for oxygen while reducing the duration of diastole— the period of greatest coronary flow.

Tachycardia:
Causes and associated findings

Major associated signs and symptoms

Common causes	Abdominal pain	Abnormal pulse pressure	Altered bowel habits	Anxiety	Bleeding tendencies	Chest pain	Cough	Crackles	Cyanosis	Decreased LOC	Diaphoresis	Dizziness	Dyspnea	Fatigue	Fever	Headache
Acute respiratory distress syndrome				•				•	•	•			•			
Adrenocortical insufficiency	•		•											•		
Alcohol withdrawal syndrome				•							•				•	
Anaphylactic shock				•			•				•		•			•
Anemia					•			•					•	•		
Anxiety						•										
Aortic insufficiency		•				•		•					•			
Aortic stenosis						•		•				•	•	•		
Cardiac arrhythmias										•	•	•	•			
Cardiac contusion						•							•			
Cardiac tamponade		•		•		•			•		•		•			
Cardiogenic shock		•		•						•	•	•				
Cholera			•													
COPD							•	•	•				•			
Diabetic ketoacidosis	•									•						
Febrile illness															•	
Heart failure		•						•					•	•		
Hyperosmolar hyperglycemic nonketotic syndrome										•						
Hypertensive crisis				•		•				•			•			•
Hypoglycemia				•						•	•	•				•

Hypertension	Hypotension	Irritability	Jugular vein distension	Lightheadedness	Murmur	Muscle cramps	Nausea & vomiting	Oliguria	Pallor	Palpitations	Pericardial friction rub	Restlessness	Rhonchi	Seizures	Skin changes	Stridor	Syncope	Tachypnea	Thirst	Weakness	Weight loss	Wheezing
													●					●				
	●	●					●										●			●	●	
		●																●				
	●						●							●	●	●						
									●													
				●			●											●				
			●			●			●	●								●				
						●				●							●					
	●									●								●		●		
										●	●											
	●		●									●						●				
	●																	●				
	●					●	●	●											●	●		
												●						●				●
	●						●											●		●		
																		●				
	●							●		●								●				
	●						●								●			●				
●		●					●								●			●				
							●								●						●	

(continued)

MAJOR ASSOCIATED SIGNS AND SYMPTOMS

COMMON CAUSES	Abdominal pain	Abnormal pulse pressure	Altered bowel habits	Anxiety	Bleeding tendencies	Chest pain	Cough	Crackles	Cyanosis	Decreased LOC	Diaphoresis	Dizziness	Dyspnea	Fatigue	Fever	Headache
Hyponatremia										●				●		●
Hypovolemia																
Hypovolemic shock		●								●	●					
Hypoxemia									●				●			
Myocardial infarction				●		●		●			●					
Neurogenic shock				●							●					
Orthostatic hypotension											●	●				
Pheochromocytoma	●			●		●					●					●
Pneumothorax						●	●		●				●			
Pulmonary embolism						●	●	●	●		●		●		●	
Septic shock			●	●						●	●	●			●	
Thyrotoxicosis		●	●	●							●		●	●		

pressure. Finally, auscultate the heart and lungs for abnormal sounds or rhythms.

Pediatric pointers

When examining a child for tachycardia, remember that the normal heart rate for a child is higher than an adult's heart rate. (See *Normal pediatric vital signs,* pages 292 and 293.) In a child, tachycardia may result from many of the adult causes described above.

MEDICAL CAUSES

See *Tachycardia: Causes and associated findings,* pages 288 to 291.
● *Acute respiratory distress syndrome (ARDS).* Besides tachycardia, ARDS causes crackles, rhonchi, dyspnea, tachypnea, nasal flaring, and grunting respirations. Other find-ings include cyanosis, anxiety, a decreased LOC, and abnormal chest X-ray findings.
● *Adrenocortical insufficiency.* With adrenocortical insufficiency, tachycardia commonly occurs with a weak pulse as well as progressive weakness and fatigue, which may become so severe that the patient requires bed rest. Other signs and symptoms include abdominal pain, nausea and vomiting, altered bowel habits, weight loss, orthostatic hypotension, irritability, bronze skin, decreased libido, and syncope. The patient may report an enhanced sense of taste, smell, and hearing.
● *Alcohol withdrawal syndrome.* Tachycardia can occur with tachypnea, profuse diaphoresis, fever, insomnia, anorexia, and anxiety. The patient is characteristically anx-

Hypertension	Hypotension	Irritability	Jugular vein distension	Lightheadedness	Murmur	Muscle cramps	Nausea & vomiting	Oliguria	Pallor	Palpitations	Pericardial friction rub	Restlessness	Rhonchi	Seizures	Skin changes	Stridor	Syncope	Tachypnea	Thirst	Weakness	Weight loss	Wheezing
	●	●				●		●				●							●	●		
	●																●		●			
	●							●				●						●	●			
																		●	●			
●	●				●		●		●			●										
							●											●				
							●		●								●					
							●			●												
																		●				
										●								●				
	●						●	●				●						●	●			
							●			●											●	

ious, irritable, and prone to visual and tactile hallucinations.

● *Anaphylactic shock.* With life-threatening anaphylactic shock, tachycardia and hypotension develop within minutes after exposure to an allergen, such as penicillin or an insect sting. Typically, the patient is visibly anxious and has severe pruritus, perhaps with urticaria and a pounding headache. Other findings may include flushed and clammy skin, cough, dyspnea, nausea, abdominal cramps, seizures, stridor, change or loss of voice associated with laryngeal edema, and urinary urgency and incontinence.

● *Anemia.* Tachycardia and bounding pulse are characteristic with anemia. Associated signs and symptoms include fatigue, pallor, dyspnea and, possibly, bleeding tendencies.

Auscultation may reveal an atrial gallop, a systolic bruit over the carotid arteries, and crackles.

● *Anxiety.* A fight-or-flight response produces tachycardia, tachypnea, chest pain, nausea, and light-headedness. The symptoms dissipate as anxiety resolves.

● *Aortic insufficiency.* Accompanying tachycardia with aortic insufficiency are a "water-hammer" bounding pulse and a large, diffuse apical heave. With severe insufficiency, widened pulse pressure occurs. Auscultation reveals a hallmark diastolic murmur that starts with S_2; is decrescendo, high-pitched, and blowing; and is heard best at the left sternal border of the second and third intercostal spaces. An atrial or ventricular gallop, an early systolic murmur, an Austin Flint

NORMAL PEDIATRIC VITAL SIGNS

This chart lists the normal resting respiratory rate, blood pressure, and pulse rate for females and males up to age 16.

VITAL SIGNS	NEONATE	2 YEARS	4 YEARS	6 YEARS	8 YEARS	10 YEARS
RESPIRATORY RATE (BREATHS/MINUTE)						
Females	28	26	25	24	24	22
Males	30	28	25	24	22	23
BLOOD PRESSURE (MM HG)						
Females	—	98/60	98/60	98/64	104/68	110/72
Males	—	96/60	98/60	98/62	102/68	110/72
PULSE RATE (BEATS/MINUTE)						
Females	130	110	100	100	90	90
Males	130	110	100	100	90	90

murmur (apical diastolic rumble), or Duroziez's murmur (heard over the femoral artery during systole and diastole) may also be heard. Other findings include angina, dyspnea, palpitations, strong and abrupt carotid pulsations, pallor, and signs of heart failure, such as crackles and jugular vein distention.

- *Aortic stenosis.* Typically, aortic stenosis causes tachycardia; a weak, thready pulse; and an atrial gallop. Its chief features, however, are exertional dyspnea, angina, dizziness, and syncope. This valvular disorder also causes a harsh, crescendo-decrescendo systolic ejection murmur that's loudest at the right sternal border of the second intercostal space. Other findings include palpitations, crackles, and fatigue.
- *Cardiac arrhythmias.* Tachycardia may occur with an irregular heart rhythm. The patient may be hypotensive and report dizziness, palpitations, weakness, and fatigue. Depending on his heart rate, he may also exhibit tachypnea, a decreased LOC, and pale, cool, clammy skin.
- *Cardiac contusion.* The result of blunt chest trauma, this contusion may cause tachycardia, substernal pain, dyspnea, and palpitations. Assessment may detect sternal ecchymoses and a pericardial friction rub.
- *Cardiac tamponade.* With life-threatening cardiac tamponade, tachycardia is commonly accompanied by paradoxical pulse, dyspnea, and tachypnea. The patient is visibly anxious and restless and has cyanotic, clammy skin and distended jugular veins. He may develop muffled heart sounds, a pericardial friction rub, chest pain, hypotension, narrowed pulse pressure, and hepatomegaly.
- *Cardiogenic shock.* Although many features of cardiogenic shock appear in other types of shock, they're usually more profound in this type. Tachycardia is accompanied by narrowing pulse pressure, hypotension, tachypnea, oliguria, restlessness, and an altered LOC. The patient will also exhibit a weak, thready pulse and cold, pale, clammy, and cyanotic skin.
- *Cholera.* Signs of cholera, an infectious disorder, include abrupt watery diarrhea and vomiting. Severe fluid and electrolyte loss leads to tachycardia, thirst, weakness, muscle cramps, decreased skin turgor, oliguria, and hypotension. Without treatment, death can occur within hours.

12 YEARS	14 YEARS	16 YEARS
20	18	16
20	16	16
114/74	118/76	120/78
112/74	120/76	124/78
90	85	80
85	80	75

symptoms, such as palpitations, narrowed pulse pressure, hypotension, tachypnea, crackles, dependent edema, weight gain, slowed mental response, diaphoresis, pallor and, possibly, oliguria. Late signs include hemoptysis, cyanosis, and marked hepatomegaly and pitting edema.

● *Hyperosmolar hyperglycemic nonketotic syndrome.* A rapidly deteriorating LOC is commonly accompanied by tachycardia, hypotension, tachypnea, seizures, oliguria, and severe dehydration with poor skin turgor and dry mucous membranes.

● *Hypertensive crisis.* Life-threatening hypertensive crisis is characterized by tachycardia, tachypnea, diastolic blood pressure that exceeds 120 mm Hg, and systolic blood pressure that may exceed 200 mm Hg. Typically, the patient develops pulmonary edema with jugular vein distention, dyspnea, and pink, frothy sputum. Related findings include chest pain, severe headache, drowsiness, confusion, anxiety, tinnitus, epistaxis, muscle twitching, seizures, nausea, and vomiting. Focal neurologic signs, such as paresthesia, may also occur.

● *Hypoglycemia.* A common sign of hypoglycemia, tachycardia is accompanied by hypothermia, nervousness, trembling, fatigue, malaise, weakness, headache, hunger, nausea, diaphoresis, and moist, clammy skin. Central nervous system effects include blurred or double vision, motor weakness, hemiplegia, seizures, and a decreased LOC.

● *Hyponatremia.* Tachycardia, although rare, is a possible effect of hyponatremia, an electrolyte imbalance. Other effects include orthostatic hypotension, headache, muscle twitching and weakness, fatigue, oliguria or anuria, poor skin turgor, thirst, irritability, seizures, nausea and vomiting, and a decreased LOC that may progress to coma. Severe hyponatremia may cause cyanosis and signs of vasomotor collapse such as a thready pulse.

● *Hypovolemia.* Tachycardia may occur with hypovolemia. Associated findings include hypotension, decreased skin turgor, sunken eyeballs, thirst, syncope, and dry skin and tongue.

● *Hypovolemic shock.* Mild tachycardia, an early sign of life-threatening hypovolemic shock, may be accompanied by tachypnea, restlessness, thirst, and pale, cool skin. As shock progresses, the patient's skin becomes clammy and his pulse becomes increasingly

● *Chronic obstructive pulmonary disease (COPD).* Although the clinical picture varies widely with COPD, tachycardia is a common sign. Other characteristic findings include cough, tachypnea, dyspnea, pursed lip breathing, accessory muscle use, cyanosis, diminished breath sounds, rhonchi, crackles, and wheezing. Clubbing and barrel chest are usually late findings.

● *Diabetic ketoacidosis (DKA).* A life-threatening disorder, DKA commonly produces tachycardia and a thready pulse. Its cardinal sign, however, is Kussmaul's respirations — abnormally rapid, deep breathing. Other signs and symptoms of DKA include fruity breath odor, orthostatic hypotension, generalized weakness, anorexia, nausea, vomiting, and abdominal pain. The patient's LOC may vary from lethargy to coma.

● *Febrile illness.* Fever can cause tachycardia. Related findings reflect the specific disorder.

● *Heart failure.* Especially common with left-sided heart failure, tachycardia may be accompanied by a ventricular gallop, fatigue, dyspnea (exertional and paroxysmal nocturnal), orthopnea, and leg edema. Eventually, the patient develops widespread signs and rapid and thready. He may also develop hypotension, narrowed pulse pressure, oliguria, subnormal body temperature, and a decreased LOC.

- *Hypoxemia.* Tachycardia may accompany tachypnea, dyspnea, and cyanosis. Confusion, syncope, and incoordination may also occur.
- *Myocardial infarction (MI).* A life-threatening disorder, an MI may cause tachycardia or bradycardia. Its classic symptom, however, is crushing substernal chest pain that may radiate to the left arm, jaw, neck, or shoulder. Auscultation may reveal an atrial gallop, a new murmur, and crackles. Other signs and symptoms include pallor, clammy skin, dyspnea, diaphoresis, nausea and vomiting, anxiety, restlessness, and increased or decreased blood pressure.
- *Neurogenic shock.* Tachycardia or bradycardia may accompany tachypnea, apprehension, oliguria, variable body temperature, a decreased LOC, and warm, dry skin.
- *Orthostatic hypotension.* Tachycardia accompanies the characteristic signs and symptoms of orthostatic hypotension, which include dizziness, syncope, pallor, blurred vision, diaphoresis, and nausea.
- *Pheochromocytoma.* Characterized by sustained or paroxysmal hypertension, pheochromocytoma is a rare tumor that may also cause tachycardia and palpitations. Other findings include headache; chest and abdominal pain; diaphoresis; pale or flushed, warm skin; paresthesia; tremors; nausea; vomiting; insomnia; and extreme anxiety—possibly even panic.
- *Pneumothorax.* Life-threatening pneumothorax causes tachycardia and other signs and symptoms of distress, such as severe dyspnea and chest pain, tachypnea, and cyanosis. Related findings include dry cough, subcutaneous crepitation, absent or decreased breath sounds, cessation of normal chest movement on the affected side, and decreased vocal fremitus.
- *Pulmonary embolism.* With pulmonary embolism, tachycardia is usually preceded by sudden dyspnea, angina, or pleuritic chest pain. Common associated signs and symptoms include weak peripheral pulses, cyanosis, tachypnea, low-grade fever, restlessness, diaphoresis, and a dry cough or a cough with blood-tinged sputum.
- *Septic shock.* Initially, septic shock produces chills, sudden fever, tachycardia,

tachypnea and, possibly, nausea, vomiting, and diarrhea. The patient's skin is flushed, warm, and dry and his blood pressure is normal or slightly decreased. Eventually, he may display a rapid, thready pulse accompanied by anxiety, restlessness, thirst, oliguria or anuria, severe hypotension, and cool, clammy, cyanotic skin. His LOC may decrease progressively, perhaps culminating in a coma.

- *Thyrotoxicosis.* Tachycardia is a classic feature of thyrotoxicosis, a thyroid disorder. Other signs and symptoms include an enlarged thyroid, nervousness, heat intolerance, weight loss despite increased appetite, diaphoresis, diarrhea, tremors, and palpitations. Although also considered characteristic, exophthalmos is sometimes absent.

Because thyrotoxicosis affects virtually every body system, its associated features are diverse and numerous. Some examples include full and bounding pulse, widened pulse pressure, dyspnea, anorexia, nausea, vomiting, altered bowel habits, hepatomegaly, and muscle weakness, fatigue, and atrophy. The patient's skin is smooth, warm, and flushed; the hair is fine and soft and may gray prematurely or fall out. The female patient may have a reduced libido and oligomenorrhea or amenorrhea; the male patient may exhibit a reduced libido and gynecomastia.

OTHER CAUSES

- *Diagnostic tests.* Cardiac catheterization and electrophysiologic studies may induce transient tachycardia.
- *Drugs and alcohol.* Various drugs affect the nervous system, circulatory system, or heart muscle, resulting in tachycardia. Examples of these include sympathomimetics; phenothiazines; anticholinergics, such as atropine; thyroid drugs; vasodilators, such as hydralazine and nifedipine; acetylcholinesterase inhibitors, such as captopril; nitrates, such as nitroglycerin; alpha-adrenergic blockers, such as phentolamine; and beta-adrenergic bronchodilators such as albuterol. Excessive caffeine intake and alcohol intoxication may also cause tachycardia.
- *Surgery and pacemakers.* Cardiac surgery and pacemaker malfunction or wire irritation may cause tachycardia.

Nursing considerations

Monitor the patient closely. Explain ordered diagnostic tests, such as a thyroid panel, electrolyte and hemoglobin levels, hematocrit, pulmonary function studies, and 12-lead ECG. If appropriate, prepare him for an ambulatory ECG.

Patient teaching

Provide information about the possibility of the tachyarrhythmia recurring. Teach the patient to take his pulse and monitor his blood pressure at home. Explain the importance of following the medication regimen as prescribed, such as thyroid medication or antiarrhythmics. Explain dietary limitations such as caffeine and alcohol.

Explain that an antiarrhythmic and an internal defibrillator or ablation therapy may be indicated for symptomatic tachycardia.

Tachypnea

A common sign of cardiopulmonary disorders, tachypnea is an abnormally fast respiratory rate — 20 or more breaths/minute. Tachypnea may reflect the need to increase minute volume — the amount of air breathed each minute. Under these circumstances, it may be accompanied by an increase in tidal volume — the volume of air inhaled or exhaled per breath — resulting in hyperventilation. Tachypnea, however, may also reflect stiff lungs or overloaded ventilatory muscles, in which case tidal volume may actually be reduced.

Tachypnea may result from reduced arterial oxygen tension or arterial oxygen content, decreased perfusion, or increased oxygen demand. Heightened oxygen demand, for example, may result from fever, exertion, anxiety, and pain. It may also occur as a compensatory response to metabolic acidosis or may result from pulmonary irritation, stretch receptor stimulation, or a neurologic disorder that upsets medullary respiratory control. Generally, respirations increase by 4 breaths/minute for every 1° F (–17.2° C) increase in body temperature.

Act now *After detecting tachypnea, quickly evaluate the patient's cardiopulmonary status; obtain a set of vital signs with oxygen saturation; and check for cyanosis, chest pain,*

dyspnea, tachycardia, and hypotension. If the patient has paradoxical chest movement, suspect flail chest and immediately splint his chest with your hands or with sandbags. Then administer supplemental oxygen by nasal cannula or face mask and, if possible, place the patient in semi-Fowler's position to help ease his breathing. Intubation and mechanical ventilation may be necessary if respiratory failure occurs. Also, insert an I.V. line for fluid and drug administration and begin cardiac monitoring.

Assessment
History

If the patient's condition permits, obtain a medical history. Find out when the tachypnea began. Did it follow activity? Has he had it before? Does the patient have a history of asthma, chronic obstructive pulmonary disease (COPD), or other pulmonary or cardiac conditions? Then have him describe associated signs and symptoms, such as diaphoresis, chest pain, and recent weight loss. Is he anxious about anything or does he have a history of anxiety attacks? Obtain a medication history, including use of prescription, over-the-counter, and illicit drug use.

Physical examination

Begin the physical examination by taking the patient's vital signs, including oxygen saturation if you haven't already done so, and observing his overall behavior. Does he seem restless, confused, or fatigued? Then auscultate the chest for abnormal heart and breath sounds. If the patient has a productive cough, record the color, amount, and consistency of sputum. Finally, check for jugular vein distention, and examine the skin for pallor, cyanosis, edema, and warmth or coolness.

Pediatric pointers

When assessing a child for tachypnea, be aware that the normal respiratory rate varies with the child's age. (See *Normal pediatric vital signs,* pages 292 and 293.)

The conditions that can lead to tachypnea in adults may also trigger tachypnea in children. This population may also develop tachypnea due to congenital heart defects, meningitis, metabolic acidosis, and cystic fibrosis. Hunger and anxiety may also cause tachypnea in children.

Geriatric pointers

Tachypnea may have many causes in elderly patients, such as pneumonia, heart failure, COPD, anxiety, or failure to take cardiac and respiratory medications appropriately. Mild increases in respiratory rate may be unnoticed in these patients.

MEDICAL CAUSES

- *Acute respiratory distress syndrome (ARDS).* With ARDS, tachypnea and apprehension may be the earliest features. Tachypnea gradually worsens as fluid accumulates in the patient's lungs, causing them to stiffen. It's accompanied by accessory muscle use, grunting expirations, suprasternal and intercostal retractions, crackles, and rhonchi. Eventually, ARDS produces hypoxemia, resulting in tachycardia, dyspnea, cyanosis, respiratory failure, and shock.
- *Alcohol withdrawal syndrome.* A late sign in the acute phase of alcohol withdrawal syndrome, tachypnea typically accompanies anorexia, insomnia, tachycardia, fever, and diaphoresis. The patient may also experience anxiety, irritability, and bizarre visual or tactile hallucinations.
- *Anaphylactic shock.* With life-threatening anaphylactic shock, tachypnea develops within minutes after exposure to an allergen, such as penicillin or insect venom. Accompanying signs and symptoms include anxiety, pounding headache, flushed skin, intense pruritus and, possibly, diffuse urticaria. The patient may exhibit widespread edema, affecting the eyelids, lips, tongue, hands, feet, and genitalia. Other findings include a rapid, thready pulse accompanied by cough, dyspnea, stridor, and cool, clammy skin. The patient may also experience change or loss of voice associated with laryngeal edema.
- *Anemia.* Tachypnea may occur with anemia, depending on its duration and severity. Associated signs and symptoms include fatigue, pallor, dyspnea, tachycardia, postural hypotension, bounding pulse, an atrial gallop, and a systolic bruit over the carotid arteries.
- *Anxiety.* Tachypnea may occur during high-anxiety states because of the fight-or-flight response. Associated signs and symptoms include tachycardia, restlessness, chest pain, nausea, and light-headedness, all of which dissipate as anxiety resolves.
- *Aspiration of a foreign body.* Life-threatening upper airway obstruction may result from aspiration of a foreign body. With a partial obstruction, the patient abruptly develops a dry, paroxysmal cough with rapid, shallow respirations. Other signs and symptoms include dyspnea, gagging or choking, intercostal retractions, nasal flaring, cyanosis, decreased or absent breath sounds, hoarseness, and stridor or coarse wheezing. Typically, the patient appears frightened and distressed. A complete obstruction may rapidly cause asphyxia and death.
- *Asthma.* Tachypnea is common with life-threatening asthma attacks, which commonly occur at night. These attacks usually begin with mild wheezing and a dry cough that progresses to mucus expectoration. Eventually, the patient becomes apprehensive and develops prolonged expirations, intercostal and supraclavicular retractions on inspiration, accessory muscle use, severe audible wheezing, rhonchi, flaring nostrils, tachycardia, diaphoresis, and flushing or cyanosis.
- *Bronchiectasis.* Although bronchiectasis may produce tachypnea, its classic sign is a chronic productive cough that produces copious amounts of mucopurulent, foul-smelling sputum and, occasionally, hemoptysis. Related findings include coarse crackles on inspiration, exertional dyspnea, rhonchi, and halitosis. The patient may also exhibit fever, malaise, weight loss, fatigue, and weakness. Clubbing is a common late sign.
- *Bronchitis (chronic).* Mild tachypnea may occur in chronic bronchitis, a form of COPD, but it isn't typically a predominant sign. Usually, if begins with a dry, hacking cough, which later produces copious amounts of sputum. Other characteristics include dyspnea, prolonged expirations, wheezing, scattered rhonchi, accessory muscle use, and cyanosis. Clubbing and barrel chest are late signs.
- *Cardiac arrhythmias.* Depending on the patient's heart rate, tachypnea may occur along with hypotension, dizziness, palpitations, weakness, and fatigue. The patient's level of consciousness (LOC) may be decreased.
- *Cardiac tamponade.* With life-threatening cardiac tamponade, tachypnea may accompany tachycardia, dyspnea, and paradoxical pulse. Related findings include muffled heart sounds, a pericardial friction rub, chest pain, hypotension, narrowed pulse pressure, and hepatomegaly. The patient is noticeably anx-

ious and restless. His skin is clammy and cyanotic, and his jugular veins are distended.

- **Cardiogenic shock.** Although many signs of cardiogenic shock appear in other types of shock, they're usually more severe in this type. Besides tachypnea, the patient commonly displays cold, pale, clammy, cyanotic skin as well as hypotension, tachycardia, narrowed pulse pressure, a ventricular gallop, oliguria, a decreased LOC, and jugular vein distention.
- **Emphysema.** A chronic pulmonary disorder, emphysema commonly produces tachypnea accompanied by exertional dyspnea. It may also cause anorexia, malaise, peripheral cyanosis, pursed-lip breathing, accessory muscle use, and a chronic productive cough. Percussion yields a hyperresonant tone; auscultation reveals wheezing, crackles, and diminished breath sounds. Clubbing and barrel chest are late signs.
- **Febrile illness.** Fever can cause tachypnea, tachycardia, and other signs depending on the underlying cause.
- **Flail chest.** Tachypnea usually appears early in life-threatening flail chest. Other findings include paradoxical chest wall movement, rib bruises and palpable fractures, localized chest pain, hypotension, and diminished breath sounds. The patient may also develop signs of respiratory distress, such as dyspnea and accessory muscle use.
- **Head trauma.** When trauma affects the brain stem, the patient may display central neurogenic hyperventilation, a form of tachypnea marked by rapid, even, and deep respirations. The tachypnea may be accompanied by other signs of life-threatening neurogenic dysfunction, such as coma, unequal and nonreactive pupils, seizures, hemiplegia, flaccidity, and hypoactive or absent deep tendon reflexes.
- **Hyperosmolar hyperglycemic nonketotic syndrome.** A rapidly deteriorating LOC occurs with tachypnea, tachycardia, hypotension, seizures, oliguria, and signs of dehydration.
- **Hypovolemic shock.** An early sign of life-threatening hypovolemic shock, tachypnea is accompanied by cool, pale skin as well as restlessness, thirst, and mild tachycardia. As shock progresses, the patient's skin becomes clammy; his pulse is increasingly rapid and thready. Other findings include hypotension, narrowed pulse pressure, oliguria, subnormal body temperature, and a decreased LOC.

- **Hypoxia.** Lack of oxygen from any cause increases the rate (and typically the depth) of breathing. Associated symptoms are related to the cause of the hypoxia.
- **Interstitial fibrosis.** With interstitial fibrosis, tachypnea develops gradually and may become severe. Associated features include exertional dyspnea, pleuritic chest pain, a paroxysmal dry cough, crackles, late inspiratory wheezing, cyanosis, fatigue, and weight loss. Clubbing is a late sign.
- **Lung abscess.** With lung abscess, tachypnea is usually paired with dyspnea and accentuated by fever. However, the chief sign is a productive cough with copious amounts of purulent, foul-smelling, usually bloody sputum. Other findings include chest pain, halitosis, diaphoresis, chills, fatigue, weakness, anorexia, weight loss, and clubbing.
- **Lung, pleural, or mediastinal tumor.** The tumor may cause tachypnea along with exertional dyspnea, cough, hemoptysis, and pleuritic chest pain. Other effects include weight loss, anorexia, and fatigue.
- **Mesothelioma (malignant).** Commonly related to asbestos exposure, this pleural mass initially produces tachypnea and dyspnea on mild exertion. Other classic symptoms are persistent, dull chest pain and aching shoulder pain that progresses to arm weakness and paresthesia. Later signs and symptoms include cough, insomnia associated with pain, clubbing, and dullness over the malignant mesothelioma.
- **Neurogenic shock.** Tachypnea is characteristic in life-threatening neurogenic shock. It's commonly accompanied by apprehension, bradycardia or tachycardia, oliguria, fluctuating body temperature, and a decreased LOC that may progress to coma. The patient's skin is warm, dry, and perhaps flushed. He may experience nausea and vomiting.
- **Plague (Yersinia pestis).** The onset of the pneumonic form of plague is usually sudden with chills, fever, headache, and myalgia. Pulmonary signs and symptoms include tachypnea, productive cough, chest pain, dyspnea, hemoptysis, and increasing respiratory distress and cardiopulmonary insufficiency.

Alert *The pneumonic form of plague may be contracted from person-to-person direct contact via the respiratory system. This would also be the form contracted in biological warfare from aerosolization and inhalation of the organism.*

- *Pneumonia (bacterial).* A common sign in bacterial pneumonia, tachypnea is usually preceded by a painful, hacking, dry cough that rapidly becomes productive. Other signs and symptoms quickly follow, including high fever, shaking chills, headache, dyspnea, pleuritic chest pain, tachycardia, grunting respirations, nasal flaring, and cyanosis. Auscultation reveals diminished breath sounds and fine crackles; percussion yields a dull tone.
- *Pneumothorax.* Tachypnea, a common sign of life-threatening pneumothorax, is typically accompanied by severe, sharp, and commonly unilateral chest pain that's aggravated by chest movement. Associated signs and symptoms include dyspnea, tachycardia, accessory muscle use, asymmetrical chest expansion, dry cough, cyanosis, anxiety, and restlessness. Examination of the affected lung reveals hyperresonance or tympany, subcutaneous crepitation, decreased vocal fremitus, and diminished or absent breath sounds. The patient with tension pneumothorax also develops a deviated trachea.
- *Pulmonary edema.* An early sign of life-threatening pulmonary edema, tachypnea is accompanied by exertional dyspnea, paroxysmal nocturnal dyspnea and, later, orthopnea. Other features include dry cough, crackles, tachycardia, and a ventricular gallop. With severe pulmonary edema, respirations become increasingly rapid and labored, tachycardia worsens, and crackles become more diffuse. The patient's cough also produces frothy, bloody sputum. Signs of shock—such as hypotension, thready pulse, and cold, clammy skin—may also occur.
- *Pulmonary embolism (acute).* Tachypnea occurs suddenly with pulmonary embolism and is usually accompanied by dyspnea. The patient may complain of angina or pleuritic chest pain. Other common characteristics include tachycardia, a dry or productive cough with blood-tinged sputum, low-grade fever, restlessness, and diaphoresis. Less common signs include massive hemoptysis, chest splinting, leg edema, and—with a large embolus—jugular vein distention and syncope. Other findings include a pleural friction rub, crackles, diffuse wheezing, dullness on percussion, diminished breath sounds, and signs of shock, such as hypotension and a weak, rapid pulse.
- *Pulmonary hypertension (primary).* With primary pulmonary hypertension, a rare dis-

order, tachypnea is usually a late sign that's accompanied by exertional dyspnea, general fatigue, weakness, and episodes of syncope. The patient may complain of angina on exertion, which may radiate to the neck. Other effects include cough, hemoptysis, and hoarseness.
- *Septic shock.* Early in septic shock, tachypnea is typically accompanied by sudden fever, chills, and flushed, warm, yet dry skin. The patient may also experience nausea, vomiting, and diarrhea, along with tachycardia and normal or slightly decreased blood pressure. As this life-threatening type of shock progresses, the patient may display a rapid, thready pulse, along with thirst, anxiety, restlessness, a decreased LOC, hypotension, and cool, clammy, and cyanotic skin. Oliguria, if present, may progress to anuria.

OTHER CAUSES
- *Salicylates.* Tachypnea may result from an overdose of these drugs.

NURSING CONSIDERATIONS
Continue to monitor the patient's vital signs closely. Be sure to keep suction and emergency equipment nearby. Prepare to intubate the patient and to provide mechanical ventilation if necessary. Prepare the patient for diagnostic studies, such as arterial blood gas analysis, blood cultures, chest X-rays, pulmonary function tests, and an electrocardiogram.

PATIENT TEACHING
Reassure the patient that slight increases in respiratory rate may be normal. Explain signs and symptoms that require immediate attention from a health care professional.

Tracheal deviation

Normally, the trachea is located at the midline of the neck—except at the bifurcation, where it shifts slightly toward the right. Visible deviation from its normal position signals an underlying condition that can compromise pulmonary function and possibly cause respiratory distress. A hallmark of life-threatening tension pneumothorax, tracheal deviation occurs with disorders that produce mediastinal shift due to asymmetrical thoracic volume or pressure. A nonlesion pneumothorax can produce tracheal deviation to the ipsilateral side. (See *Detecting slight tracheal deviation*.)

Act now *Monitor the patient with tracheal deviation for signs and symptoms of respiratory distress (tachypnea, dyspnea, decreased or absent breath sounds, stridor, nasal flaring, accessory muscle use, asymmetrical chest expansion, restlessness, and anxiety). If possible, place him in semi-Fowler's position to aid respiratory excursion and improve oxygenation. Give supplemental oxygen, and intubate the patient if necessary. Insert an I.V. line for fluid and drug administration. In addition, palpate for subcutaneous crepitation in the neck and chest, a sign of tension pneumothorax. Chest tube insertion may be necessary to release trapped air or fluid and to restore normal intrapleural and intrathoracic pressure gradients.*

ASSESSMENT
History
If the patient isn't in distress, obtain his medical history, noting pulmonary or cardiac disorders, surgery, trauma, or infection. If he smokes, determine smoking habits. Ask about associated signs and symptoms, especially breathing difficulty, pain, and cough.

Physical examination
Assess the patient's vital signs. Perform a complete cardiopulmonary assessment with careful attention to the auscultation of breath sounds. Observe for respiratory distress.

Pediatric pointers
Keep in mind that respiratory distress typically develops more rapidly in children than in adults.

Geriatric pointers
In elderly patients, tracheal deviation to the right commonly stems from an elongated, atherosclerotic aortic arch, which isn't considered abnormal.

MEDICAL CAUSES
● *Atelectasis.* Extensive lung collapse can produce tracheal deviation toward the affected side. Respiratory findings include dys-

---

DETECTING SLIGHT TRACHEAL DEVIATION

Although gross tracheal deviation is visible, detection of slight deviation requires palpation and perhaps even an X-ray. Try palpation first.

With the tip of your index finger, locate the patient's trachea by palpating between the sternocleidomastoid muscles. Then compare the trachea's position to an imaginary line drawn vertically through the suprasternal notch. Any deviation from midline is usually considered abnormal.

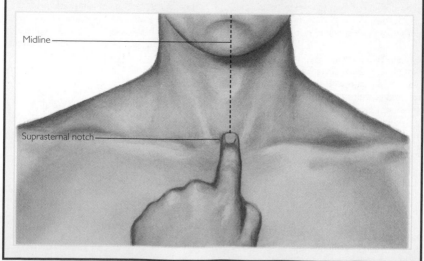

Midline

Suprasternal notch

pnea, tachypnea, pleuritic chest pain, dry cough, dullness on percussion, decreased vocal fremitus and breath sounds, inspiratory lag, and substernal or intercostal retraction.

● *Hiatal hernia.* Intrusion of abdominal viscera into the pleural space causes tracheal deviation toward the unaffected side. The degree of attendant respiratory distress depends on the extent of herniation. Other effects include pyrosis, regurgitation or vomiting, and chest or abdominal pain.

● *Kyphoscoliosis.* Kyphoscoliosis can cause rib cage distortion and mediastinal shift, producing tracheal deviation toward the compressed lung. Respiratory effects include dry cough, dyspnea, asymmetrical chest expansion and, possibly, asymmetrical breath sounds. Backache and fatigue are also common.

● *Mediastinal tumor.* Commonly asymptomatic in its early stages, a mediastinal tumor, when large, can press against the trachea and nearby structures, causing tracheal deviation and dysphagia. Other late findings include stridor, dyspnea, brassy cough, hoarseness, and stertorous respirations with suprasternal retraction. The patient may experience shoulder, arm, or chest pain as well as neck, face, or arm edema. His neck and chest wall veins may be dilated.

● *Pleural effusion.* A large pleural effusion can shift the mediastinum to the contralateral side, producing tracheal deviation. Related effects include dry cough, dyspnea, pleuritic pain, a pleural friction rub, tachypnea, decreased chest motion, decreased or absent breath sounds, egophony, flatness on percussion, decreased tactile fremitus, fever, and weight loss.

● *Pulmonary fibrosis.* Asymmetrical fibrosis can cause tracheal deviation as the mediastinum shifts toward the affected side. Associated findings reflect the underlying condition and pattern of fibrosis. Dyspnea, cough, clubbing, malaise, and fever commonly occur.

● *Pulmonary tuberculosis.* With a large cavitation, tracheal deviation toward the affected side accompanies asymmetrical chest excursion, dullness on percussion, increased tactile fremitus, amphoric breath sounds, and inspiratory crackles. Insidious early effects include fatigue, anorexia, weight loss, fever, chills, and night sweats. Productive cough, hemoptysis, pleuritic chest pain, and dyspnea develop as pulmonary tuberculosis progresses.

● *Retrosternal thyroid.* An anatomic abnormality, retrosternal thyroid can displace the trachea. The gland is felt as a movable neck mass above the suprasternal notch. Dysphagia, cough, hoarseness, and stridor are common. Signs of thyrotoxicosis may be present.

● *Tension pneumothorax.* Acute, life-threatening tension pneumothorax produces tracheal deviation toward the unaffected side. It's marked by a sudden onset of respiratory distress with sharp chest pain, dry cough, severe dyspnea, tachycardia, wheezing, cyanosis, accessory muscle use, nasal flaring, air hunger, and asymmetrical chest movement. Restless and anxious, the patient may also develop subcutaneous crepitation in the neck and upper chest, decreased vocal fremitus, decreased or absent breath sounds on the affected side, jugular vein distention, and hypotension.

● *Thoracic aortic aneurysm.* Thoracic aortic aneurysm usually causes the trachea to deviate to the right. Highly variable associated findings may include stridor, dyspnea, wheezing, brassy cough, hoarseness, and dysphagia. Edema of the face, neck, or arm may occur with distended chest wall and jugular veins. The patient may also experience substernal, neck, shoulder, or lower back pain, possibly with paresthesia or neuralgia.

NURSING CONSIDERATIONS

Because tracheal deviation usually signals a severe underlying disorder that can cause respiratory distress at any time, monitor the patient's respiratory and cardiac status constantly and make sure that emergency equipment is readily available. Prepare the patient for diagnostic tests, such as chest X-rays, bronchoscopy, an electrocardiogram, and arterial blood gas analysis.

PATIENT TEACHING

Teach the patient the techniques required to perform coughing and deep-breathing exercises. Explain the signs and symptoms of respiratory difficulty that require immediate attention.

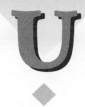

Urticaria

Urticaria is a vascular skin reaction characterized by the eruption of transient pruritic wheals — smooth, slightly elevated patches with well-defined erythematous margins and pale centers of various shapes and sizes (hives). It's produced by the local release of histamine or other vasoactive substances as part of a hypersensitivity reaction. (See *Recognizing common skin lesions,* pages 302 and 303.)

Acute urticaria evolves rapidly and usually has a detectable cause, commonly hypersensitivity to certain drugs, foods, insect bites, inhalants, or contactants. Emotional stress or environmental factors may also trigger urticaria. Although individual lesions usually subside within 12 to 24 hours, new crops of lesions may erupt continuously, thus prolonging the attack.

Urticaria lasting longer than 6 weeks is classified as chronic. The lesions may recur for months or years, and the underlying cause is usually unknown. Occasionally, a diagnosis of psychogenic urticaria is made.

Angioedema, or giant urticaria, is characterized by the acute eruption of wheals involving the mucous membranes and, occasionally, the arms, legs, or genitals.

Act now In an acute case of urticaria, quickly evaluate the patient's respiratory status and take his vital signs. Ensure patent I.V. access if you note respiratory difficulty or signs of impending anaphylactic shock. Also, as appropriate, give local epinephrine or apply ice to the affected site to decrease absorption through vasoconstriction. Clear and maintain the patient's airway, give oxygen as needed, and institute cardiac monitoring. Have resuscitation equipment at hand, and be prepared to begin cardiopulmonary resuscitation. Intubation or a tracheostomy may be required.

ASSESSMENT
History
If the patient isn't in distress, obtain his medical history. Does he have known allergies? Does urticaria follow a seasonal pattern? Do certain foods or drugs seem to aggravate it? Is there a relationship to physical exertion? Is the patient routinely exposed to chemicals on the job or at home? Has the patient recently changed or used new skin products? Obtain a detailed drug history, including prescription and over-the-counter drugs. Note a history of chronic or parasitic infection, skin disease, or GI disorder.

Physical examination
Obtain the patient's vital signs. Perform a complete cardiopulmonary assessment, noting signs and symptoms of shock or respiratory distress. Assess for urticaria in other areas because new crops may continue to appear.

Pediatric pointers
Pediatric forms of urticaria include acute papular urticaria (usually after insect bites) and urticaria pigmentosa (rare). Hereditary angioedema may be causative.

MEDICAL CAUSES
● *Anaphylaxis.* An acute reaction, anaphylaxis is marked by the rapid eruption of diffuse urticaria and angioedema, with wheals ranging from pinpoint to palm-size or larger.

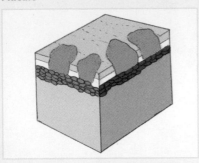
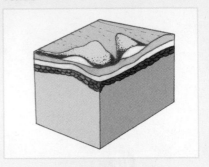
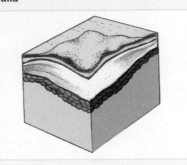
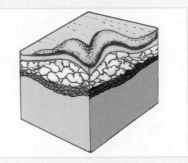
Lesions are usually pruritic and stinging; paresthesia commonly precedes their eruption. Other acute findings include profound anxiety, weakness, diaphoresis, sneezing, shortness of breath, profuse rhinorrhea, nasal congestion, dysphagia, and warm, moist skin.

● *Hereditary angioedema.* An autosomal dominant disorder, cutaneous involvement is manifested by nonpitting, nonpruritic edema of an extremity or the face. Respiratory mucosal involvement can produce life-threatening acute laryngeal edema.

● *Lyme disease.* Although not diagnostic of this tick-borne disease, urticaria may result from the characteristic skin lesion (erythema chronicum migrans). Later effects include constant malaise and fatigue, intermittent headache, fever, chills, lymphadenopathy, neurologic and cardiac abnormalities, and arthritis.

OTHER CAUSES

● *Drugs.* Many drugs can cause urticaria; the most common include aspirin, atropine, codeine, dextran, immune serums, insulin,

Wheal

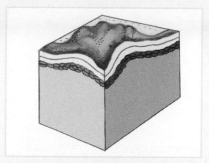

A slightly raised, firm lesion of variable size and shape, surrounded by edema; skin may be red or pale

Papule

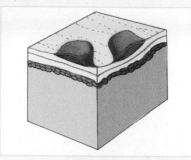

A small, solid, raised lesion less than 1 cm in diameter, with red to purple skin discoloration

Nodule

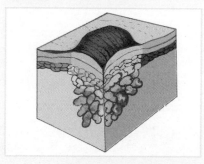

A small, firm, circumscribed, elevated lesion 1 to 2 cm in diameter with possible skin discoloration

Tumor

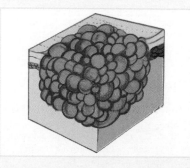

A solid, raised mass usually larger than 2 cm in diameter with possible skin discoloration

morphine, penicillin, quinine, sulfonamides, and vaccines. In addition, radiographic contrast medium commonly produces urticaria, especially when administered intravenously.

NURSING CONSIDERATIONS

To help relieve the patient's discomfort, apply a bland skin emollient or one containing menthol and phenol. Expect to give an antihistamine, a systemic corticosteroid or, if stress is a suspected contributing factor, a tranquilizer. Tepid baths and cool compress-es may also enhance vasoconstriction and decrease pruritus.

PATIENT TEACHING

Teach the patient to avoid the causative stimulus, if appropriate. Emphasize the importance of wearing a medical alert bracelet that identifies his allergies. Explain the risks of delayed symptoms and which signs and symptoms to report. Discuss methods and techniques to prevent anaphylaxis. Instruct the patient on the proper use of an anaphylaxis kit and epinephrine administration.

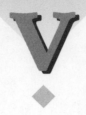

Vision loss

The inability to perceive visual stimuli, vision loss can be sudden or gradual and temporary or permanent. The deficit can range from a slight impairment of vision to total blindness. It can result from an ocular, neurologic, or systemic disorder or from trauma or the use of certain drugs. The ultimate visual outcome may depend on early, accurate diagnosis and treatment.

Act now *Sudden vision loss can signal central retinal artery occlusion or acute angle-closure glaucoma — ocular emergencies that require immediate intervention. If the patient reports sudden vision loss, immediately notify an ophthalmologist for an emergency examination, and perform the following interventions.*

For a patient with suspected central retinal artery occlusion, perform light massage over his closed eyelid. Increase his carbon dioxide level by administering a set flow of oxygen through a Venturi mask, or have the patient rebreathe in a paper bag to retain exhaled carbon dioxide. These steps will dilate the artery and, possibly, restore blood flow to the retina.

For a patient with suspected acute angle-closure glaucoma, measure intraocular pressure (IOP) with a tonometer. IOP can also be estimated without a tonometer by placing a finger over the patient's closed eyelid. A rock-hard eyeball usually indicates increased IOP. Instill timolol drops and administer I.V. acetazolamide to assist in decreasing IOP.

ASSESSMENT
History
Sudden vision loss can signal an ocular emergency. Don't touch the eye if the patient has perforating or penetrating ocular trauma.

If the patient's vision loss occurred gradually, ask him if it developed over hours, days, or weeks. Does it affect one eye or both? Does it affect all or part of the visual field? Is the vision loss transient or persistent? What's the patient's age? Ask whether he has experienced photosensitivity, and ask him about the location, intensity, and duration of eye pain. Obtain an ocular history, including history of eye problems or systemic diseases that may lead to eye problems, such as infections, cancer, hypertension, diabetes mellitus, and thyroid, rheumatic, or vascular disease.

Physical examination
Assess visual acuity and determine the best available vision correction in each eye. (See *Testing visual acuity.*)

Carefully inspect both eyes, noting edema, foreign bodies, drainage, or conjunctival or scleral redness. Observe whether lid closure is complete or incomplete, and check for ptosis. Using a flashlight, examine the cornea and iris for scars, irregularities, and foreign bodies. Evaluate extraocular muscle function by testing the six cardinal fields of gaze. (See *Testing extraocular muscles,* page 306.) Observe the size, shape, and color of the pupils, and test the direct and consensual light reflex and the effect of accommodation. (See *Vision loss: Causes and associated findings,* pages 308 and 309.)

TESTING VISUAL ACUITY

Use a Snellen letter chart to test visual acuity in the literate patient older than age 6. Have the patient sit or stand 20′ (6 m) from the chart. Then, tell him to cover his left eye and read aloud the smallest line of letters that he can see. Record the fraction assigned to that line on the chart (the numerator indicates distance from the chart; the denominator indicates the distance at which a normal eye can read the chart). Normal vision is 20/20. Repeat the test with the patient's right eye covered.

If the patient can't read the largest letter from a distance of 20′, have him approach the chart until he can read it. Then, record the distance between him and the chart as the numerator of the fraction. For example, if he can see the top line of the chart at a distance of 3′ (1 m), record the test result as 3/20.

Use a Snellen symbol chart to test children ages 3 to 6 and illiterate patients. Follow the same procedure as for the Snellen letter chart, but ask the patient to indicate the direction of the E's fingers as you point to each symbol.

Snellen letter chart

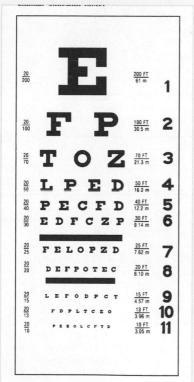

Snellen symbol chart

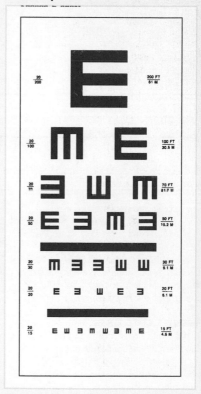

Pediatric pointers

Children who complain of slowly progressive vision loss may have an optic nerve glioma (a slow-growing, usually benign tumor) or retinoblastoma (a malignant tumor of the retina). Congenital rubella and syphilis may cause vision loss in infants. Retrolental fibroplasia may cause vision loss in premature infants. Other congenital causes of vi-

TESTING EXTRAOCULAR MUSCLES

The coordinated action of six muscles controls eyeball movements. To test the function of each muscle and the cranial nerve (CN) that innervates it, ask the patient to look in the direction controlled by that muscle. The six directions you can test make up the cardinal fields of gaze. The patient's inability to turn the eye in the designated direction indicates muscle weakness or paralysis.

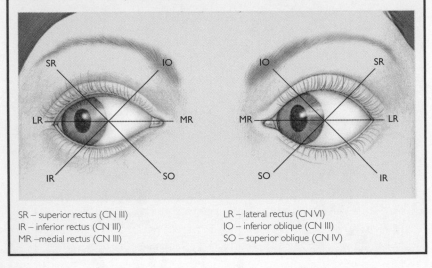

SR – superior rectus (CN III)
IR – inferior rectus (CN III)
MR –medial rectus (CN III)

LR – lateral rectus (CN VI)
IO – inferior oblique (CN III)
SO – superior oblique (CN IV)

---

sion loss include Marfan syndrome, retinitis pigmentosa, and amblyopia.

Geriatric pointers

In elderly patients, reduced visual acuity may be caused by morphologic changes in the choroid, pigment epithelium, and retina or by decreased function of the rods, cones, and other neural elements. Elderly patients commonly have difficulty turning their eyes upward. IOP also increases with age.

MEDICAL CAUSES

- *Amaurosis fugax.* With this amaurosis fugax, recurrent attacks of unilateral vision loss may last from a few seconds to a few minutes. Vision is normal at other times. Transient unilateral weakness, hypertension, and elevated IOP in the affected eye may also occur.
- *Cataract.* Typically, painless and gradual blurred vision precedes vision loss. As the cataract progresses, the pupil turns milky white.
- *Concussion.* Immediately or shortly after blunt head trauma, vision may be blurred, double, or lost. Generally, vision loss is temporary. Other findings include headache, anterograde and retrograde amnesia, transient loss of consciousness, nausea, vomiting, dizziness, irritability, confusion, lethargy, and aphasia.
- *Diabetic retinopathy.* Retinal edema and hemorrhage lead to blurred vision, which may progress to blindness.
- *Endophthalmitis.* Typically, endophthalmitis, an intraocular inflammation, follows penetrating trauma, I.V. drug use, or intraocular surgery, causing possibly permanent unilateral vision loss; a sympathetic inflammation may affect the other eye.
- *Glaucoma.* Glaucoma produces gradual blurred vision that may progress to total blindness. Findings are the rapid onset of unilateral inflammation and pain, pressure over the eye, moderate pupil dilation, nonreactive pupillary response, a cloudy cornea, reduced visual acuity, photophobia, and perception of blue or red halos around lights. Nausea and vomiting may also occur.

Alert *Acute angle-closure glaucoma is an ocular emergency that may produce blindness within 3 to 5 days.*

Chronic angle-closure glaucoma has a gradual onset and usually produces no symptoms, although blurred or halo vision may occur. If untreated, it progresses to blindness and extreme pain.

Chronic open-angle glaucoma is usually bilateral, with an insidious onset and a slowly progressive course. It causes peripheral vision loss, aching eyes, halo vision, and reduced visual acuity (especially at night).

- **Hereditary corneal dystrophies.** Some dystrophies cause vision loss with associated pain, photophobia, tearing, and corneal opacities.

- **Herpes zoster.** When herpes zoster affects the nasociliary nerve, bilateral vision loss is accompanied by eyelid lesions, conjunctivitis, skin lesions that usually appear on the nose, and ocular muscle palsies.

- **Hyphema.** Blood in the anterior chamber can reduce vision to light perception only. Most hyphemas are the direct result of blunt trauma to the normal eye.

- **Keratitis.** An inflammation of the cornea, keratitis may lead to complete unilateral vision loss. Other findings include an opaque cornea, increased tearing, irritation, and photophobia.

- **Ocular trauma.** Following eye injury, sudden unilateral or bilateral vision loss may occur. Vision loss may be total or partial and permanent or temporary. The eyelids may be reddened, edematous, and lacerated; intraocular contents may be extruded.

- **Optic atrophy.** Degeneration of the optic nerve, optic atrophy can develop spontaneously or follow inflammation or edema of the nerve head, causing irreversible loss of the visual field with changes in color vision. Pupillary reactions are sluggish, and optic disk pallor is evident.

- **Optic neuritis.** An umbrella term for inflammation, degeneration, or demyelinization of the optic nerve, optic neuritis usually produces temporary but severe unilateral vision loss. Pain around the eye occurs, especially with movement of the globe. This may occur with visual field deficits and a sluggish pupillary response to light. Ophthalmoscopic examination commonly reveals hyperemia of the optic disk, blurred disk margins, and filling of the physiologic cup.

- **Paget's disease.** Bilateral vision loss may develop as a result of bony impingements on the cranial nerves. This occurs with hearing loss, tinnitus, vertigo, and severe, persistent bone pain. Cranial enlargement may be noticeable frontally and occipitally, and headaches may occur. Sites of bone involvement are warm and tender, and impaired mobility and pathologic fractures are common.

- **Papilledema.** Papilledema is characterized by swelling of the optic disk from increased intracranial pressure; both optic disks are affected. Acute papilledema may lead to momentary blurring or transiently obscured vision, whereas chimeric papilledema may lead to vision loss.

- **Pituitary tumor.** As a pituitary adenoma grows, blurred vision progresses to hemianopia and, possibly, unilateral blindness. Double vision, nystagmus, ptosis, limited eye movement, and headaches may also occur.

- **Retinal artery occlusion (central).** A painless ocular emergency, retinal artery occlusion causes sudden unilateral vision loss, which may be partial or complete. Pupil examination reveals a sluggish direct pupillary response and a normal consensual response. Permanent blindness may occur within hours.

- **Retinal detachment.** Depending on the degree and location of detachment, painless vision loss may be gradual or sudden and total or partial. Macular involvement causes total blindness.

With partial vision loss, the patient may describe visual field deficits or a shadow or curtain over the visual field as well as visual floaters.

- **Retinal vein occlusion (central).** Most common in elderly patients, retinal vein occlusion is a painless disorder that causes a unilateral decrease in visual acuity with variable vision loss. IOP may be elevated in both eyes.

- **Rift Valley fever.** A viral disease, Rift Valley fever causes inflammation of the retina and may result in some permanent vision loss. Typical signs and symptoms include fever, myalgia, weakness, dizziness, and back pain. A small percentage of patients may develop encephalitis or may progress to hemorrhagic fever that can lead to shock and hemorrhage.

(Text continues on page 310.)

Vision loss:
Causes and associated findings

Major associated signs and symptoms

Common causes	Aphasia	Blurred vision	Bone pain	Color vision change	Confusion	Conjunctivitis	Corneal opacities	Decreased night vision	Dizziness	Double vision	Elevated IOP	Eye inflammation	Eye muscle changes	Eye pain	Eye tearing
Amauroses fugax											●				
Cataract		●		●											
Concussion	●	●			●					●					
Diabetic retinopathy		●													
Endophthalmitis												●			
Glaucoma							●							●	
Hereditary corneal dystrophies							●							●	●
Herpes zoster						●							●		
Keratitis							●					●			●
Optic atrophy															
Optic neuritis												●		●	
Paget's disease			●												
Papilledema		●													
Pituitary tumor		●								●					
Retinal artery occlusion (central)															
Retinal vein occlusion (central)		●									●				
Rift Valley fever									●				●		
Senile macular degeneration		●						●							
Stevens-Johnson syndrome						●	●							●	
Temporal arteritis		●			●										
Trachoma						●								●	●
Uveitis		●				●								●	
Vitreous hemorrhage				●											

Fever	Headache	Hypertension	Loss of consciousness	Myalgia	Nausea & vomiting	Nystagmus	Optic disk changes	Peripheral visual field loss	Photophobia	Ptosis	Pupil dilation	Pupil reaction changes	Retinal edema	Retinal hemorrhage	Skin lesions	Tinnitus	Vertigo	Visual floaters	Visual halos	Weakness	Weight loss	White lens
		●																		●		
																						●
	●		●		●																	
													●	●								
					●			●	●			●							●			
									●													
															●							
									●													
							●	●				●										
								●				●										
	●															●	●					
							●															
	●					●					●											
												●										
●				●																●		
●				●	●										●							
●	●			●																●	●	
									●						●							
									●		●								●			
																	●					

- *Senile macular degeneration.* Occurring in elderly patients, senile macular degeneration causes painless blurring or loss of central vision. Vision loss may proceed slowly or rapidly, eventually affecting both eyes. Visual acuity may be worse at night.
- *Stevens-Johnson syndrome.* Corneal scarring from associated conjunctival lesions produces marked vision loss. Purulent conjunctivitis, eye pain, and difficulty opening the eyes occur. Additional findings include widespread bullae, fever, malaise, cough, drooling, an inability to eat, sore throat, chest pain, vomiting, diarrhea, myalgia, arthralgia, hematuria, and signs of renal failure.
- *Temporal arteritis.* Vision loss and visual blurring with a throbbing, unilateral headache characterize temporal arteritis. Other findings include malaise, anorexia, weight loss, weakness, low-grade fever, generalized muscle aches, and confusion.
- *Trachoma.* A rare disorder, trachoma may initially produce varying vision loss and a mild infection resembling bacterial conjunctivitis. Conjunctival follicles, red and edematous eyelids, pain, photophobia, tearing, and exudation also occur. After about 1 month, conjunctival follicles enlarge into inflamed yellow or gray papillae.
- *Uveitis.* Inflammation of the uveal tract may result in unilateral vision loss. Anterior uveitis produces moderate to severe eye pain, severe conjunctival injection, photophobia, and a small, nonreactive pupil. Posterior uveitis may produce an insidious onset of blurred vision, conjunctival injection, visual floaters, pain, and photophobia. Associated posterior scar formation distorts the shape of the pupil.
- *Vitreous hemorrhage.* With vitreous hemorrhage, sudden unilateral vision loss may result from intraocular trauma, ocular tumors, or systemic disease (especially diabetes, hypertension, sickle cell anemia, or leukemia). Visual floaters and partial vision with a reddish haze may occur. The vision loss may be permanent.

OTHER CAUSES

- *Drugs.* Chloroquine therapy may cause patchy retinal pigmentation that typically leads to blindness. Phenylbutazone may cause vision loss and increased susceptibility to retinal detachment. Digoxin, indomethacin, ethambutol, quinine sulfate, and

methanol toxicity may also cause visual disturbances and possibly vision loss.

NURSING CONSIDERATIONS

Any degree of vision loss can be extremely frightening. To ease the patient's fears, orient him to his environment and make sure that it's safe. Announce your presence each time you approach him. If the patient reports photophobia, darken the room and suggest that he wear sunglasses during the day. Obtain cultures of any drainage, and instruct him not to touch the unaffected eye with anything that has come in contact with the affected eye. If necessary, prepare him for surgery.

PATIENT TEACHING

Discuss safety measures to prevent injury. Emphasize the importance of frequent hand washing and to avoid rubbing the eyes. If the loss is progressive or permanent, refer the patient to the appropriate social service agencies, community support services, and related associations for assistance with adaptation and equipment.

Vomiting

Vomiting is the forceful expulsion of gastric contents through the mouth. Characteristically preceded by nausea, vomiting results from a coordinated sequence of abdominal muscle contractions and reverse esophageal peristalsis.

A common sign of GI disorders, vomiting also occurs with fluid and electrolyte imbalances, infections, and metabolic, endocrine, labyrinthine, central nervous system (CNS), and cardiac disorders. It can also result from drug therapy, surgery, or radiation.

Vomiting occurs normally during the first trimester of pregnancy, but its subsequent development may signal complications. It can also result from stress, anxiety, pain, alcohol intoxication, overeating, or ingestion of distasteful food or liquid.

Act now Immediate action is required if the patient's vomiting has lead to dehydration or is resulting in significant blood loss. Immediate response includes instituting I.V. fluid or blood replacement. Obtain blood samples to assess electrolyte level, renal studies, liver function tests, and a complete blood count. *Assess the patient's vital signs frequently until he's stable. Administer an antiemetic as ordered. Offer supportive care during vomiting episodes, and provide meticulous mouth care afterward.*

Assessment

History
Ask the patient to describe the onset, duration, and intensity of his vomiting. What started the vomiting? What makes it subside? If possible, collect, measure, and inspect the character of the vomitus. (See *Vomitus: Characteristics and causes.*) Explore associated complaints, particularly nausea, abdominal pain, anorexia and weight loss, changes in bowel habits or stools, excessive belching or flatus, and bloating or fullness.

Obtain a medical history, noting GI, endocrine, and metabolic disorders; recent infections; and cancer, including chemotherapy or radiation therapy. Ask about current medication use and alcohol consumption. If the patient is a female of childbearing age, ask if she is or could be pregnant. Ask which contraceptive method she's using.

Physical examination
Inspect the abdomen for distention, and auscultate for bowel sounds and bruits. Palpate for rigidity and tenderness, and test for rebound tenderness. Next, palpate and percuss the liver for enlargement. Assess other body systems as appropriate.

During the examination, keep in mind that projectile vomiting unaccompanied by nausea may indicate increased intracranial pressure (ICP), a life-threatening emergency. If this occurs in a patient with a CNS injury, you should quickly check his vital signs. Stay alert for widened pulse pressure or bradycardia.

Pediatric pointers
In a neonate, pyloric obstruction may cause projectile vomiting, whereas Hirschsprung's disease may cause fecal vomiting. Intussusception may lead to vomiting of bile and fecal matter in an infant or toddler. Because an infant may aspirate vomitus as a result of his immature cough and gag reflexes, position him on his side or abdomen and clear any vomitus immediately.

VOMITUS: CHARACTERISTICS AND CAUSES

When you collect a sample of the patient's vomitus, observe it carefully for clues to the underlying disorder. Here's what vomitus may indicate:

BILE-STAINED (GREENISH) VOMITUS
Obstruction below the pylorus, as from a duodenal lesion

BLOODY VOMITUS
Upper GI bleeding (if bright red, may result from gastritis or a peptic ulcer; if dark red, from esophageal or gastric varices)

BROWN VOMITUS WITH A FECAL ODOR
Intestinal obstruction or infarction

BURNING, BITTER-TASTING VOMITUS
Excessive hydrochloric acid in gastric contents

COFFEE-GROUND VOMITUS
Digested blood from slowly bleeding gastric or duodenal lesion

UNDIGESTED FOOD
Gastric outlet obstruction such as from gastric tumor or ulcer

---

Geriatric pointers
Although elderly patients can develop several of the disorders mentioned earlier, always rule out intestinal ischemia first—it's especially common in patients of this age-group and it has a high mortality.

Medical causes
- *Adrenal insufficiency.* Common GI findings with adrenal insufficiency include vomiting, nausea, anorexia, and diarrhea. Other findings include weakness, fatigue, weight loss, bronze skin, orthostatic hypotension, and a weak, irregular pulse.
- *Anthrax (GI).* Initial signs and symptoms after eating contaminated meat from an infected animal include vomiting, loss of appetite, nausea, and fever. Signs and symp-

toms may progress to abdominal pain, severe bloody diarrhea, and hematemesis.

- **Appendicitis.** Vomiting and nausea may follow or accompany abdominal pain. Pain typically begins as vague epigastric or periumbilical discomfort and rapidly progresses to severe, stabbing pain in the right lower quadrant. The patient generally has a positive McBurney sign — severe pain and tenderness on palpation about 2″ (5 cm) from the right anterior superior spine of the ilium, on a line between that spine and the umbilicus. Associated findings usually include abdominal rigidity and tenderness, anorexia, constipation or diarrhea, cutaneous hyperalgesia, fever, tachycardia, and malaise.
- **Bulimia.** Most common in females ages 18 to 29, bulimia is characterized by polyphagia that alternates with self-induced vomiting, fasting, or diarrhea. It's commonly accompanied by anorexia. The patient typically weighs less than what is considered healthy but has a morbid fear of obesity. Self-induced vomiting may be evidenced by calloused knuckles.
- **Cholecystitis (acute).** With acute cholecystitis, nausea and mild vomiting commonly follow severe right upper quadrant pain that may radiate to the back or shoulders. Associated findings include abdominal tenderness and, possibly, rigidity and distention, fever, and diaphoresis.
- **Cholelithiasis.** Nausea and vomiting accompany severe unlocalized right upper quadrant or epigastric pain after eating fatty foods. Other findings include abdominal tenderness and guarding, flatulence, belching, epigastric burning, pyrosis, tachycardia, and restlessness.
- **Cholera.** Signs and symptoms include vomiting and abrupt watery diarrhea. Severe water and electrolyte loss leads to thirst, weakness, muscle cramps, decreased skin turgor, oliguria, tachycardia, and hypotension. Without treatment, death can occur within hours.
- **Cirrhosis.** Insidious early signs and symptoms of cirrhosis typically include nausea and vomiting, anorexia, aching abdominal pain, and constipation or diarrhea. Later findings include jaundice, hepatomegaly, and abdominal distention.
- **Escherichia coli O157:H7.** The signs and symptoms of E. coli O157:H7 infection include vomiting, watery or bloody diarrhea, nausea, fever, and abdominal cramps. In chil-

dren younger than age 5 and in elderly people, hemolytic uremic syndrome may develop in which the red blood cells are destroyed, and this may ultimately lead to acute renal failure.

- **Ectopic pregnancy.** Vomiting, nausea, vaginal bleeding, and lower abdominal pain occur in ectopic pregnancy, a potentially life-threatening disorder.
- **Electrolyte imbalances.** Such disturbances as hyponatremia, hypernatremia, hypokalemia, and hypercalcemia commonly cause nausea and vomiting. Other effects include arrhythmias, tremors, seizures, anorexia, malaise, and weakness.
- **Food poisoning.** Vomiting is a common finding in food poisoning, caused by preformed toxins produced by bacteria typically found in foods, such as *Bacillus cereus, Clostridium,* and *Staphylococcus.* Diarrhea and fever also usually occur.
- **Gastric cancer.** This rare cancer may produce mild nausea, vomiting (possibly of mucus or blood), anorexia, upper abdominal discomfort, and chronic dyspepsia. Fatigue, weight loss, melena, and altered bowel habits are also common.
- **Gastritis.** Nausea and vomiting of mucus or blood are common with gastritis, especially after ingestion of alcohol, aspirin, spicy foods, or caffeine. Epigastric pain, belching, and fever may also occur.
- **Gastroenteritis.** Gastroenteritis causes nausea, vomiting (commonly of undigested food), diarrhea, and abdominal cramping. Fever, malaise, hyperactive bowel sounds, and abdominal pain and tenderness may also occur.
- **Heart failure.** Nausea and vomiting may occur, especially with right-sided heart failure. Associated findings include tachycardia, ventricular gallop, fatigue, dyspnea, crackles, peripheral edema, and jugular vein distention.
- **Hepatitis.** Vomiting commonly follows nausea as an early sign of viral hepatitis. Other early findings include fatigue, myalgia, arthralgia, headache, photophobia, anorexia, pharyngitis, cough, and fever.
- **Hyperemesis gravidarum.** Unremitting nausea and vomiting that last beyond the first trimester characterize hyperemesis gravidarum, a disorder of pregnancy. Vomitus contains undigested food, mucus, and small amounts of bile early in the disorder; later, it has a coffee-ground appearance. Associated

findings include weight loss, headache, and delirium. Thyroid dysfunction may be associated with this condition.

- **Increased ICP.** Projectile vomiting that isn't preceded by nausea is a sign of increased ICP. The patient may exhibit a decreased level of consciousness (LOC) and Cushing's triad (bradycardia, hypertension, and respiratory pattern changes). He may also have headache, widened pulse pressure, impaired motor movement, vision disturbances, pupillary changes, and papilledema.
- **Infection.** Acute localized or systemic infection may cause vomiting and nausea. Other common findings include fever, headache, malaise, and fatigue.
- **Intestinal obstruction.** Nausea and vomiting (bilious or fecal) are common with intestinal obstruction, especially of the upper small intestine. Abdominal pain is usually episodic and colicky but can become severe and steady. Constipation occurs early in large intestinal obstruction and late in small intestinal obstruction. Obstipation, however, may signal complete obstruction. In partial obstruction, bowel sounds are typically high pitched and hyperactive; in complete obstruction, hypoactive or absent. Abdominal distention and tenderness also occur, possibly with visible peristaltic waves and a palpable abdominal mass.
- **Labyrinthitis.** Nausea and vomiting commonly occur with labyrinthitis, an acute inner ear inflammation. Other findings include severe vertigo, progressive hearing loss, nystagmus and, possibly, otorrhea.
- **Listeriosis.** After eating food contaminated with the bacterium *Listeria monocytogenes,* vomiting, fever, myalgia, abdominal pain, nausea, and diarrhea occur. If the infection spreads to the nervous system, meningitis may develop. Signs and symptoms may include fever, headache, nuchal rigidity, and change in the patient's LOC. The food-borne illness primarily affects pregnant females, neonates, and those with weakened immune systems.
- **Ménière's disease.** Ménière's disease causes sudden, brief, recurrent attacks of nausea and vomiting, dizziness, vertigo, hearing loss, tinnitus, diaphoresis, and nystagmus.
- **Mesenteric artery ischemia.** A life-threatening disorder, mesenteric artery ischemia may cause nausea and vomiting and severe, cramping abdominal pain, especially after meals. Other findings include diarrhea or constipation, abdominal tenderness and bloating, anorexia, weight loss, and abdominal bruits.
- **Mesenteric venous thrombosis.** An insidious or an acute onset of nausea, vomiting, and abdominal pain occur with mesenteric venous thrombosis and may be accompanied by diarrhea or constipation, abdominal distention, hematemesis, and melena.
- **Metabolic acidosis.** Metabolic acidosis is an imbalance that may produce nausea, vomiting, anorexia, diarrhea, Kussmaul's respirations, and a decreased LOC.
- **Migraine headache.** Nausea and vomiting are prodromal signs and symptoms, with fatigue, photophobia, light flashes, increased noise sensitivity and, possibly, partial vision loss and paresthesia.
- **Motion sickness.** Nausea and vomiting may be accompanied by headache, vertigo, dizziness, fatigue, diaphoresis, and dyspnea.
- **Myocardial infarction.** Nausea and vomiting may occur, but the cardinal symptom is severe substernal chest pain, which may radiate to the left arm, jaw, or neck. Dyspnea, pallor, clammy skin, diaphoresis, and restlessness also occur.
- **Pancreatitis (acute).** Vomiting, usually preceded by nausea, is an early sign of pancreatitis. Associated findings include steady, severe epigastric or left upper quadrant pain that may radiate to the back, abdominal tenderness and rigidity, hypoactive bowel sounds, anorexia, vomiting, and fever. Tachycardia, restlessness, hypotension, skin mottling, and cold, sweaty extremities may occur in severe cases.
- **Peptic ulcer.** Nausea and vomiting may follow sharp, burning or gnawing epigastric pain, especially when the stomach is empty or after the ingestion of alcohol, caffeine, or aspirin. Attacks are relieved by eating or taking antacids. Hematemesis or melena may also occur.
- **Peritonitis.** Nausea and vomiting usually accompany acute abdominal pain in the area of inflammation. Other findings include abdominal distention, rigidity, and tenderness as well as high fever with chills, tachycardia, hypoactive or absent bowel sounds, weakness, and pale, cold skin. The patient may also experience diaphoresis, hypotension, signs of dehydration, and shallow respirations.
- **Preeclampsia.** Nausea and vomiting are common with preeclampsia, a disorder of

pregnancy. Rapid weight gain, epigastric pain, generalized edema, elevated blood pressure, oliguria, severe frontal headache, and blurred or double vision also occur.

● *Q fever.* Signs and symptoms of Q fever, a rickettsial infection, include vomiting, fever, chills, severe headache, malaise, chest pain, nausea, and diarrhea. Fever may last up to 2 weeks. In severe cases, the patient may develop hepatitis or pneumonia.

● *Renal and urologic disorders.* Cystitis, pyelonephritis, calculi, and other disorders of this system can cause vomiting. Accompanying findings reflect the specific disorder. Persistent nausea and vomiting are typical findings in patients with acute or worsening chronic renal failure.

● *Rhabdomyolysis.* Signs and symptoms of rhabdomyolisis include vomiting, muscle weakness or pain, fever, nausea, malaise, and dark urine. Acute renal failure is the most commonly reported complication. It results from renal structure obstruction and injury during the kidney's attempt to filter myoglobin from the bloodstream.

● *Thyrotoxicosis.* Nausea and vomiting may accompany the classic findings of severe anxiety, heat intolerance, weight loss despite increased appetite, diaphoresis, diarrhea, tremors, tachycardia, and palpitations. Other findings include exophthalmos, ventricular or atrial gallop, and an enlarged thyroid gland.

● *Typhus.* Typhus is a rickettsial disease transmitted to humans by fleas, mites, or body lice. Initial symptoms include headache, myalgia, arthralgia, and malaise, followed by an abrupt onset of vomiting, nausea, chills, and fever. A maculopapular rash may be present in some cases.

● *Ulcerative colitis.* Vomiting, nausea, and anorexia may occur, but the most common sign is recurrent diarrhea with blood, pus, and mucus. Fever, chills, and weight loss are also common.

OTHER CAUSES

● *Drugs.* Drugs that commonly cause vomiting include antineoplastics, opiates, ferrous sulfate, levodopa, oral potassium, chloride replacements, estrogens, sulfasalazine, antibiotics, quinidine, anesthetics, and overdoses of cardiac glycosides and theophylline. Syrup of ipecac, a mixture of ipecac fluid extract, glycerin, and syrup, is used to treat overdoses by inducing vomiting.

● *Radiation and surgery.* Radiation therapy may cause nausea and vomiting if it disrupts the gastric mucosa. Postoperative nausea and vomiting are common, especially after abdominal surgery.

NURSING CONSIDERATIONS

Draw blood to determine fluid, electrolyte, and acid-base balance. (Prolonged vomiting can cause dehydration, electrolyte imbalances, and metabolic alkalosis.) Have the patient breathe deeply to ease his nausea and help prevent further vomiting. Keep his room fresh and clean smelling by removing bedpans and emesis basins promptly after use. Elevate his head or position him on his side to prevent aspiration of vomitus. Continuously monitor his vital signs and intake and output (including vomitus and liquid stools). If necessary, administer I.V. fluids or have the patient sip clear liquids to maintain hydration.

Because pain can precipitate or intensify nausea and vomiting, administer pain medications promptly. If possible, give these by injection or suppository to prevent exacerbating associated nausea. If an opioid is used to treat pain, monitor bowel sounds and flatus and bowel movements carefully because they slow down GI motility and may exacerbate vomiting. If you administer an antiemetic, be alert for abdominal distention and hypoactive bowel sounds, which may indicate gastric retention. If this occurs, insert a nasogastric tube.

PATIENT TEACHING

Advise the patient to replace fluid losses to avoid dehydration. Inform the patient suffering from migraine headaches that vomiting may be a prodromal symptom; advise him to take antimigraine medication should vomiting occur.

WXYZ

Wheezing

Wheezes are adventitious breath sounds with a high-pitched, musical, squealing, creaking, or groaning quality. They're caused by air flowing at a high velocity through a narrowed airway. When they originate in the large airways, they can be heard by placing an unaided ear over the chest wall or at the mouth. When they originate in smaller airways, they can be heard by placing a stethoscope over the anterior or posterior chest. Unlike crackles and rhonchi, wheezes can't be cleared by coughing.

Usually, prolonged wheezing occurs during expiration when bronchi are shortened and narrowed. Causes of airway narrowing include bronchospasm; mucosal thickening or edema; partial obstruction from a tumor, a foreign body, or secretions; and extrinsic pressure, such as in tension pneumothorax or goiter. With airway obstruction, wheezing occurs during inspiration.

Act now *Assess the degree of the patient's respiratory distress. Is he responsive? Is he restless, confused, anxious, or afraid? Are his respirations abnormally fast, slow, shallow, or deep? Are they irregular? Can you hear wheezing through his mouth? Does he exhibit increased accessory muscle use; increased chest wall motion; intercostal, suprasternal, or supraclavicular retractions; stridor; or nasal flaring? Take his other vital signs, noting hypotension or hypertension, decreased oxygen saturation, and an irregular, weak, rapid, or slow pulse.*

Help the patient relax, and administer humidified oxygen by face mask and encourage slow, deep breathing. Have endotracheal intubation and emergency resuscitation equipment readily available. Call the respiratory therapy department to supply intermittent positive-pressure breathing and nebulization treatments with bronchodilators. Insert an I.V. line for administration of drugs, such as diuretics, steroids, bronchodilators, and sedatives. Perform the abdominal thrust maneuver, as indicated, for airway obstruction.

ASSESSMENT
History

If the patient isn't in respiratory distress, obtain his medical history. What provokes his wheezing? Does he have asthma or allergies? Does he smoke or have a history of a pulmonary, cardiac, or circulatory disorder? Does he have cancer? Ask about recent surgery, illness, or trauma or changes in appetite, weight, exercise tolerance, or sleep patterns. Obtain a drug history. Ask about exposure to toxic fumes or respiratory irritants. If he has a cough, ask how it sounds, when it starts, and how often it occurs. Does he have paroxysms of coughing? Is his cough dry, sputum producing, or bloody?

Ask the patient about chest pain. If he reports pain, determine its quality, onset, duration, intensity, and radiation. Does it increase with breathing, coughing, or certain positions?

Physical examination

Examine the patient's nose and mouth for congestion, drainage, or signs of infection such as halitosis. If he produces sputum, obtain a sample for examination. Check for cyanosis, pallor, clamminess, masses, tenderness, swelling, jugular vein distention, and enlarged lymph nodes. Inspect his chest for

EVALUATING BREATH SOUNDS

Diminished or absent breath sounds indicate some interference with airflow. If pus, fluid, or air fills the pleural space, breath sounds will be quieter than normal. If a foreign body or secretions obstruct a bronchus, breath sounds will be diminished or absent over distal lung tissue. Increased thickness of the chest wall, such as with a patient who's obese or extremely muscular, may cause breath sounds to be decreased, distant, or inaudible. Absent breath sounds typically indicate loss of ventilation power.

When air passes through narrowed airways or through moisture, or when the membranes lining the chest cavity become inflamed, adventitious breath sounds will be heard. These include crackles, rhonchi, wheezes, and pleural friction rubs. Usually, these sounds indicate pulmonary disease.

Follow the auscultation sequences shown to assess the patient's breath sounds. Have him take full, deep breaths, and compare sound variations from one side to the other. Note the location, timing, and character of abnormal breath sounds.

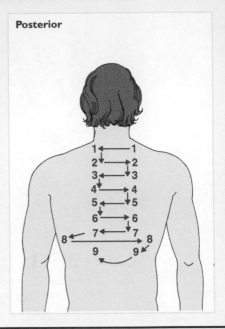

Posterior

---

abnormal configuration and asymmetrical motion, and determine if the trachea is midline. (See *Detecting slight tracheal deviation,* page 299.) Percuss for dullness or hyperresonance, and auscultate for crackles, rhonchi, or a pleural friction rub. Note absent or hypoactive breath sounds, abnormal heart sounds, gallops, or murmurs. (See *Evaluating breath sounds.*) Also note arrhythmias, bradycardia, or tachycardia. (See *Wheezing: Causes and associated findings,* pages 318 and 319.)

Pediatric pointers

Primary causes of wheezing in children include bronchospasm, mucosal edema, and accumulation of secretions, which may occur with such disorders as cystic fibrosis, aspiration of a foreign body, acute bronchiolitis, and pulmonary hemosiderosis.

Children are especially susceptible to wheezing because their small airways allow rapid obstruction.

MEDICAL CAUSES
● *Anaphylaxis.* An allergic reaction, anaphylaxis can cause tracheal edema or bronchospasm, resulting in severe wheezing and stridor. Initial signs and symptoms include fright, weakness, sneezing, dyspnea, nasal pruritus, urticaria, erythema, and angioedema. Respiratory distress occurs with nasal flaring, accessory muscle use, and intercostal retractions. Other findings include nasal edema and congestion with profuse, watery rhinorrhea as well as chest or throat tightness and dysphagia. Cardiac effects include arrhythmias and hypotension.
● *Aspiration of a foreign body.* Partial obstruction by a foreign body produces the sudden onset of wheezing and possibly stridor; a dry, paroxysmal cough; gagging; and hoarseness. Other findings include tachycardia, dyspnea, decreased breath sounds and, possibly, cyanosis. A retained foreign body may cause inflammation leading to fever, pain, and swelling.
● *Aspiration pneumonitis.* With aspiration pneumonitis, wheezing may accompany tachypnea, marked dyspnea, cyanosis, tachycardia, fever, a productive (eventually purulent) cough, and pink, frothy sputum.

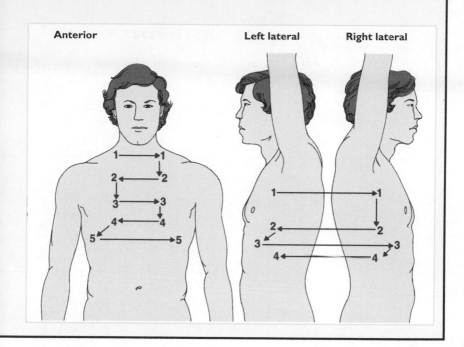

Anterior   Left lateral   Right lateral

- **Asthma.** Wheezing is an initial and cardinal sign of asthma. It's heard at the mouth during expiration. An initially dry cough later becomes productive with thick mucus. Other findings include apprehension, prolonged expiration, intercostal and supraclavicular retractions, rhonchi, accessory muscle use, nasal flaring, and tachypnea. Asthma also produces tachycardia, diaphoresis, and flushing or cyanosis.
- **Bronchial adenoma.** An insidious disorder, bronchial adenoma produces unilateral, possibly severe wheezing. Common features are chronic cough and recurring hemoptysis. Symptoms of airway obstruction may occur later.
- **Bronchiectasis.** Excessive mucus commonly causes intermittent and localized or diffuse wheezing. A copious, foul-smelling, mucopurulent cough is classic. It's accompanied by hemoptysis, rhonchi, and coarse crackles. Weight loss, fatigue, weakness, exertional dyspnea, fever, malaise, halitosis, and late-stage clubbing may also occur.
- **Bronchitis (chronic).** Chronic bronchitis causes wheezing that varies in severity, loca-

tion, and intensity. Associated findings include prolonged expiration, coarse crackles, scattered rhonchi, and a hacking cough that later becomes productive. Other effects include dyspnea, accessory muscle use, barrel chest, tachypnea, clubbing, edema, weight gain, and cyanosis.
- **Bronchogenic carcinoma.** Obstruction may cause localized wheezing. Typical findings include a productive cough, dyspnea, hemoptysis (initially blood-tinged sputum, possibly leading to massive hemorrhage), anorexia, and weight loss. Upper extremity edema and chest pain may also occur.
- **Chemical pneumonitis (acute).** Mucosal injury causes increased secretions and edema, leading to wheezing, dyspnea, orthopnea, crackles, malaise, fever, and a productive cough with purulent sputum. The patient may also have signs of conjunctivitis, pharyngitis, laryngitis, and rhinitis.
- **Emphysema.** Mild to moderate wheezing may occur with emphysema, a form of chronic obstructive pulmonary disease. Related findings include dyspnea, tachypnea, diminished breath sounds, peripheral cya-

WHEEZING:
CAUSES AND ASSOCIATED FINDINGS

MAJOR ASSOCIATED SIGNS AND SYMPTOMS

COMMON CAUSES	Accessory muscle use	Anorexia	Anxiety	Arrhythmias	Chest pain	Cough	Crackles	Cyanosis	Decreased breath sounds	Diaphoresis	Dysphagia	Dyspnea	Epistaxis	Fatigue
Anaphylaxis				●	●						●	●		
Aspiration of a foreign body						●		●	●			●		
Aspiration pneumonitis						●		●				●		
Asthma	●		●			●				●		●		
Bronchial adenoma						●								
Bronchiectasis						●	●					●		●
Bronchitis, chronic	●					●	●	●				●		
Bronchogenic carcinoma					●	●						●		
Chemical pneumonitis						●	●					●		
Emphysema	●	●				●		●	●			●		
Inhalation in jury						●	●							
Pneumothorax	●		●		●	●		●	●			●		
Pulmonary coccidioidomycosis		●				●	●							
Pulmonary edema				●		●	●	●		●		●		
Pulmonary embolus					●			●				●		
Pulmonary tuberculosis		●				●	●	●						●
Thyroid goiter											●			
Tracheobronchitis						●	●	●						
Wegener's granulomatosis						●	●					●	●	

nosis, pursed-lip breathing, anorexia, and malaise. Accessory muscle use, barrel chest, a chronic productive cough, and clubbing may also occur.

● *Inhalation injury.* Wheezing may eventually occur. Early findings include hoarseness and coughing, singed nasal hairs, orofacial

	Fever	Headache	Hemoptysis	Hoarseness	Hypotension	Malaise	Nasal flaring	Night sweats	Orthopnea	Prolonged expiration	Restlessness	Rhonchi	Sinusitis	Skin lesions	Stridor	Tachycardia	Tachypnea	Weakness	Weight loss
					●		●							●	●			●	
				●											●	●			
	●															●	●		
							●			●		●				●	●		
			●																
			●			●						●						●	●
										●		●					●		
			●																●
	●					●			●										
																	●		
				●								●							
											●					●	●		
	●	●				●						●	●					●	
					●				●							●	●		
	●					●		●											●
	●											●	●						
														●					

burns, and soot-stained sputum. Later effects are crackles, rhonchi, and respiratory distress.

● *Pneumothorax (tension).* A life-threatening disorder, tension pneumothorax causes respiratory distress with possible wheezing, dyspnea, tachycardia, tachypnea, and sudden, severe, sharp chest pain (commonly unilateral). Other findings include a dry cough, cyanosis, accessory muscle use, asymmetrical chest wall movement, anxiety, and restlessness. Examination reveals hyperresonance or tympany and diminished or absent breath sounds on the affected side, subcutaneous crepitation, decreased vocal fremitus, and tracheal deviation.

- *Pulmonary coccidioidomycosis.* Pulmonary coccidiodomycosis may cause wheezing and rhonchi along with cough, fever, chills, pleuritic chest pain, headache, weakness, malaise, anorexia, and a macular rash.
- *Pulmonary edema.* Wheezing may occur with pulmonary edema, a life-threatening disorder. Other signs and symptoms include coughing, exertional and paroxysmal nocturnal dyspnea and, later, orthopnea. Examination reveals tachycardia, tachypnea, dependent crackles, and a diastolic gallop. Severe pulmonary edema produces rapid, labored respirations and a productive cough with frothy, bloody sputum. The patient may also exhibit diffuse crackles, arrhythmias, hypotension, a thready pulse, and cold, clammy, cyanotic skin.
- *Pulmonary embolus.* Rarely, diffuse, mild wheezing occurs in pulmonary embolus. The condition is characterized by dyspnea, chest pain, and cyanosis.
- *Pulmonary tuberculosis.* In late stages, fibrosis causes wheezing. Common findings include a mild to severe productive cough with pleuritic chest pain and fine crackles, night sweats, anorexia, weight loss, fever, malaise, dyspnea, and fatigue. Other features are dullness on percussion, increased tactile fremitus, and amphoric breath sounds.
- *Thyroid goiter.* Thyroid goiter may be asymptomatic, or it may cause wheezing, dysphagia, and respiratory difficulty related to a compressed airway.
- *Tracheobronchitis.* Auscultation may detect wheezing, rhonchi, and crackles. The patient also has cough, slight fever, sudden chills, muscle and back pain, and substernal tightness.
- *Wegener's granulomatosis.* Wegener's granulomatosis may cause mild to moderate wheezing if it compresses major airways. Other findings include cough (possibly bloody), dyspnea, pleuritic chest pain, hemorrhagic skin lesions, and progressive renal failure. Epistaxis and severe sinusitis are common.

NURSING CONSIDERATIONS

Prepare the patient for diagnostic tests, such as chest X-rays, arterial blood gas analysis, pulmonary function tests, and sputum culture.

Ease the patient's breathing by placing him in semi-Fowler's position and repositioning him frequently. Perform pulmonary physiotherapy as necessary.

Administer an antibiotic to treat infection, a bronchodilator to relieve bronchospasm and maintain a patent airway, a steroid to reduce inflammation, and a mucolytic or expectorant to increase the flow of secretions. Provide humidification to thin secretions.

PATIENT TEACHING

If appropriate, encourage increased activity to promote drainage and prevent pooling of secretions. Encourage regular deep breathing and coughing. Explain the importance of drinking fluids to liquefy secretions and prevent dehydration.

TOXIC DRUG-DRUG INTERACTIONS

DANGEROUS HERB-DRUG INTERACTIONS

POTENTIAL AGENTS OF BIOTERRORISM

SELECTED REFERENCES

INDEX

TOXIC DRUG-DRUG INTERACTIONS

◆

INTERACTION	DRUG	INTERACTING DRUGS
Decreased corticosteroid effects	*Corticosteroids* (betamethasone, cortisone, dexamethasone, fludrocortisone, hydrocortisone, methylprednisolone, prednisolone, prednisone, triamcinolone)	*Rifamycins* (rifabutin, rifampin, rifapentine)
Digoxin toxicity and arrhythmias	*Digoxin* (Lanoxin)	*Tetracyclines* (demeclocycline, doxycycline, minocycline, tetracycline) *Thiazide diuretics* (chlorothiazide, hydrochlorothiazide, indapamide, methyclothiazide, metolazone, polythiazide, trichlormethiazide) *Verapamil* (Calan)
Hearing loss	*Aminoglycosides* (amikacin, gentamicin, kanamycin, neomycin, netilmicin, streptomycin, tobramycin)	*Loop diuretics* (bumetanide, ethacrynic acid, furosemide, torsemide)
Increased bleeding	*Warfarin* (Coumadin)	*Alteplase* (Activase, tPA) *Androgens* [17-alkyl] (danazol, fluoxymesterone, methyltestosterone, oxandrolone) *Cimetidine* (Tagamet) *Fibric acids* (clofibrate, fenofibrate, gemfibrozil) *Cranberry juice* *Salicylates* (aspirin, methylsalicylate) *Amiodarone* (Cordarone, Pacerone) *Azole antifungals* (fluconazole, itraconazole, ketoconazole, miconazole, voriconazole) *Macrolide antibiotics* (azithromycin, clarithromycin, erythromycin) *Metronidazole* (Flagyl) *Quinine derivatives* (quinidine, quinine) *Sulfinpyrazone* (Anturane) *Sulfonamides* (sulfasalazine, sulfisoxazole, cotrimoxazole) *Thyroid hormones* (levothyroxine, liothyronine, liotrix, thyroid) *Vitamin E*

Nursing considerations

◆ Avoid use together, if possible.
◆ Effects may persist for 2 to 3 weeks after discontinuation.

◆ Use together cautiously.
◆ Monitor digoxin serum concentrations. The therapeutic range for digoxin is 0.8 to 2 ng/ml.
◆ Effects of tetracyclines on digoxin may persist for several months after the antibiotic is stopped.
◆ Monitor serum potassium and magnesium levels if taking both thiazide diuretics and digoxin.
◆ Monitor the patient for signs of digoxin toxicity including arrhythmias (such as bradycardia, atrio-ventricular [AV] block, ventricular ectopy), lethargy, drowsiness, confusion, hallucinations, headaches, syncope, vision disturbances, nausea, anorexia, vomiting, or diarrhea.

◆ Use together cautiously.
◆ Patients with renal insufficiency are at a greater risk.
◆ Irreversible hearing loss is more likely with this combination than when either drug is used alone.

◆ Use together is contraindicated.

◆ Avoid use together, if possible.
◆ If use together is unavoidable, monitor coagulation parameters carefully; the dosage require-ments for warfarin will be decreased.
◆ Suggest the use of a different histamine-2 antagonist.
◆ Aspirin doses of 500 mg or more daily are associated with a greater risk.

◆ Use together cautiously.
◆ Monitor prothrombin time and International Normalized Ratio closely when starting or stopping any of these medications.
◆ Bleeding effects may persist after interacting drug is stopped.
◆ Typically, a reduction of the warfarin dose is needed.

◆ Vitamin E doses of less than 400 mg daily may not have this effect.

INTERACTION	DRUG	INTERACTING DRUGS
Increased potassium level	*Potassium-sparing diuretics* (amiloride, spironolactone, triamterene)	*Angiotensin-converting enzyme (ACE) inhibitors* (benazepril, captopril, enalapril, fosinopril, lisinopril, moexipril, perindopril, quinapril, ramipril, trandolapril) *Angiotensin II receptor antagonists* (candesartan, eprosartan, irbesartan, losartan, olmesartan, telmisartan, valsartan) *Potassium preparations* (potassium acetate, potassium phosphate, potassium bicarbonate, potassium chloride, potassium citrate, potassium gluconate, potassium iodine, potassium phosphate)
Increased risk of pregnancy, breakthrough bleeding	*Barbiturates* (amobarbital, butabarbital, pentobarbital, phenobarbital, primidone, secobarbital)	*Hormonal contraceptives* (Ortho-Evra, Yasmin-28)
Life-threatening hypertension	*Clonidine* (Catapres)	*Beta-adrenergic blockers* (acebutolol, atenolol, betaxolol, carteolol, esmolol, metoprolol, nadolol, penbutolol, pindolol, propranolol, timolol) *Tricyclic antidepressants (TCAs)* (amitriptyline, amoxapine, clomipramine, desipramine, doxepin, imipramine, nortriptyline, protriptyline, trimipramine)
	Monoamine oxidase (MAO) inhibitors (isocarboxazid, phenelzine, tranylcypromine)	*Anorexiants* (amphetamine, benzphetamine, dextroamphetamine, methamphetamine, phentermine) *Methylphenidate* (dexmethylphenidate, Concerta)
Methotrexate toxicity	*Methotrexate* (Rheumatrex, Trexall)	*Nonsteroidal anti-inflammatory drugs (NSAIDs)* (diclofenac, etodolac, fenoprofen, flurbiprofen, ibuprofen, indomethacin, ketoprofen, ketorolac, meclofenamate, nabumetone, naproxen, oxaprozin, piroxicam, sulindac, tolmetin) *Penicillins* (amoxicillin, ampicillin, carbenicillin, cloxacillin, dicloxacillin, nafcillin, oxacillin, penicillin G, penicillin V, piperacillin, ticarcillin)
Reduced penicillin effectiveness	*Penicillins* (amoxicillin, ampicillin, carbenicillin, cloxacillin, dicloxacillin, nafcillin, oxacillin, Penicillin G, Penicillin V, piperacillin, ticarcillin)	*Tetracyclines* (demeclocycline, doxycycline, minocycline, tetracycline)

◆ Use together cautiously.
◆ High-risk patients include those with renal impairment, type 2 diabetes, decreased renal perfusion, and elderly patients.
◆ Don't use potassium preparations and potassium-sparing diuretics unless the patient has severe hypokalemia that isn't responding to either drug class alone.
◆ Monitor the patient's potassium level; also monitor for palpitations, chest pain, nausea and vomiting, paresthesia, and muscle weakness.

◆ Use together cautiously.
◆ Suggest use of an alternative barrier form of contraception while on both drugs.

◆ Use together cautiously.
◆ Monitor blood pressure closely when starting and stopping clonidine and beta-adrenergic blockers simultaneously; discontinue beta-adrenergic blocker first.

◆ Use together is contraindicated.

◆ Avoid using these drugs together, if possible.
◆ Several deaths have occurred as a result of hypertensive crisis leading to cerebral hemorrhage.
◆ Monitor the patient for hypertension, hyperpyrexia, and seizures.
◆ Hypertensive reaction may occur for several weeks after stopping an MAO inhibitor.

◆ Use together is contraindicated.

◆ Use together cautiously.
◆ Monitor the patient for mouth sores, hematemesis, diarrhea with melena, nausea and weakness, and bone marrow suppression.
◆ Methotrexate toxicity is less likely to occur with weekly low-dose methotrexate regimens for rheumatoid arthritis and other inflammatory diseases.
◆ Longer leucovorin rescue should be considered when giving NSAIDs and methotrexate at antineoplastic doses.
◆ Obtain methotrexate levels twice weekly for the first 2 weeks of concurrent penicillin and methotrexate therapy.

◆ Avoid use together, if possible.

INTERACTION	DRUG	INTERACTING DRUGS
Rhabdomyolysis and myopathy	*HMG-CoA reductase inhibitors* (atorvastatin, fluvastatin, lovastatin, pravastatin, rosuvastatin, simvastatin)	*Cyclosporine* (Neoral) *Gemfibrozil* (Lopid) *Protease inhibitors* (amprenavir, atazanavir, indinavir, lopinavir/ritonavir, nelfinavir, ritonavir, saquinavir) *Macrolide antibiotics* (azithromycin, clarithromycin, erythromycin)
Serious cardiac events	Quinidine	*Verapamil* (Calan)
Serotonin syndrome	*Selective serotonin reuptake inhibitors (SSRIs)* (fluoxetine, paroxetine, sertraline)	*Risperidone* (Risperdal)
	SSRIs (citalopram, fluoxetine, fluvoxamine, nefazodone, paroxetine, sertraline, venlafaxine)	*Selective 5-HT$_1$ receptor agonists* (almotriptan, eletriptan, frovatriptan, naratriptan, rizatriptan, sumatriptan, zolmitriptan)
	Serotonin reuptake inhibitors (citalopram, escitalopram, fluoxetine, fluvoxamine, nefazodone, paroxetine, sertraline, venlafaxine)	*MAO inhibitors* (isocarboxazid, phenelzine, selegiline, tranylcypromine) *Sibutramine* (Meridia) *Sympathomimetics* (amphetamine, dextroamphetamine, methamphetamine, phentermine)

◆ Use of nelfinavir and simvastatin is contraindicated.
◆ Avoid use together, if possible.
◆ Monitor patient on an HMG-CoA reductase inhibitor and gemfibrozil for signs of acute renal failure, including decreased urine output, elevated blood urea nitrogen and creatinine, edema, dyspnea, tachycardia, distended jugular veins, nausea, vomiting, weakness, fatigue, confusion, and agitation.
◆ Monitor the patient for fatigue, muscle aches and weakness, joint pain, unintentional weight gain, seizures, dramatically increased serum creatine kinase level, and dark, red, or cola-colored urine.

◆ Use together cautiously.
◆ Monitor the patient for rhabdomyolysis, especially 5 to 21 days after initiating the macrolide antibiotic.

◆ Use together only when there are no other alternatives.
◆ Monitor the patient for hypotension, bradycardia, ventricular tachycardia, and AV block.
◆ Tell the patient to report diaphoresis, dizziness, or blurred vision as well as palpitations, shortness of breath, dizziness or fainting, and chest pain.
◆ Complications of this interaction may be noticed in a little as 1 day or as long as 5 months of concomitant therapy.

◆ Monitor the patient carefully if an SSRI is started or stopped or if dosage is changed while on risperidone therapy— risperidone levels may be increased.
◆ Assess the patient for central nervous system (CNS) irritability, increased muscle tone, muscle twitching or jerking, and changes in level of consciousness (LOC).
◆ Although average doses of fluoxetine and paroxetine may cause this interaction, higher doses of sertraline (greater than 100 mg daily) are needed.

◆ Avoid coadministration of these drugs if possible.
◆ If concurrent use can't be avoided, start with the lowest dosages possible and observe the patient closely.
◆ Stop the selective 5-HT$_1$ receptor agonist at the first sign of interaction. Begin an antiserotonergic agent such as cyproheptadine (Periactin).
◆ Some patients may note increased frequency of migraine and reduced effectiveness of antimigraine agents if a serotonin reuptake inhibitor is begun.
◆ Monitor the patient for symptoms of serotonin syndrome, including CNS irritability, motor weakness, shivering, muscle twitching, and altered LOC.

◆ Don't use these drugs together.
◆ Allow 1 week after stopping nefazodone or venlafaxine before giving an MAO inhibitor.
◆ Allow 2 weeks after stopping citalopram, escitalopram, fluvoxamine, paroxetine, or sertraline before giving an MAO inhibitor.
◆ Allow 5 weeks after stopping fluoxetine before giving an MAO inhibitor.
◆ Allow 2 weeks after stopping an MAO inhibitor before giving any serotonin reuptake inhibitor.
◆ Serotonin syndrome effects include CNS irritability, motor weakness, shivering, myoclonus, and altered LOC.
◆ The selective MAO type-B inhibitor selegiline has been given with fluoxetine, paroxetine, or sertraline to patients with Parkinson disease without negative effects.

◆ Don't use these drugs together, if possible.
◆ If this combination must be used, carefully monitor the patent for adverse effects, which require immediate medical attention.
◆ Monitor the patient closely for increased CNS effects, such as anxiety, jitteriness, agitation, and restlessness, plus dizziness, nausea, vomiting, motor weakness, shivering, myoclonus, and altered LOC.

INTERACTION	DRUG	INTERACTING DRUGS
Severe arrhythmias	Cisapride (Propulsid)	Phenothiazines (chlorpromazine, fluphenazine, mesoridazine, perphenazine, prochlorperazine, promethazine, thioridazine, trifluoperazine) Thiazide diuretics (chlorothiazide, hydrochlorothiazide, indapamide, methyclothiazide, metolazone, polythiazide, trichlormethiazide) TCAs (amitriptyline, amoxapine, clomipramine, desipramine, doxepin, imipramine, nortriptyline, protriptyline, trimipramine) Quinolones (gatifloxacin, levofloxacin, moxifloxacin) Loop diuretics (bumetanide, ethacrynic acid, furosemide, torsemide)
	Dofetilide (Tikosyn)	Thiazide diuretics (chlorothiazide, hydrochlorothiazide, indapamide, methyclothiazide, metolazone, polythiazide, trichlormethiazide) Verapamil (Calan)
	Pimozide (Orap)	SSRIs (citalopram, sertraline)
	Quinolones (gatifloxacin, levofloxacin, moxifloxacin, sparfloxacin)	Antiarrhythmics (amiodarone, bretylium, disopyramide, procainamide, quinidine, sotalol) Erythromycin (E-mycin, Eryc) Phenothiazines (chlorpromazine, fluphenazine, mesoridazine, perphenazine, prochlorperazine, promethazine, thioridazine) TCAs (amitriptyline, amoxapine, clomipramine, desipramine, doxepin, imipramine, nortriptyline, trimipramine) Ziprasidone (Geodon)
	Thioridazine (Mellaril)	Fluoxetine (Prozac)
Severe hypotension	Nitrates (amyl nitrite, isosorbide dinitrate, isosorbide mononitrate, nitroglycerin)	Sildenafil (Viagra) Tadalafil (Cialis) Vardenafil (Levitra)
	Protease inhibitors (amprenavir, indinavir, nelfinavir, ritonavir, saquinavir)	Sildenafil (Viagra) Tadalafil (Cialis) Vardenafil (Levitra)
Severe muscular depression	Cholinesterase inhibitors (ambenonium, edrophonium, neostigmine, pyridostigmine)	Corticosteroids (betamethasone, corticotrophin, cortisone, cosyntropin, dexamethasone, fludrocortisone, hydrocortisone, methylprednisolone, prednisolone, prednisone, triamcinolone)

- Use together is contraindicated,
- Pharmacologic effects of the quinolone drug may be increased.
- Cisapride is only available through a limited access program to patients who don't respond to all other standard treatments and who meet strict eligibility criteria.
- Patients receiving cisapride have experienced prolongation of the QT interval, torsades de pointes, cardiac arrest, and sudden death.

- Use together cautiously.
- Cisapride is only available through a limited access program to patients who don't respond to all other standard treatments and who meet strict eligibility criteria.
- Patients receiving cisapride have experienced prolongation of the QT interval, torsades de pointes, cardiac arrest, and sudden death.
- Monitor serum electrolyte level due to risk of rapid potassium loss.

- Use together is contraindicated.
- In the event of inadvertent use together, monitor electrocardiogram for excessive prolongation of the QT_c interval or the development of ventricular arrhythmias.
- Use of a thiazide diuretic increases potassium excretion.
- Monitor renal function and QT_c interval every 3 months during dofetilide and verapamil therapy.

- Use together is contraindicated.
- Life-threatening risk is due to prolongation of the QT_c interval.

- Use of sparfloxacin with antiarrhythmics, erythromycin, phenothiazines, or TCAs is contraindicated.
- Use of class IA or III antiarrhythmics, erythromycin, phenothiazines, or TCAs with levofloxacin should be avoided.
- Gatifloxacin and moxifloxacin may be used with caution and increased monitoring with phenothiazines and TCAs but should be avoided with antiarrhythmics and erythromycin.

- Use together is contraindicated.

- Use together is contraindicated.
- Risk increases proportional to increased dose of thioridazine.

- Use together is contraindicated.
- Determine if the patient with chest pain has taken an erectile drug during the previous 24 to 48 hours before giving a nitrate.

- Use together is contraindicated.
- Tell the patient to take sildenafil exactly as prescribed. Dosage may be reduced to 25 mg and an interval of at least 48 hours between drugs may be needed.

- If used concomitantly in a patient with myasthenia gravis, monitor for severe muscle deterioration unresponsive to cholinesterase inhibitor therapy.
- Be prepared to provide respiratory support and mechanical ventilation, as needed.
- Be aware of the potential for long-term benefits from corticosteroid therapy in patients with myasthenia gravis.

DANGEROUS HERB-DRUG INTERACTIONS

◆

HERB	DRUG	POSSIBLE EFFECTS
Aloe (dried juice from leaf [latex])	Antiarrhythmics, digoxin	May lead to hypokalemia, which in turn may potentiate digoxin and antiarrhythmics
	Thiazide drugs, other potassium-wasting drugs such as cortico-steroids	May cause additive effect of potassium wasting
	Stimulant laxatives	May increase risk of potassium loss
Bilberry	Anticoagulants, antiplatelets	Decreases platelet aggregation
	Hypoglycemics, insulin	May increase insulin level, causing hypo-glycemia; additive effect with antidiabetics
Capsicum	Anticoagulants, antiplatelets	Decreases platelet aggregation and increas-es fibrinolytic activity, prolonging bleeding time
	Antihypertensives	May interfere with antihypertensives by in-creasing catecholamine secretion
	Central nervous system (CNS) depressants, such as barbiturates, benzodiazepines, opioids	Increases sedative effect
	Cocaine	May increase effects of drug and risk of ad-verse effects, including death (Interaction may occur with exposure to capsicum in pepper spray.)
	Theophylline	Increases absorption of theophylline, possi-bly leading to higher drug level or toxicity
Chamomile	Anticoagulants	Warfarin constituents in herb may enhance drug therapy and prolong bleeding time
	Drugs with sedative properties such as benzodiazepines	May cause additive effects and adverse ef-fects
Echinacea	Hepatotoxic drugs	Hepatotoxicity may increase with drugs known to elevate liver enzyme levels

Herb	Drug	Possible effects
Echinacea (continued)	Warfarin	Increases bleeding time without increased International Normalized Ratio (INR)
Evening primrose oil	Anticonvulsants	Lowers seizure threshold
	Anticoagulants, antiplatelets	Increases risk of bleeding and bruising
Feverfew	Anticoagulants, antiplatelets	May decrease platelet aggregation and increase fibrinolytic activity
	Methysergide	May potentiate drug
Garlic	Antihypertensives	May cause additive hypotension
	Cyclosporine	May decrease efficacy of drug; may induce metabolism and decrease drug level to subtherapeutic; may cause organ rejection
	Insulin, other drugs causing hypoglycemia	May increase insulin level, causing hypoglycemia, an additive effect with these drugs
Ginger	Anticoagulants, antiplatelets	Inhibits platelet aggregation by antagonizing thromboxane synthetase and enhancing prostacyclin, leading to prolonged bleeding time
	Antidiabetics	May interfere with diabetes therapy because of hypoglycemic effects
	Barbiturates	May enhance drug effects
	Calcium channel blockers	May increase calcium uptake by myocardium, leading to altered drug effects
	Histamine-2 blockers, proton pump inhibitors	May decrease efficacy because of increased acid secretion by herb
Ginkgo	Anticonvulsants	May decrease efficacy of drugs
	Drugs known to lower seizure threshold	May further reduce seizure threshold
	Insulin	May alter insulin secretion and metabolism, affecting glucose level (ginkgo leaf)
	Thiazide diuretics	May increase blood pressure (ginkgo leaf)
Ginseng	Anabolic steroids, hormones	May potentiate effects of drugs; estrogenic effects of herbs may cause vaginal bleeding and breast nodules
	Anticoagulants, antiplatelets	Decreases platelet adhesiveness
	Antidiabetics	May enhance glucose-lowering effects
	Antipsychotics	CNS stimulant; avoid use with these drugs

Herb	Drug	Possible effects
Ginseng (continued)	Digoxin	May falsely elevate drug level
	Furosemide	May decrease diuretic effect of drug
	Immunosuppressants	May interfere with drug therapy
	Monoamine oxidase (MAO) inhibitors	Potentiates action of MAO inhibitors; may cause insomnia, headache, tremors, and hypomania
	Stimulants	May potentiate drug effects
	Warfarin	Causes antagonism of warfarin, resulting in decreased INR
Goldenseal	Antihypertensives	May interfere with blood pressure control with large amounts of herb
	CNS depressants, such as barbiturates, benzodiazepines, opioids	Increases sedative effect
	General anesthetics	May potentiate hypotensive action of drugs
Grapeseed	Warfarin	Increases effects and INR because of tocopherol content of herb
Green tea	Albuterol, isoproterenol, metaproterenol, terbutaline	May increase cardiac inotropic effect of these drugs
	Clozapine	May cause acute worsening of psychotic symptoms
	Disulfiram	Increases risk of adverse effects of caffeine; decreases clearance and increases half-life of caffeine
	Ephedrine	Increases risk of agitation, tremors, and insomnia
	Hormonal contraceptives	Decreases clearance by 40% to 65%; increases effects and adverse effects
	Lithium	Abrupt caffeine withdrawal increases drug level; may cause lithium tremor
	MAO inhibitors	May precipitate hypertensive crisis with large amounts of herb
	Mexiletine	Decreases caffeine elimination by 50%; increases effects and adverse effects
	Verapamil	Increases caffeine level by 25%; increases effects and adverse effects
Hawthorn berry	Cardiovascular drugs	May potentiate or interfere with conventional therapies used for heart failure, hypertension, angina, and arrhythmias

Herb	Drug	Possible effects
Hawthorn berry (continued)	CNS depressants	Causes additive effects
	Coronary vasodilators	Causes additive vasodilator effects when used with theophylline, caffeine, papaverine, sodium nitrate, adenosine, and epinephrine
	Digoxin	Causes additive positive inotropic effect with potential for drug toxicity
Kava	Alcohol	Potentiates depressant effect of alcohol and other CNS depressants
	Benzodiazepines	Use with these drugs may cause comalike states
	CNS depressants or stimulants	May hinder therapy with CNS stimulants
	Hepatotoxic drugs	May increase risk of liver damage
Licorice	Antihypertensives	Decreases effect of drug therapy; sodium and water retention and hypertension with large amounts of herb
	Corticosteroids	Causes additive and enhanced effects of drugs
	Digoxin	Predisposes to drug toxicity due to hypokalemia with herb use
	Hormonal contraceptives	Increases fluid retention and potential for increased blood pressure due to fluid overload
	Hormones	Interferes with estrogen or antiestrogen therapy
	Insulin	Causes hypokalemia and sodium retention
Ma huang (ephedra)	Caffeine	Increases risk of stimulatory adverse effects of ephedra and caffeine; increases risk of hypertension, myocardial infarction, stroke, and death
	Caffeine, CNS stimulants, theophylline	Causes additive CNS stimulation
	Digoxin	Increases risk of arrhythmias
	MAO inhibitors	Potentiates drugs
	Oxytocin	May cause hypertension
	Theophylline	May increase risk of stimulatory effects
Melatonin	CNS depressants, such as barbiturates, benzodiazepines, opioids	Increases sedative effect

Herb	Drug	Possible effects
Melatonin (continued)	Immunosuppressants	May stimulate immune function and interfere with drug therapy
	Nifedipine	May decrease efficacy of drug; increases heart rate
Milk thistle	Drugs causing diarrhea	Increases bile secretion and often causes loose stools; may increase effect of other drugs commonly causing diarrhea
	Indinavir	May decrease trough level of drug, reducing virologic response
Nettle	Anticonvulsants	May increase sedative adverse effects; may increase risk of seizure
	Anxiolytics, hypnotics, opioids	May increase sedative adverse effects
Passion flower	CNS depressants, such as barbiturates, benzodiazepines, opioids	Increases sedative effect
St. John's wort	5-hydroxytriptamin₁ agonists (triptans)	Increases risk of serotonin syndrome
	Alcohol, opioids	Enhances sedative effect of drugs
	Anesthetics	May prolong effect of drugs
	Cyclosporine	Decreases drug level below therapeutic levels, threatening transplanted organ rejection
	Digoxin	May reduce drug level, which decreases therapeutic effects
	Hormonal contraceptives	Increases breakthrough bleeding; decreases level and efficacy of drugs
	Human immunodeficiency virus protease inhibitors, indinavir, nonnucleotide reverse transcriptase inhibitors	Induces cytochrome P-450 metabolic pathway, which may decrease therapeutic effects of drugs using the pathway for metabolism; subtherapeutic antiretroviral level and insufficient virologic response could lead to resistance or class cross-resistance
	MAO inhibitors, nefazodone, selective serotonin reuptake inhibitors (SSRIs), trazodone	Causes additive effects with MAO inhibitors, SSRIs, and other antidepressants, potentially leading to serotonin syndrome, especially when combined with SSRIs
	Photosensitizing drugs	Increases photosensitivity
	Reserpine	Antagonizes effects of drug
	Sympathomimetic amines such as pseudoephedrine	Causes additive effects and increases risk of adverse effects

Herb	Drug	Possible effects
St. John's wort (continued)	Theophylline	May decrease drug level, which reduces drug efficacy
Valerian	Alcohol	May be risk of increased sedation
	CNS depressants, sedative hypnotics	Enhances effects of drugs

POTENTIAL AGENTS OF BIOTERRORISM

Here are examples of biological agents that may be used as biological weapons and the major signs and symptoms for each.

AGENT (CONDITION)	MAJOR ASSOCIATED SIGNS AND SYMPTOMS										
	Abdominal pain	Back pain	Blood pressure, decreased	Chest pain	Chills	Cough	Diarrhea, bloody	Diplopia	Dysarthria	Dysphagia	Dyspnea
Bacillus anthracis (anthrax)	●		●	●	●	●	●				●
Clostridium botulinum (botulism)								●	●	●	●
Francisella tularensis (tularemia)				●	●	●					●
Variola major (smallpox)	●	●									
Yersinia pestis (pneumonic plague)				●	●	●					●

	Fever	Headache	Hematemesis	Hemoptysis	Lymphadenopathy	Malaise	Myalgia	Nausea	Oliguria	Papular rash (skin lesions)	Ptosis	Stridor	Tachypnea	Vomiting	Weakness
	●	●	●		●	●		●		●		●		●	●
											●				●
	●	●					●								
	●	●				●				●					
	●	●		●			●		●				●		

SELECTED REFERENCES

◆

Fultz, J., and Sturt, P.A. *Mosby's Emergency Nursing Reference,* 3rd ed. St. Louis: Mosby–Year Book, Inc., 2005.

Huether, S.E., and McCance, K.L. *Understanding Pathophysiology,* 3rd ed. St. Louis: Mosby–Year Book, Inc., 2004.

Hughes, B.W., et al. "Pathophysiology of Myasthenia Gravis," *Seminars in Neurology* 24(1):21-30, March 2004.

Ignatavicius, D.D., and Workman, L. *Medical-Surgical Nursing: Critical Thinking for Collaborative Care,* 5th ed. Philadelphia: W.B. Saunders Co., 2006.

Kenny, P.E. "The Changing Face of AIDS," *Nursing* 34(8):56-63, August 2004.

Koennecke, H.C. "Secondary Prevention of Stroke: A Practical Guide to Drug Treatment," *CNS Drugs* 18(4):221-41, 2004.

Kuwabara, S. "Guillain-Barré Syndrome: Epidemiology, Pathophysiology and Management," *Drugs* 64(6):597-610, 2004.

Levi, M., et al. "New Treatment Strategies for Disseminated Intravascular Coagulation Based on Current Understanding of the Pathophysiology," *Annals of Medicine* 36(1):41-49, 2004.

Meduri, G.U., and Yates, C.R. "Systemic Inflammation-associated Glucocorticoid Resistance and Outcome of ARDS," *Annals of the New York Academy of Sciences* 1024:24-53, June 2004.

"Methylprednisolone: Life-saving in SARS?" *Inpharma Weekly* 1444(1):11, July 2004.

Nurse's Quick Check: Signs & Symptoms. Philadelphia: Lippincott Williams & Wilkins, 2006.

Pathophysiology: A 2-in-1 Reference for Nurses. Philadelphia: Lippincott Williams & Wilkins, 2005.

Perry, S.E., et al. *Maternal Child Nursing Care,* 3rd ed. St. Louis: Mosby–Year Book, Inc., 2006.

Pillitteri, A. *Maternal & Child Health Nursing: Care of the Childbearing and Childrearing Family,* 4th ed. Philadelphia: Lippincott Williams & Wilkins, 2003.

Porth, C. *Pathophysiology: Concepts of Altered Health States,* 7th ed. Philadelphia: Lippincott Williams & Wilkins, 2005.

Price, S.A., and Wilson, L.M. *Pathophysiology: Clinical Concepts of Disease Processes,* 6th ed. St. Louis: Mosby–Year Book, Inc., 2003.

Professional Guide to Diseases, 8th ed. Philadelphia: Lippincott Williams & Wilkins, 2005.

"SARS Coronavirus in Tears," *Journal of Clinical Pathology* 57(9):979, September 2004.

Signs & Symptoms: A 2-in-1 Reference for Nurses. Philadelphia: Lippincott Williams & Wilkins, 2005.

INDEX

i refers to an illustration; t refers to a table.

i refers to an illustration; t refers to a table.

i refers to an illustration; t refers to a table.

---

i refers to an illustration; t refers to a table.

Gastrointestinal disorders *(continued)*
    fecal breath odor in, 66-67
    hematemesis in, 162, 164
    hematochezia in, 166, 167
    hyperactive bowel sounds in, 60-61, 60t
    melena in, 203
    vomiting in, 312, 313, 314
Glomerulonephritis
    anuria in, 24
    epistaxis in, 133
    flank pain in, 151-152
Gout, erythema in, 138
Guillain-Barré syndrome
    ataxia in, 35
    dyspnea in, 121, 122-123t
    fasciculations in, 146
    paralysis in, 228
    shallow respirations in, 261

Head and neck cancer, jaw pain in, 189
Head trauma
    aphasia in, 28
    decorticate posture in, 105
    decreased level of consciousness in, 197
    hyperpnea in, 175
    ocular deviation in, 220-221
    paralysis in, 228
    seizures in, 272
    tachypnea in, 297
    vision loss in, 306
Heart failure
    abdominal pain in, 5, 6-7t
    blood pressure decrease in, 50
    Cheyne-Stokes respirations in, 84
    costal and sternal retractions in, 266
    cyanosis in, 100
    dyspnea in, 121, 122-123t
    edema in, 131
    grunting respirations in, 253
    jugular vein distention in, 191-192
    tachycardia in, 293
    vomiting in, 312
Heart sounds, 157i, 158-159t
Heat dissipation, impaired, hyperthermia and, 178
Heat syndromes
    anhidrosis in, 21
    clammy skin in, 275
    decreased level of consciousness in, 198
Heavy metal poisoning, hematochezia in, 167
Hematemesis, 161-164
Hematochezia, 164-167, 202i
Hemolytic-uremic syndrome, anuria in, 24
Hemoptysis, 167-171
Hemothorax, asymmetrical chest expansion in, 73
Hepatic disorders
    abdominal pain in, 4, 5, 6-7t, 8-9t, 10
    bradypnea in, 64
    edema in, 131
    epistaxis in, 133
    splenomegaly in, 278-279
    vomiting in, 312
Hepatocerebral degeneration, ataxia in, 35
Herbal remedies
    blood pressure increase and, 57
    diarrhea in, 109
    erythema and, 139
    facial edema in, 129

Herbal remedies *(continued)*
    palpitations and, 226
Herb-drug interactions, 330-335t
Hereditary angioedema, urticaria in, 302
Hereditary hemorrhagic telangiectasia, epistaxis
        in, 133
Hernia
    chest pain in, 78-79t, 79
    scrotal swelling in, 268
    tracheal deviation in, 300
Herniated disk
    fasciculations in, 146
    Kernig's sign in, 194
    neck pain in, 216
Herpes zoster
    abdominal pain in, 8-9t, 10
    chest pain in, 78-79t, 79
    facial edema in, 128
    pupillary changes in, 249-250
    vision loss in, 307
Histoplasmosis, splenomegaly in, 279
Hodgkin's disease, neck pain in, 216
Homans' sign, 171-173
Horner's syndrome, anhidrosis in, 21
Hyperaldosteronism, orthostatic hypotension
        in, 180
Hyperemesis gravidarum, vomiting in, 312-313
Hyperosmolar hyperglycemic nonketotic syndrome
    blood pressure decrease in, 50
    decreased level of consciousness in, 198
    tachycardia in, 293
    tachypnea in, 297
Hyperpnea, 173-176
Hypersplenism, splenomegaly in, 279
Hypertension
    atrial gallop in, 159
    blood pressure increase in, 56
    dizziness in, 111
    epistaxis in, 133
    palpitations in, 225
Hyperthermia
    ataxia in, 35
Hyperthermia, 176-179
Hyperventilation syndrome
    decreased level of consciousness in, 198
    dizziness in, 111
    hyperpnea in, 175
Hypervolemia, jugular vein distention in, 192
Hypoglycemia
    clammy skin in, 275
    dizziness in, 111
    palpitations in, 225
    seizures in, 272
    tachycardia in, 293
Hypotension, orthostatic, 179-180, 182
Hypothermia, 62, 182-183, 198
Hypothyroidism
    bradycardia in, 62
    muscle spasms in, 210
Hypovolemia
    dizziness in, 111
    orthostatic hypotension in, 180
Hypoxemia
    blood pressure decrease in, 51
    hyperpnea in, 175
    syncope in, 286

---

i refers to an illustration; t refers to a table.

i refers to an illustration; t refers to a table.

i refers to an illustration; t refers to a table.

Plummer-Vinson syndrome, dysphagia in, 119
Pneumonia
  abdominal pain in, 8-9t, 12
  abdominal rigidity in, 16
  asymmetrical chest expansion in, 73
  chest pain in, 80-81t, 82
  crackles in, 94t, 95
  cyanosis in, 101
  dyspnea in, 122-123t, 123
  hemoptysis in, 170
  pleural friction rub in, 236-237
  productive cough in, 87t, 90
Pneumothorax
  abdominal pain in, 8-9t, 12
  asymmetrical chest expansion in, 73
  chest pain in, 80-81t, 82
  cyanosis in, 101
  dyspnea in, 122-123t, 123-124
  subcutaneous crepitation in, 96-97
Poisoning
  ataxia in, 35
  decreased level of consciousness and, 200
  myoclonus in, 212
  seizures in, 273
Poliomyelitis
  asymmetrical chest expansion in, 73
  dyspnea in, 124, 124-125t
  fasciculations in, 146
  paralysis in, 232
Polyarteritis nodosa, ataxia in, 35
Polycystic kidney disease, blood pressure increase
    in, 56
Polycythemia vera
  cyanosis in, 101
  epistaxis in, 134
  mottled skin in, 276-277
  splenomegaly in 280-281
Polyneuropathy, ataxia in, 35-36
Pontine hemorrhage, decreased level of conscious-
    ness in, 199
Popliteal cyst, Homans' sign in, 172
Porphyria
  ataxia in, 36
  seizures in, 272
Postconcussion syndrome, dizziness in, 111
Posterior fossa tumor, ataxia in, 36
Preeclampsia
  blood pressure increase in, 56
  facial edema in, 129
  vomiting in, 313-314
Prickly heat, anhidrosis in, 21
Prostate cancer
  back pain in, 40
  bladder distention in, 45, 46-47t
Prostatitis
  abdominal pain in, 8-9t, 12
  bladder distention in, 45, 46-47t
Pseudomembranous enterocolitis, diarrhea in, 108
Psittacosis
  chest pain in, 80-81t, 82
  crackles in, 94t, 95
  productive cough in, 87t, 90
Pulmonary disorders
  apnea in, 30
  chest pain in, 78-79t, 79, 80-81t, 82-83
  crackles in, 93-94, 94t, 95
  dyspnea in, 124-125t, 125

Pulmonary disorders *(continued)*
  hemoptysis in, 170-171
  pleural friction rub in, 236, 237
  productive cough in, 87t, 90-91
  shallow respirations in, 260, 262
Pulmonary edema
  crackles in, 94t, 95
  cyanosis in, 101
  dyspnea in, 124, 124-125t
  hemoptysis in, 170
  productive cough in, 87t, 90
  shallow respirations in, 262
  tachypnea in, 298
  wheezing in, 320
Pulmonary embolism
  asymmetrical chest expansion in, 73
  atrial gallop in, 159
  blood pressure decrease in, 51
  chest pain in, 80-81t, 82
  crackles in, 94t, 95
  cyanosis in, 101
  dyspnea in, 124, 124-125t
  hemoptysis in, 170
  pleural friction rub in, 237
  productive cough in, 87t, 90
  pulsus paradoxus in, 248
  shallow respirations in, 262
  tachycardia in, 294
  tachypnea in, 298
  wheezing in, 320
Pulse pressure, widened, 238, 240
Pulse rhythm abnormality, 240-241
Pulsus paradoxus, 241, 244-245, 247-248
Pupillary changes, 248-251
Pyelonephritis
  abdominal pain in, 8-9t, 12
  back pain in, 40

Q fever
  chest pain in, 80-81t, 83
  diarrhea in, 109
  fever in, 149
  vomiting in, 314

Rabies
  dysphagia in, 119
  paralysis in, 232
Raynaud's disease
  cyanosis in, 101
  erythema in, 139
  pallor in, 223
Rebound tenderness, eliciting, 4i
Reiter's syndrome, back pain in, 40
Renal calculi
  abdominal pain in, 8-9t, 12
  back pain in, 40
Renal disorders
  bradypnea in, 65
  Cheyne-Stokes respirations in, 85
  edema in, 131
  epistaxis in, 134
  flank pain in, 151-152, 153-154
  hyperpnea in, 175-176
  seizures in, 271
  vomiting in, 314
Renal vein occlusion, anuria in, 25

---

i refers to an illustration; t refers to a table.

Renovascular stenosis, blood pressure increase in, 56
Respirations
  costal and sternal, 264-266
  grunting, 252-253
  shallow, 256-263
  stertorous, 263-264
Respiratory disorders
  bradypnea in, 65
  costal and sternal retractions in, 265-266
  dyspnea in, 121, 122-123t, 124-125, 124-125t
  epistaxis in, 134
  fever in, 149
  grunting respirations in, 253
  shallow respirations in, 257, 260-261, 262
  stridor in, 282-283, 284
  tachycardia in, 290, 294
  tachypnea in, 296, 297, 298
  tracheal deviation in, 299-300
  wheezing in, 316-320
Respiratory therapy
  productive cough and, 91
  subcutaneous crepitation in, 97
Rhabdomyolysis
  fever in, 149
  vomiting in, 314
Rhinitis, facial edema in, 129
Rift Valley fever
  back pain in, 40
  dizziness in, 111-112
  fever in, 149
  vision loss in, 307
Rubella, erythema in, 139

Sacroiliac strain, back pain in, 40
Sarcoidosis
  crackles in, 94t, 95
  epistaxis in, 134
  seizures in, 272
  splenomegaly in, 281-282
Scleroma, epistaxis in, 134
Scrotal swelling, 267-269
Seizure disorders
  decreased level of consciousness in, 199
  myoclonus in, 211
  paralysis in, 232
  seizures in, 272
Seizures, generalized tonic-clonic, 269-273
Sepsis
  dyspnea in, 124, 124-125t
  hyperpnea in, 176
Shock
  blood pressure decrease in, 50, 51
  clammy skin in, 275
  cyanosis in, 101
  decreased level of consciousness in, 199
  dyspnea in, 124-125t, 125
  edema in, 131
  hyperpnea in, 176
  mottled skin in, 276
  tachycardia in, 291, 292, 293-294
  tachypnea in, 296, 297, 298
Shy-Drager syndrome
  anhidrosis in, 21
  dysarthria in, 114-115t, 115
  orthostatic hypotension in, 180
Sialolithiasis, jaw pain in, 190

Sickle cell crisis
  abdominal pain in, 8-9t, 12
  chest pain in, 80-81t, 83
Sick sinus syndrome, palpitations in, 225
Skin
  clammy, 273-275
  mottled, 275-277
Skin disorders
  erythema in, 137-138, 139
  mottled skin in, 276
Skin lesions, recognizing, 302-303i
Skull fracture
  Battle's sign in, 43
  epistaxis in, 134, 136
Sleep apnea
  apnea in, 30
  cyanosis in, 101
  stertorous respirations in, 264
Smallpox
  abdominal pain in, 8-9t, 12-13
  back pain in, 40, 42
  fever in, 149-150
Spasmodic croup, barking cough in, 86
Spinal cord injury or disorders
  analgesia in, 20
  anhidrosis in, 21
  back pain in, 42
  bladder distention in, 45, 46-47t
  fasciculations in, 146
  Kernig's sign in, 192
  muscle spasms in, 210
  neck pain in, 215-216
  paralysis in, 232
  shallow respirations in, 262
Spinocerebellar ataxia, ataxia in, 36
Splenic infarction, abdominal pain in, 10-11t, 13
Splenic rupture, splenomegaly in, 282
Splenomegaly, 277-282
Spondylolisthesis, back pain in, 42
Stridor, 282-284
Stroke
  aphasia in, 28
  apraxia in, 32-33, 32t
  ataxia in, 36
  decorticate posture in, 105-106
  decreased level of consciousness in, 199
  dysarthria in, 114-115t, 115
  ocular deviation in, 221
  paralysis in, 232
  seizures in, 272-273
Subarachnoid hemorrhage
  Kernig's sign in, 192
  neck pain in, 216
  paralysis in, 232
Subdural hematoma
  decreased level of consciousness in, 199-200
  eye pain in, 144
Superior vena cava obstruction, jugular vein distention in, 192
Superior vena cava syndrome, facial edema in, 129
Surgery
  absent bowel sounds in, 58
  epistaxis and, 136
  facial edema and, 130
  shallow respirations and, 262
  subcutaneous crepitation in, 97
  tachycardia and, 294

i refers to an illustration; t refers to a table.

i refers to an illustration; t refers to a table.